Nursing & Healthcare Ethics

SIXTH EDITION

Nursing & Healthcare Ethics

SIMON ROBINSON

Professor of Applied and Professional Ethics (Emeritus)
Leeds Beckett University
Hon Fellow in Theology
University of Leeds

OWEN DOODY

Senior Lecturer
Department of Nursing and Midwifery
University of Limerick
Ireland

ELSEVIER

ISBN: 978-0-7020-7904-7

Content Strategist: Poppy Garraway
Content Development Specialist: Denise Roslonski
Publishing Services Manager: Shereen Jameel
Project Manager: Aparna Venkatachalam
Design: Amy Buxton

Printed in Poland

Last digit is the print number: 9 8 7 6 5 4 3 2 1

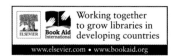

Working together
to grow libraries in
developing countries

www.elsevier.com • www.bookaid.org

*We dedicate this book to the memory of Barbie Birchall and
Fiona Stewart, two remarkable women who faced terminal
cancer remaining true to themselves and their families,
and to all the remarkable people in health services who remain
true to their calling to practice and sustain healthcare for all.*

Nursing Ethics has for decades been at the forefront of developing a carefully reasoned and highly practical approach to professional ethics. Unfortunately, this is very rarely recognised. As with the practice of medicine itself, the ethical concerns of the medical profession have dominated the literature and caught the attention of the public through extensive media coverage of both breakthroughs and scandals in health care. It must seem that the image of the nurse as the doctor's handmaiden (though of course in reality many nurses are male) lingers on!

Even a cursory glance at the history of healthcare ethics will show how mistaken is this view of the relative attention paid to ethics by the two professions. It is true that in 1949 the World Medical Association adopted an updated version of the Hippocratic Oath, the Geneva Convention Code of Medical Ethics, this being a response to the shocking revelations in the Nuremberg Trials of medical atrocities. But, like the Oath itself, the Code is highly generalised and – perhaps deliberately - vague on detail. By contrast, the International Council of Nurses adopted in 1953 the International Code of Nursing Ethics, a highly detailed account of the ethical requirements of nursing practice. The same was true of professional education in ethics. In the 1960s the Royal College of Nursing instituted a theoretically rich course in ethics for its senior nurses (my efforts to teach this course led to the publication of my first book, *Moral Dilemmas in Medicine* in 1972 and at the publisher's suggestion, the draft of the book was altered to make it a coursebook for both nurses and doctors, but the clinical examples all came from my nursing students.) Ethics in medical education, on the other hand, took many years to gain a foothold in the curriculum, and only after strong lobbying by the Society for the Study of Medical Ethics.

Given this history, it is really no surprise to find that this volume is rich in theory, but also totally relevant to the painful dilemmas of profession practice, of which the current challenge of the Covid19 pandemic is but one vivid example. To face such dilemmas health care professionals need, not just a knowledge of ethical theory, though this is important, but also an understanding of both personal integrity, stemming from Virtue Ethics, and a hard-nosed political realism, which can confront the institutional and political failures that undercut the best intentioned efforts of nurses to act in a clinically responsible manner. This volume provides all of this and more, with a full complement of references and sources for further reflection and study. Such theoretical richness and practical realism are exactly what the field requires.

Alastair V. Campbell
Emeritus Director
Centre for Biomedical Ethics
National University of Singapore

This book builds on Thompson's Nursing Ethics and we acknowledge a massive debt to Ian Thompson and his co-authors who worked on the previous five editions. The writing of this book occurs during a time of great change for the healthcare system, as it faces a growing population of older persons, persons with dementia and those living with chronic conditions, and crises in the practice of clinical governance, not least the seminal scandal of the Mid Staffs Hospital Trust. In recognition of these issues, chapters within this book address issues relating to healthcare practice and service provision. Existing chapters were updated, some chapters underwent major revisions, and some new chapters were added to connect better to the challenges faced by healthcare practitioners and organisation in the 21ˢᵗ century. Central to supporting the readers understanding and engagement with the topic area this book addresses issues across the lifespan, practice environments and populations. To support engagement, the authors, identify ethical theory and principles as the foundation so readers can analyse current and future issues in their practice based on ethics theory and principles. Building on this foundation the authors throughout the book present cases from practice and pause for thought moments to allow the reader to consider and apply to their own practice. Within this process, the authors emphasise the importance of continual dialogue with self, a critical companion, clinical supervisor or mentor, the profession, the organisation, and the classroom. While this edition is an update the authors cannot fully predict the practice issues in the coming years. However, the reader can apply the theories and principles of ethics to their situation as it arises and that the reader continues to ask themselves 'ethically is this the best decision to make' and 'how do I know this is the best decision' through out their professional career.

We want to thank Fiona Conn and Poppy Garraway Smith for their care, patience and push, and family and colleagues who have enabled time to be discovered. We apologize for the shortcomings in the book but do not apologise for our shared determination to focus on how professional ethics shapes identity and thus our shared responsibility for care.

Simon Robinson. Professor of Applied and Professional Ethics (emeritus), Leeds Beckett University, Hon Fellow in Theology, University of Leeds.

Educated at Oxford and Edinburgh Universities, Robinson became a psychiatric social worker before entering the Church of England priesthood in 1978. He entered university chaplaincy in Edinburgh and Leeds, developing research and lecturing in areas of spirituality ethics and care, applied ethics and business ethics. In 2004 he joined Leeds Metropolitan (now Beckett) University working across Healthcare, Business and Social Sciences.

He has worked with business and the professions, including nursing, medicine, engineering and the police on the practice and teaching of ethics, and has written and researched extensively in business ethics, corporate social responsibility, the nature and dynamics of responsibility, equality, ethics and culture, and ethics and care. Books include: *Agape, Moral Meaning and Pastoral Counselling*; *Their Rights, Advanced Directives*; *Case Histories in Business Ethics*; *Spirituality and the Practice of Healthcare*; *Values in Higher Education*; *The Teaching and Practice of Professional Ethics*; *Employability and Ethics*; *Engineering, Business and Professional Ethics*; *Spirituality, Ethics and Care*; *Ethics for Living and Working*; *Ethics and the Alcohol Industry*; *Leadership Responsibility*; *The Practice of Integrity in Business*; *The Spirituality of Responsibility*.

Owen Doody. Senior Lecturer, Department of Nursing and Midwifery, University of Limerick, Ireland.

Owen is a registered intellectual disability nurse who worked as a staff nurse with children with intellectual disability and their families. Following which he moved into nurse management of a unit for adults with intellectual disability and disturbed behaviour. During his staff and management years, Owen continued his education to complete a BSc at the University of Limerick and MSc with the Royal College of Nursing – Manchester University (UK). Following which Owen moved into nurse education and began his PhD with the University of Ulster. Currently Owen is a Senior Lecturer in the Department of Nursing and Midwifery in the University of Limerick. Owen's teaching areas focus on intellectual disability, research and practice development in nursing and midwifery. Owen's research interests relate to specialist practice, community living for persons with an intellectual disability, supporting families and in working with and supporting practice staff in research and publications. Owen's passion is to make nursing practice visible through practice-based evidence/publications.

CONTENTS

There are many books pertaining to healthcare, and professional and nursing ethics. Some claim to have cornered the meaning and practice of applied ethics. The authors of this book do not claim that, for two reasons. Firstly, we believe that ethics is the responsibility of all healthcare professionals and organizations who represent them. Secondly, we believe that ethics involves an ongoing learning process of reflecting on how the profession is viewed, how society and healthcare is viewed, and how we view ourselves. Nobody at a professional level, management level or leadership level in healthcare in the Mid Staffs Hospital Trust scandal believed they were unethical (our opening case in chapter one). Public opinion would have us assume that doctors, nurses and other healthcare professions are the 'good guys', because these roles are a vocation. But the case shows clearly that even the good guys are not always aware of what they are doing, crossing the ethical red lines without realizing it. Whatever ethics is, it has to involve reflection on our personal and professional identity and seeing if we really do practice what we and the profession believes in. A good example of such reflections is found in the book *The Road* by Cormac McCarthy start now a DVD (*The Road* 2010, Icon Home Entertainment http://www.youtube.com/watch?v=JaYvISSTyG4&feature=related).

A man and his son are on journey to the south in the USA. It is a time of chaos after a nuclear disaster, and they hope that the south will provide safety. Along the way the boy asks his father, 'are we still the good guys?' His father believes they are, and that for him this involves defending his son at all costs against some very scary people, but his son wants to know where he will draw the line, and why he no longer helps people in need who he meets. Has he crossed the line?

The message of history is that it is very easy, and quite common, to cross the line and not to realize it. Our capacity to rationalize tells us that we are still the good guys even though our practice is anything but good. If this book achieves anything in practice it will help the healthcare professionals to reflect on practice and develop ways of challenging themselves and others about what they think they are doing. In pursuit of this aim we have three objectives, to provide:

- Key tools for understanding and practising ethics in your profession. These will help you to talk confidently about ethical values and interrogate and develop practice effectively in light of those values.
- Critical reflection on how to practice ethical deliberation and judgement in key areas of the healthcare ethical environment. This will include attention to ways of thinking and to ethical and other virtues that will provide the muscle for the practice of ethics.
- Ways of practising ethics in coordination with different professions and in the context of a complex organisational environment.

To achieve these objectives, the book will focus on ethical decision-making frameworks, ethical and professional codes, and broader vision and values statements. However, these are of little use without professionals at every level of the organisation taking responsibility for the meaning and practice of ethics. Hence, this book focuses on the practice of ethical judgement and challenge, and while codes and frameworks provide a useful discipline for developing ethical responsibility, they cannot replace it. The authors recognize that different healthcare professions must work and collaborate together with a range of different stakeholders; patients/clients, families, other professions, one's own profession and the healthcare organisation (hospital or community). In this collaborative working approach, each person brings different ethical narratives that have to be creatively engaged and focused in dialogue as part of the ethical dynamic of professional practice; where individual and corporate responsibility for profession and overall care is shared. It is precisely because of the complexity of ethical practice that we will begin the book with the complex case of the Mid Staffs Healthcare Trust. We have not done this to show nursing or healthcare in a bad light. On the contrary, we use this case which is just one of many across all sectors which have shown how difficult it is to engage ethical practice consistently. Secondly, Mid Staffs shows us something about how professional ethics is linked directly to identity, who we are and who we think we are. However, before we present this case in chapter one it is important to examine different conceptions of ethics.

Conceptions of Ethics

There are several misconceptions of what ethics involves, including: preaching, theorizing, specialising and being kind. *Preaching.* Ethics is often seen as a series of prescriptions, telling people what they should and should not do. Not surprisingly, this leads to the argument that this does not respect the freedom of the ordinary person. In this light some argue that it is wrong to try to teach ethics. Teaching would be telling people what to think when the task of education should be to enable critical thinking and dialogue that develops reflective practice.

Theorizing. Ethicists, especially philosophers, do not know anything about the issues faced by people in practice. As Vardy (1989, 196) puts it, they 'live in a secure and problem free environment removed from professional realities'. Lurking beneath this argument is a large gap between theory and practice. The ethicist is seen as someone who will work in theoretical and even ideal terms, while the healthcare professional is someone who must get his/her hands dirty on occasions.

Specialising. Ethics is a specialism. It involves having to learn a whole set of new ideas including handling complex concepts. Considering that it is sometimes felt that professionals simply do not have the time to get involved. A variation of this is the argument in Higher Education that healthcare ethics is itself a disciplinary specialism, and not one essential to the practice or teaching of professional practice. Hence, healthcare ethics might be at best an option in the curriculum.

Being kind. This is an argument that starts with the view that ethics is really about altruism, putting the other first. In this view, self-interest is by definition bad.

These misconceptions set up false dichotomies; ethics is either one thing of the other. This book focuses on the complexity of ethics. Strictly speaking ethics is the systematic study of how to behave in the right way and how we decide what is right in a situation. Nursing and healthcare ethics is a form of applied ethics which focuses on decisions made and practice conducted. Nursing and healthcare ethics thus involves exploration of:

- The underlying ethical values of the healthcare professions, including managers and leaders of the organization. It is important to hear and understand the different ethical perspectives that may be held by these different groups.
- How any values might be embodied in the profession and the health organization. This includes the development of codes of ethics.
- Underlying ethical theories that seek to explain the basis of what is ethically good. This involves descriptive theories and normative theories; theories that try to explain how we make ethical decisions and theories about how we ought to make ethical decisions.
- Underlying values, worldviews, and different social and cultural contexts of the areas in which practice operates. Any of these may affect our view of what is ethically right or wrong.
- How to make ethical decisions as a part of everyday practice decision making in a variety of contexts.
- How to make an ethical argument and engage in ethical dialogue. Ethics is not just about asserting an opinion. Any argument must be crafted and coherent if it is to justify actions. The better the healthcare professional is at this the better he/she will be at making and handling challenges.
- How to develop the capacities to make such decisions? It is one thing working out what to do and another thing having the capacity to put this into practice.

The dichotomy between theory and practice is false. Whilst it is possible to distinguish theory from practice, the term theory is about a belief or principle that guides action or assists comprehension or judgment, or about a set of statements or principles devised to explain a group of facts or phenomena. In other words, theory is devised to make sense of practice, experience, or phenomena. Hence, the root of the word is 'to see'. The test of any theory then is that it should help you make sense of practice. Theory about ethics then, should help the nurse and other healthcare practitioners to make sense of their practice.

INTRO.1: PAUSE FOR THOUGHT

The dichotomy between theory and practice: philosophical perspective

Consider the gap between theory and practice parallels that of the gap between intellect and practical skills. So, what is the intellect, and do you have one?

Aristotle, philosopher of ancient Greece (384-322 BCE) saw the intellect as connected directly to practice. Hence, he argued there were five intellectual virtues or capacities (Aristotle 2004):
- scientific knowledge (*episteme*), or empirical understanding.
- artistic or technical knowledge (*techne*), knowledge of how to make or do things.
- intuitive reason (*nous*), the capacity to discern first principles of understanding, sometimes referred to as common sense.
- practical wisdom (*phronesis*), the capacity to reflect on the good and act in accordance with that.
- philosophic wisdom (*sophia*), a combination of intuitive and scientific knowledge.

While one may tend to assume that intellect is not related to practice, all of these are at the centre of professional practice and are interconnected. Theory is developed to guide practice but practice grounds theory. Thereby they both work hand in hand and not in opposition with one another and cannot be seen in isolation. Without practice there would be no theory and without theory practice would be blind, not evidence based, inconsistent and without development (Lloyd 2017).

ETHICAL THINKING AS PART OF EVERYDAY LIFE

So, when did you last mull over an ethical theory? In a philosophy of social science course? In a bible study? The truth is that we are involved in ethical thinking throughout our lives. As your child demands a larger portion of pudding, your response will begin to work out why he should not have so much. You might argue that such large portions will make him greedy, and so affect both his character, and his weight. You might argue that the guiding principle of this family is equality; we all get the same portion, young or old. This then sparks off an ethical debate about the nature and application of justice. Is it fair to give grandma the same portion as a growing boy who needs more energy?

The subsequent dialogue can then begin to establish that 'this is how and why we do these things in this family'. Ideas like justice, fairness and freedom are common in day to day dialogue, often without us realizing that these are ethical values that help us to decide what is right or wrong. All power to your elbow, parents, if you do take them through the reasons for how you decided portion size, and avoid the 'because I know best school of ethics', a variation of the 'do as you are told approach'. Many believe that their personal values are formed in the family, and there must be some truth in this. So, the question then would be, are ethical principles and values formed because you were told to follow them or because your family spent time showing what they meant and why they are important?

We make ethical decisions every day. Take a moment to consider the pause for thought present in intro 2.

INTRO. 2: PAUSE FOR THOUGHT

Ethical decisions

Consider the decisions you made in the last twenty-four hours, were any of them an ethical decision?
Did you realize at the time that you were taking an ethical decision?
How often do you make ethical decisions?
How do you make these decisions?

Such values are also commonly used in the any organizations, not least universities, as a student or practitioner take a moment to consider the pause for thought present in table 1.

Being part of higher education involves core ethical issues and values including:

- The problem of plagiarism. The root of this word is to kidnap. It is wrong to use someone else's ideas or words as if they are yours. Principles such as truth and respect are involved.
- Fairness in marking. There are many efforts to ensure that student assignments are fairly marked, including anonymous scripts, double marking, moderation, and external examiners. Principles such as justice and impartiality are involved.
- Fair recruitment. How do we decide between accepting students for university who have similar qualifications?
- Ethics in research. For instance, are research participants able to give informed consent for their involvement?

Without concern for fairness, academic freedom and other values, the very project of higher education would collapse. Hence, applied ethics are not extra to the job of universities, they are rather at its heart. The point is that we are not always aware that we are thinking about and practicing ethics. The issue then is not whether we think about ethics but rather how best are we to think ethically. This means being clear and being able to justify the view of ethics that we have.

In this light the idea of ethics as a specialism, additional to professional practice, makes no sense. Actively reflecting on ethics and how we practice it simply helps us to do our job better, and to integrate ethics more effectively into everyday life. Core to this activity is making connections around ideas, values and practice. Far from healthcare ethics being a narrow sub-discipline, it connects to many different but related areas, including:

- Different views of what ethics means, and what are important underlying values.
- Different roles and functions that may have particular perspectives on ethics, e.g. professional bodies, CEO, Trust Board, leaders across the project, and so on.
- Related ideas, including corporate social responsibility, health and safety, diversity.

In turn, this relates to different areas of ethics, such as: communication ethics, leadership ethics, and corporate ethics. All of these are connected, and we shall attempt to make some of those connections. A good leader, for instance, needs to be a good communicator, and needs to be aware of the complexity of the organization and how it relates to society. This means that ethics cannot be confined to a narrow area of 'ethical dilemmas', difficult ethical choices. It is at the heart of all professional

---

TABLE 1 ■ **Higher education / Organisation values**

Higher education	Health Organization
What do you consider are the core ethical values of higher education?	What are the values that are part of your institution?
How are these values discussed in your institution?	How are such values talked about or expressed in workplace conversation?
Are the values referred to on your institution's website?	Are values referred to on your organization's website?

and personal decisions that we make. This is partly why we wanted to extend this edition from simply nursing ethics to include healthcare ethics. Nursing ethics is a professional ethics (the word ethics is singular). Healthcare ethics refers the practice of applied ethics in every aspect of healthcare, including nursing, medicine, physiotherapy, support staff, board directors, HR directors, to accountants (who are represented by their own professional bodies, with their own ethical stances). In this book we have focused on nursing and the wider organizational ethics, the culture of which affects all the different professions who are part of the healthcare project. It is easy to think of the nurse as responsible for care and the board director as responsible for tough things like governance. They have different roles, but both are responsible for care, and both share a responsibility for ethical practice.

Key ideas

VALUES AND PRINCIPLES

These are the 'big ideas' of ethics, and include principles such as equal respect, justice, and human rights. We will show how such principles must be addressed in every aspect of professional life, whatever the size. Justice, for instance, is a key part of human resources, focusing especially on procedural justice - where practices in any organization must be seen to be fair. It is also a key part of working globally. Justice is also part of personal development and the virtues, and how one develops the capacity for justice. It is important to know how to handle the concept and practice of justice across the working environment.

PRACTICE

Ethics is focused in practice. Ethical theory is only useful if it explains what we can see. Hence, we want to see what ethics looks like. We will provide examples of how ethical practised has been successfully and unsuccessfully developed. The use of cases and pause for thoughts exercises will show how one might think about and practice ethics, aiming to develop your own ethical perspective. All behaviour that we see reflects some view of values. The key question is, do we know what that is, and can we effectively justify it?

DIFFERENCE

The ethical big ideas will always lead to debate. This is partly to do with the perspective of different cultures and partly different views within one's own culture. The differences become more marked the more we get down to details of ethical practice. So, we have to decide how we deal with those differences. One culture might argue that it is best to put the interest of families first - with family as a key value. Another culture may argue the importance equal treatment for all, regardless of family or national links.

One argument is that we should tolerate different views just because they are different. Another argument says that some things are more important than difference, such as human rights and justice. Good ethical practice finds a way of working through these issues. A theme throughout the book is that of the ambiguity of difference. It is important to respect the humanity of the different other, but their value system might be problematic and need to be challenged, as might ours. Difference is also important in ethics as a function of learning. Engaging different values causes us to reflect on, challenge and develop our own understanding and practice.

JOINED UP ETHICS

If ethical values are focused in practice, it is important to see the connections that ethics makes across different areas. First, ethical decision-making shares much the same framework as other decision-making frameworks in professional practice. Second, healthcare ethics links up through the category of responsibility with 'cognate' areas such as citizenship (civic responsibility), volunteering, employability (with core ethical virtues relating to workplace skills), enterprise (with capabilities such as creativity), and sustainability. Third, professional ethics connects to other areas of ethics and wider philosophical concerns, from political ethics to social and global ethics. This bridges the gap between personal, professional, and political. Fourth, the same ethical tools are relevant to individual and corporate decision making. There may be different stresses, but it is still about embodying responsibility in the context of different environments. All of this demands synoptic thinking, the capacity to see the overarching picture and how the different aspects connect.

ETHICAL MAPPING

The image of making a map is very apposite for ethics. In one sense maps are always developing over time, in response to differences in the physical terrain and to the sense we make of that terrain. The general shape of the ethical map may remain much the same, but there are also many different perspectives, depending on culture, context, role, and function. Professional ethics involves a continual task of mapping ethical meaning, working out what is of value and how we embody that value, and thus enabling others to take the ethical journey.

ETHICAL DECISION MAKING

The book will offer a framework of ethical decision making, with a focus on understanding the context, including the key relationships, of any decision. A lot of ethical judgements tend to be knee-jerk responses. Ethical deliberation, careful decision making, takes time and critical attention.

RESPONSIBILITY

Perhaps the central ethical category in any applied ethics is responsibility. It involves the practice of:
  - Ethical agency. Being responsible as an individual and organization for what we think and value, and how that affects out practice and the wider social environment. This means that responsibility is both about an awareness of the environment, of our effect on it, and the values that cause us to respond to it.
  - Accountability. This involves both knowing who we are accountable to and how to give a critical account to them.
  - Positive responsibility. This involves working through shared responsibility for our social and physical environment, and planning for that. This requires the exercise of the 'moral imagination', the capacity to develop creative ethical planning. The more responsibility is shared and effectively negotiated the more possibilities multiply. Even just a lack of awareness of the social environment can lead to poor strategic decisions and significant negative effects on that environment, as the Mid Staffs scandal showed.

Throughout the book we will note that that responsibility is never simple. Any professional is responsible for his/her particular practice, and accountable to many different people and organizations. Leadership in those organizations is also focused in responsibility for the management of core values and practice and accountability to many different stakeholders. A recurring theme will be the problems of negative responsibility and the fear of being blamed, and how this can prevent good ethical decision making.

SUSTAINABILITY

Many people would see environmental sustainability as the key ethical principle of our time. We argue that whilst it is a principle which demands immediate attention, it is not the primary principle. Sustaining the environment is, in effect, taking responsibility for the future of mankind. Hence, Jonas (1984) sees responsibility as the primary imperative. We have not then included sustainability in the ethical principles which inform decision making. We have focused on it in the chapters on leadership and governance, not least to stress the importance of reporting which includes the practice of this principle. The six capitals of reporting in chapter nine involve other areas which also need sustaining, including the social environment and, within that, the project of healthcare.

GROWN UP ETHICS

At various points in the book we note that ethics is focused in critical rational reflection. This involves not only intellectual reflection but also awareness of the underlying relational dynamics, which often involve strong feelings. There are three areas that may involve such feelings. The first is around the taking of responsibility. Associated with this is the fear of standing out or taking risks. We will note research that confirms that most people prefer to deny or avoid responsibility. The second is associated with the dynamics of ethical critique. Often, questioning one's values is seen as a threat to identity, thus questioning the worth of the organisation or person. This is associated with the early stages of human development, where the child is unable to distinguish between the self (with associated personal worth) and the actions of the self. A third area is not so much where we must control or handle negative feelings, but where positive feelings reinforce practice. This is often focused on the good feelings associated with service or success. In contrast to the child dynamic is the adult response, involving an awareness of the underlying dynamic, a focus on action rather than person, cultivating virtues that enable responsibility to be taken, and developing the capacity to question, challenge, and accept questions about values and practice.

Such grown up ethics confirms that ethics is not simply about altruism, but rather about mutuality, caring for each other. Much of ethics is about self-care and organizational sustainability, keeping the caring organization going. Without self-care it is hard to see how any concern for others can be fulfilled. Self-interest as such is not unethical. The issue is what is proper concern for institutional sustainability, and how can self-care be balanced with wider care.

THE DANGERS OF CLOSED ETHICS

Related to the issues of difference are closed ethics. By this we mean ethics that are based and operate in the boundaries of a particular organisation and take no account of wider ethics. Such organisations tend to avoid critical questioning and deny wider responsibilities. Hence, throughout the book we note the importance of guarding against the imposition of a closed ethical viewpoint, requiring rather critical dialogue that can test what we think and are aware of, and which can generate creative and imaginative responses to the wider environment.

Reflective Practise and ethics

This book aims to be the basis of a learning experience that exercises some of the core ethical capacities. Hence, learning in this book is based in reflective practice, and thus the idea of a learning cycle, where we reflect on practice, the context of that practice, the underlying values and purposes used in such practice and then how we can develop that practice in the light of those values. Some chapters begin with practice or a history of practice and an analysis of the values and how they can be embodied or how there was a failure to identify or embody them. Hence, dotted around the text are boxes that invite you to practice one or more of these things. These include:
  - *Pause for thought*. This usually focuses on underlying values or value conflicts.
  - *Case studies*. These may be in the form of scenarios are larger case histories

If you work through the different pause for thought exercises and cases presented this will offer practice in:

- knowing what you think, and what values you and your profession and organisation hold, and the capacity to question these.
- awareness of the social and physical environment, and the effect of you and your profession and organisation's actions on these.
- giving an account of values and how they are embodied in practice.
- developing plans for shared responsibility to be put into practice.

The capacities associated with the practice of responsibility include: critical thinking, synoptic thinking, practical wisdom (the capacity to reflect on the good), empathy (deeper awareness and understanding of the self, others and the wider environment), accountability, the capacity to plan and negotiate responsibility, and the moral imagination (the capacity to see how the common good can be embodied in practice).

Central to learning in practice is narrative. The process of telling the story of nursing and healthcare practice informs and affirms the value of that practice, the principles underlying it, and with that identity of the practitioner. Principles become part of who we are, not dusty prescriptions. The wider story of any case also opens the imagination and empathy for those involved. Hence, we would urge readers to look for stories, of patients/clients and staff, to bring to the class, and to find stories in books and the wider media which spark that imagination. Films especially are a useful focus for reflection. We have appended to this introduction a few that you might consider.

Reflection is a leading characteristic of professional development and essential for professional competence and is recognised in work integrated learning to bridge the gap between theory and practice (Patrick et al., 2008). Reflection as a process involves reviewing an experience to describe, analyse, evaluate and inform ones learning and practice. Affording the healthcare practitioner, the opportunity to understand and generalise experiences both during (reflection in) and after (reflection on) action (Schön, 1983). Thereby, reflection has a role not only in academic learning but also in skills development and lifelong learning (Harvey et al., 2010). Engaging in reflection enables the healthcare practitioner to incorporate not just the 'collecting experiences' but also the thinking, active learning and behavioural change based on their reflections (Chamber et al., 2011). Thus, reflective practices build self-awareness, critical thinking and reasoning skills, and skills for decision making within the professional environment (Donaghy and Morss, 2007). In healthcare professional education reflection is valued and this sets the scene for a lifetime of professional reflection. This process which is supported in the academic and clinical environment has a knock-on effect of supporting existing practitioners in their own reflection development as they are guided and supported to facilitate students.

In addition, the use of a clinical supervision, critical companion or mentor enables healthcare practitioners reflect on behaviours and decisions to improve standards of care and the culture of care within organisations. These three terms (clinical supervision, critical companion, or mentor) all encompass the aspect of supporting the healthcare practitioners and are best delivered in a bottom up approach rather that a top down approach. Although these are not a new phenomenon, they are approaches that can assist healthcare practitioners to critically reflect on behaviours. As a process, they are all a forum for learning which can enhance; practice, staff development and support, professional well-being, and standards of care, as these are central to their purpose and philosophy (Tomlinson, 2015; Hardiman and Dewing, 2014; Department of Health – DoH, 2010). In this way, these supportive mechanisms provide opportunities for healthcare practitioners to critically review and transform their beliefs and values, behaviours, decisions and identify opportunities for further learning and development.

We recommend involvement of different professions in the teaching. For instance, one enterprising nursing ethics module invited members of the board, including accountants, to get involved in seminars, enabling mutual challenge, and learning around the meaning of care and the practice of ethics.

Talking about ethics

Research suggests that if you do not talk about ethics then you do not think about ethics, and often avoid taking responsibility for ethical practice (Gentile, 2010). The quote attributed to E.M. Forster sums this up 'How can I tell what I think until I have seen what I say'. Strictly speaking this is less about seeing and more about listening. How can I know what I think if I have not heard those thoughts? If thoughts are not articulated, then assumptions are not questioned. This is so at every level of the healthcare project, from boardroom to the individual professional. Talking about ethics means confronting the misconceptions, identifying the ethical dynamics in our practice, and listening to others views of ethics in practice. All this demands dialogue, and this must be at the core of the development and practice of ethics. It is not anticipated that healthcare professionals are without personal beliefs, opinions or values however, they are expected to engage in a process of self-examination so as they can be appraised, grappled with, and ultimately settled against the standards of the profession (Mintz et al., 2009). Although didactic information about codes of ethics, ethical principles, ethical decision-making models, and legal issues must be presented, significant emphasis must also be placed on increasing healthcare professionals' awareness of their own values, motivations, and behaviours (Remley and Herlihy 2016). This may be accomplished by engaging in dialogue with peers and through reflection.

Overview

The first part of the book (chapters one to three) will examine professional identity and practice and how ethics emerges from that. This involves chapters on the nursing profession, ethical decision making and principles, the nature of responsibility and related professional virtues.

The second part (chapters four to seven) will explore key areas of ethics in nursing practice and healthcare research. This includes ethical dilemmas that arise in daily practice, addressing one's responsibility as a healthcare professional but also the responsibilities and rights of patients/clients. Also, within this section conflicting demands within patient/client groups and environment are considered.

The third part (chapters eight to ten) explores the ethical dynamics of leadership and management in healthcare at all levels. This includes chapters on leadership of nurses and other healthcare professions, clinical governance and shared responsibility, and the social ethics of public health and political leadership.

The book ends with a chapter on normative ethical theory as a way of reflecting on the practice discussed within the book. This sums up an ethics of care as the basis of practice in healthcare, applicable as much to governance and leadership as it is to nursing and healthcare.

References

Aristotle (2004). *Nicomachean Ethics*. Penguin: London.

Chamber, S., Brosnan, C., & Hassell, A. (2011). Introducing medical students to reflective practice. *Education for Primary Care, 22*, 100–105.

Department of Health (2010) *Preceptorship framework for newly registered nurses, midwives and allied health professionals*. London: Department of Health. Online available: https://www.networks.nhs.uk/nhs-networks/ahp-networks/documents/dh_114116.pdf.

Donaghy, M., & Morss, K. (2007). An evaluation of a framework for facilitating and assessing physiotherapy students' reflection on practice. *Physiotherapy Theory and Practice, 23*(2), 83–94.

Gentile, M. (2010). *Giving Voice to Values*. New Haven:: Yale University Press.

Hardiman, M., & Dewing, J. (2014). Critical ally and critical friend: Stepping stones to facilitating practice development. *International Practice Development Journal, 4*(1), 3.

Harvey, M., Coulson, D., Mackaway, J., & Winchester-Seeto, T. (2010). Aligning reflection in the cooperative education curriculum. *Asia Pacific Journal of Coopertive Education, 11*(3), 137–152.

Jonas, H. (1984). *The imperative of responsibility*. Chicago:: Chicago University Press.

Lloyd, H.A. (2017) Theory without practice is empty; Practice without theory is blind: The inherent inseparability of doctrine and skills. In: Edwards, L.H. The doctrine skills divide: legal education's self-inflicted wound. (pp.77-90). North Carolina: Carolina Academic Press, Durham. Online available: https://philarchive.org/archive/LLOTWP.

Mintz, L. B., Jackson, A. P., Neville, H. A., Illfelder-Kaye, J., Winterowd, C. L., & Loewy, M. I. (2009). The need for a counselling psychology model training values statement addressing diversity. *The Counseling Psychologist*, *37*, 644–675.

Patrick, C., Peach, D., Pocknee, C., Webb, F., Fletcher, M., & Pretto, G. (2008). *The WIL Report: A national scoping study of Work Integrated Learning*. Brisbane:: Australian Learning and Teaching Council.

Remley, T. P., & Herlihy, B. (2016). *Ethical, legal, and professional issues in counselling* (Fifth Edition.). Upper Saddle River, NJ:: Pearson Education.

Schön, D. (1983). *The reflective practitioner: How professionals think in action*. New York:: Basic Books.

Tomlinson, J. (2015). Using clinical supervision to improve the quality and safety of patient care: a response to Berwick and Francis. *BMC Medical Education*, *15*, 103.

Vardy, P. (1989). *Business Morality People and Profit*. London:: Harper Collins.

Films related to healthcare ethics

A Private Matter (1992) Focusing on abortion and principlism: autonomy vs. paternalism.

Whose Life is it anyway? (1981) Focusing on patient's right to end life. Patient with quadriplegia wants to end his life: principlism, virtues, autonomy.

The Diving Bell and the Butterfly Patient (2007) Focusing on a patient with "Locked in Syndrome", Principlism (Self-determination) v. utilitarianism.

Extreme Measures (1996) Secret human medical experimentation for treating spinal cord injuries; Homeless men used as research subjects. Utilitarianism, informed consent; atonement.

Miss Evers' Boys (1997) The infamous Tuskegee Syphilis Study, involving deception in medical research. Participants were told they were receiving treatment for syphilis when, in reality, their condition was simply being monitored.

Lorenzo's Oil. (1992). Involving a child with a progressive neurological condition, and the parents struggle to search for a cure. The focus is on consequences and the nature of person.

John Q (2002). Involving a child with terminal illness in need of organ transplant that is unaffordable. This focuses on distributive justice and worth of human life.

Damaged Care (2002) Involving a doctor who blows the whistle on inappropriate denials of treatment. This covers conflicts of Interest; Virtue Ethics; Hippocratic Oath; Distributive J.

The Sea Inside (2004) The factual story of Ramon Sampedro who fought for euthanasia and his own right to die, exploring complex relationships and different views of value and principles.

The Farewell (2019) A gentle and funny reflection on conflicting cultural views of death, and how families make sense of dying.

Henry V (1989) Shakespeare's play is not about healthcare but is about leadership, dialogue and authentic communication. See especially the St Crispin's Day speech (act four) and the dialogue with troops the night before.

The Nature of Healthcare Ethics

The Nursing Profession: Its Value and Values

LEARNING OUTCOMES

When you have read and worked through this chapter, you should be able to:

- Critically reflect on the Mid Staffs case, is essentially about professional ethics
- Examine the vision and purpose of a profession
- Consider the tension in professional bodies between servicing society and protecting its members
- Examine the basis of professional ethics
- Examine the social identity of the nursing profession
- Examine the key ethical values of the nursing profession and how they relate to the core vision
- Examine the complex institutional context of nursing

Introduction

The exploration of nursing and healthcare ethics begins with a reflection on what it means to be a member of the nursing and healthcare professions. The focus of that reflection will be the case history which has challenged the identity and purpose of these professions, that of the Mid Staffordshire (Mid Staffs) National Health Service (NHS) Trust. This was not the first time that healthcare professions have been questioned regarding their professional ethics and will not be the last. Other scandals include: The Winterbourne View Report (Department of Health and Social Care 2012), the Liverpool Care Pathway Review (Department of Health and Social Care 2013), and most recently, the Shrewsbury Case (Campbell 2018). However, the different reports into the Mid Staffordshire scandal have offered an opportunity to reflect on how some members of the nursing profession, along with all the other professionals and groups in this case, could have practised the opposite of what they professed. It is fair to say that, in the UK at least, the case has prompted a re-evaluation of the nursing and healthcare professions. The questions raised include:

- What is the vision and purpose of any profession?
- Are the caring professions and professional bodies built on the idea of service to society or to protect power and status of its members?
- What is the social identity of the nursing profession, and how has it developed from nurturer, to servant, to 'angel', to qualified practitioner?
- What are key ethical values of the nursing profession and how do they relate to the core vision of purpose?
- What is the institutional context of nursing, including relationships between the nursing profession and different value narratives including: institutional sustainability, medicine, healthcare policy, patient/client and family, and wider health service?

This chapter will explore these questions and also what caused many nurses in the Mid Staffs case to operate blindly, without questioning their actions. Was it a failure of individual character, a failure of professional oversight or other regulation, a failure of leadership at organisational and political level, or ineffective organisational culture? What developments are needed to focus on nursing practice across any health service? Beginning to address these questions will set the context for what follows in this book, an exploration of the ethical dimension of professional practice in nursing.

The Mid Staffordshire Healthcare Trust

The scandal of the Mid Staffs Healthcare Trust came to light in mid-2007. The Healthcare Commission (HCC), the then Healthcare regulator, flagged data which highlighted abnormally high death rates in the Trust. By 2008 the HCC had noted seven different patient/client safety alerts. The hospital's response was to suggest that the data involved 'coding errors' and the HCC commissioned the first of five reports to inquire into the situation/circumstances. A full public inquiry was then constituted led by Robert Francis (2010). This was the first of two reports by Francis and it set out a litany of poor hospital care which would haunt the surviving patients/clients and families. This included:

- Patients/clients were left in excrement in soiled bed clothes for lengthy periods;
- Assistance was not provided with feeding for patients/clients who could not eat without help;
- Water was left out of patients'/clients' reach;
- Patients/clients were not assisted with their toileting needs in spite of persistent requests for help;
- Wards and toilet facilities were left in a filthy condition, including littered with used bandages and dressings;
- Patients'/clients' families often had to take on the task of cleaning these areas;
- Privacy and dignity, even in dying and death, was denied;
- Triage in the accident and emergency department was undertaken by untrained staff;
- Treatment of patients/clients and those close to them with what appeared to be callous indifference;
- Misdiagnosis was common.

It is estimated that up to 1200 patients/clients died because of such poor care in the 50 months between January 2005 and March 2009. As Campling (2015, p. 2) suggests, this presents 'us with the reality that healthcare organisations and healthcare workers within them are capable of neglectful and abusive behaviour that can justifiably be described as cruel'.

The second report (Francis 2013) focused on the leadership and governance of the Mid Staffs Hospital Trust. This report further revealed the stark disconnect between the values and meaning espoused by the organisation and the actual practice. Just how extraordinary is not clear, as the report itself suggests that many of the problems were likely to be more widespread than just in the Mid Staffs hospital. The report suggests that there were many voices involved in a complex situation, but little valuing of these, little dialogue, and little shared meaning or sense of shared responsibility. What meaning there was seemed to be fragmented or detached, with individual employees left to establish their own sense of meaning from their work, all leading to lack of critical awareness of the core values and purpose of the whole project, and the complex relational network of healthcare. Key findings from the Francis (2013) report were summed up as:

- A culture of fear predominated, which focused on doing the system's business, expressed in terms of key targets;
- An institutional culture which ascribed more weight to positive information about the service than to information capable of implying cause for concern;
- When monitoring occurred, it was often felt more important to get the best story across, to give the regulator what it was thought they wanted to hear. In practice this included, in some cases, clinical notes being altered or forged (Mastracci 2017), and patients/clients being released before it was safe to do so, in order to achieve time targets. This was because institutional survival was predicated on successful achievement of management targets;
- Standards and methods of measuring compliance did not focus on the effect of a service on patients/clients;
- An acceptance and a degree of tolerance of poor standards and risk to patients/clients;
- A failure to communicate between the many agencies and to share their knowledge of concerns;
- Assumptions that monitoring, performance management, or intervention was the responsibility of someone else;
- A failure to tackle challenges to the building up of a positive culture, in nursing in particular but also within the medical profession;
- A failure to appreciate the risk of disruptive loss of corporate memory and focus. This occurred because of the repeated, multi-level reorganisation initiated;
- In order to achieve the financial targets necessary, the board issued swinging cuts which negatively affected the service.

One emergency room doctor in the first Francis Report elaborated on the effects of chronic crisis on nurses (Francis 2010, p. 190): 'the nurses were so under resourced they were working extra hours; they were desperately moving from place to place to try to give adequate care to patients/clients. If you are in that environment for long enough, what happens is you become immune to the sound of pain. You either become immune to the sound of pain or you walk away. You cannot feel people's pain, you cannot continue to want to do the best you possibly can when the system says no to you, you can't do the best you can. And the system in the hospital said "no" to the nursing staff doing the best they could and to the doctors, but I think the nursing staff probably feel that more acutely'.

HOW COULD THIS HAPPEN?

The board, management, and different professions, including the nursing profession, operated in a teleopathic way, defined by Goodpaster as, 'the unbalanced pursuit of purpose in either individuals or organisations, the mindset or condition is a key stimulus to which ethics is a practical response' (Goodpaster 2007, p. 28). Goodpaster suggests that the key symptoms of teleopathy are fixation, rationalisation, and detachment. Fixation in the Mid Staffs case focused on the key purpose of the organisational sustainability. This brought the Trust close to what Bauman (1989) and others refer to as instrumental rationality, involving focus on means, efficient or cost-effective, rather than on the value of the end. Fixation demands rationalisation, that is some sense of justifying action in terms of underlying value. In the case of Mid Staffs, this led to a focus on identity seen in terms of achieving targets and financial/organisational status, expressed in the aim of capturing Foundation Trust status. The benefits of becoming a Foundation Trust included governance and financial autonomy, and clearer accountability to their local community (King's Fund 2016).

Foundation trusts were then based in key values, not least that of freedom to organise themselves, and local accountability. The Mid Staffs Trust also retained the core values of care. Indeed, the focus of practice was the NHS Constitution (NHS 2015), involving seven principles, including: 'the NHS aspires to the highest standards of excellence and professionalism and the patient/client will be at the heart of everything the NHS does'. The rationalisation in the Mid Staffs Trust was that such values could not be fully sustained if the foundation status was not achieved. The tests to achieve this status were, however, 'unforgiving', demanding key financial and governance targets be achieved. There was also a narrative of competition with other trusts, which was set up by the UK Government (Campbell 2013).

Fixation on targets, and rationalisation in terms of the underlying principles of organisational sustainability, led to detachment from wider meaning and purpose, other related organisations, other professions and colleagues, and from patients/clients and families. Ironically, this led to detachment from the core values espoused by the Trust. As the Board was rewarding staff with vouchers (Campbell 2013) for the successful foundation status application, the moves toward developing investigations into the practice of the Trust were in process. Markey et al. (2019) argue that nurses become indifferent and accepting of substandard care, which is sustained through a culture of self-rationalising and of blaming organisational constraints and unsupportive caring environments. Bandura et al. (1996) suggests that moral disengagement occurs when individuals engage in habitual self-regulatory behaviour when intentionally detaching themselves from a situation. Detachment also leads to polarisation, both of values and people, viewing these different groups as 'problems', in this case getting in the way of achieving Foundation Trust status. Hence, complaints from families were not listened to. Staff whistle-blowers and new nurses who questioned practice were bullied and harassed by supervisors and co-workers (Mastracci 2017). In one case, an elderly patient/client was chastised by a senior nurse for a suicide attempt, which she said was a 'selfish act' (Francis 2010, p. 155). Another patient/client was mocked for carrying a Bible (Francis 2010, p. 156).

All this suggests a form of self-deception at personal, professional, and institutional levels. The dynamic for much of the organisation was one of denial:

- Denial of injury or problem, arguing that things are not as bad as they seemed. Witnesses to the first Francis Report frequently noted that staff justified their actions by arguing that the same practice went on across the NHS.
- Denial of responsibility, often arguing that problems were due primarily to a lack of resources and that nothing can be done. Regulators and practitioners alike saw any problems as the responsibility of other persons or professions.
- Condemning the condemners, seeing criticisms as coming from people and groups who do not fully understand the situation.

It is worth noting that this kind of thinking is often based in logical fallacies, not least variants of the ad hominem fallacy, where the issues are ignored and the focus is on problems with the other persons or groups. Logical fallacies, as we will show in the next chapter, can be an indicator of ethical problems.

RECOMMENDATIONS

The Francis (2013) Report's recommendations included:

- Government changes in the National Health Service should be cut down. Frequent change serves to focus on the changes and related actions, not the core purpose.

- All practice has to focus around the patient/client, particularly in terms of standards, possibly through tighter codes. The Report uses strong phrases such as the need for 'a relentless focus' on the patient's/client's interests and the obligation to keep patients/clients safe and protected from substandard care, requiring that the patient/client must be first in everything that is done, and that there must be no tolerance of substandard care.
- A more open and positive culture has to be developed, not focused on narrow targets and not based in fear. This should include clarity about core values across the institution.
- Leadership should be reinforced and shared amongst the different professions.
- There should be clearer standards and guidance on compliance. There should be no tolerance of non-compliance and the rigorous policing of fundamental standards. Information about compliance should be accessible and useable by all, allowing effective comparison of performance.
- The need to develop thinking laterally across boundaries; more shared leadership with managerial, clinical, and board leaders working together; and greater transparency and willingness to give and accept challenge.
- There was a lack of attention to responsibility at all levels, the reluctance to critically examine and address unconscious models of leadership that are embedded in organisations, and evidence that better performing hospitals had more devolved power and shared responsibility.

The King's Fund (2011) report on leadership in the Health Service echoes much of this, arguing for greater attention to the narratives of patients/clients and staff. At the heart of these arguments were five key demands which looked to establish responsibility for meaning and practice at both corporate and individual levels:

- A 'common culture' was required throughout the Health Service;
- A key aspect of this was to be safety, including an awareness of and responsibility for the effects of any action or lack of action;
- An organisation should have shared values from top management to frontline staff;
- The NHS should develop strong, consistent leadership to motivate and empower staff to take responsibility for practice. Mastracci (2017) notes the way in which nursing management often discouraged and eroded such leadership by encouraging trainee nurses not to raise questions about practice;
- Everyone employed by the NHS should have a 'questioning attitude, a rigorous approach and good communication skills'. This sets responsibility in some sense on everybody to understand professional practice and to challenge poor examples.

The Francis Report (2013) is light in its treatment of the UK government. It acknowledges the importance of the Government's stewardship of healthcare and thus the need to cut back on some of the spending on health (Francis Report Executive Summary 2013, p. 54), and therefore does not fully include politicians in the critique. Against that, it could be argued that Government bear equal responsibility, not least because the stress on measurable targets has come originally from them. By implication, if a Government is tied to targets then it has an investment in reinforcing a narrow perspective based on such targets. There is some evidence that politicians either do not themselves focus on the underlying vision of health services, or that they have uncritical assumption that there is a worked-out philosophy of care behind such targets. The Report did acknowledge that the UK Government was responsible over time for instituting too many major changes in practice and process, with the effect of focusing professional attention further on process and targets, rather than on the overall shared purposes of care. Well intended action thus still had the effect of reinforcing dissociative behaviour.

Organisational Breakdown

The Mid Staffs case can be characterised as a breakdown of meaning (of values and practice) and relationships. Care practitioners who ignored patients/clients in sometimes extreme need were literally not in their 'right mind', and did not even think to practise the broader sense of accountability. There was no engagement with the complexity of narratives in the Trust, and with that, a lack of awareness of how distinct professional narratives could effectively work together to share responsibility. The term breakdown intentionally suggests pathology. McKenna and Rooney (2011) have argued that organisational breakdowns of this sort are actually a form of institutional schizophrenia, in the sense of multiple personality. In fact, they mischaracterise the term. Multiple personality or dissociative identity disorder refers to a clinical condition where distinct personalities are unconsciously created to avoid either guilt or memory of earlier trauma (Brand et al. 2014). Schizophrenia rather refers to a 'breaking down' of the mind, losing touch with reality, often involving a paranoid view of the world. It literally involves a breakdown in the person's capacity to make shared and realistic meaning in relation to their social network. This analogy fits better Mid Staffs and other governance crises across all sectors in the last two decades, such as the credit crisis (see Ferguson 2010), involving: a breakdown of meaning and relational connection such that there is no sense of the significance of the organisation in relation to the wider social and physical environments (dissociation); a defensiveness which sees external relations as some form of threat; and a breakdown in awareness and connection to the social history and responsibility of the organisation – a form of organisational paranoia. It is ironical that psychosis is often associated with 'hearing voices' (Robinson 2013), something characterised as negative. In fact, the breakdown in Mid Staffs was precisely because the many voices were not 'heard', their meaning was not understood. The voices of the different professions, the key regulators, the nurses, the families, and, above all, the patients/clients, were deemed to be not part of reality.

It should come as no surprise then that such breakdowns occur. At one level, meaning, as we have argued, is more than rational, conceptual, or practical. It involves identity and worth in relation to the social network, and values, and thus feelings and emotions, and a narrow internal culture can lead to a real disconnection with reality. This breakdown connects directly to the fragmentation of organisations (Rozuel 2011). This underscores two key points: first, significant meaning is socially constructed, and second, we are all responsible for articulating and sustaining that meaning. Leadership which does not attend to these core levels of meaning (conceptual and practical) on a regular basis always runs the risk of breakdown. In the Mid Staffs case, there was a corporate disintegration of meaning, based on power and the fear of the leaders.

1.1 PAUSE FOR THOUGHT

Considering Mid Staffs

If the Mid Staffs scandal was about a breakdown in organisation, what has ethics got to do with it? Can't we just get the organisation right and all will be well? Some would argue that this is a matter of sociology not ethics. In fact, the picture shows many different players, each in different ways faced by ethical challenges.

As a student nurse should you raise your doubts with someone in authority? You don't want to be seen as a trouble maker, but this practice seems wrong.

As a middle manager, should you raise what you hear from some of the nurses, in conversation, with the directors? They have been under stress recently and are not going to thank you.

As a Trust leader should you look more closely into the reports about stress?

All of these questions and others involve taking responsibility for judging if something is right or wrong, and what you or I ought to do about it.

None of them occur free from the stress or tension of dealing with other different voices which demand different things from us.

What would you have done as a student nurse, or nurse manager faced by poor standards of care, and what would be the basis of your decision?

Nursing and Mid Staffs

Ethical issues and meaning ran throughout the Mid Staffs scandal. This was partly about the organisation. At one level it was about the practice of responsibility in the organisation. A whole series of people in management and in the professions chose not to take responsibility for what they were doing. Key to avoiding and denying responsibility was the giving of responsibility to others, including responsibility for setting meaning and purpose. This negative view of responsibility then poses the question as to what actually is your job. At both organisational and professional level, much of the ethical decisions were based in the question of the purpose of one job. What is purpose and value of what you do? The answer to that question will tell you what matters to you as a professional and will begin to shape any ethical decision that you make. Ethical practice in this sense begins to emerge from one's professional identity.

The Francis Reports focused on the governance of the whole of the Trust and the wider health service. It also focused on nursing practice in this tragedy, raising major questions about the role and identity of the nursing profession. The questions were about the role of the professional bodies as such and about the professional practice. Francis was critical of the Royal College of Nursing (RCN), referring to it as 'ineffective', arguing that little was done to uphold professional standards among nursing staff or to address concerns and problems faced by its members. In particular, he argued that RCN staff colluded with the Trust management to ensure whistle-blower concerns in A&E were not addressed. Francis argued that the nursing voice, at individual level and professional body level, was needed to challenge unethical practices. Key to the diminution of this voice, was the tension in the RCN between its role as professional body, responsible for maintaining professional standards of ethics and competency, and its role as trades union (Francis 2013). Francis argued that the trades union role, defending members, dominated the core role of focusing on the purpose of care, losing any impartiality.

1.2 PAUSE FOR THOUGHT

Consider Your Professional Body

How do you see the purpose of your professional body?
  Is it about serving interests or encouraging responsibility?
  Was Francis fair in focusing on the profession of nursing as failing in Mid Staffs?
  Why would the other professions, from medicine, to directors, to accountancy be any different, or have less responsibility?

Francis' claim led to an ongoing debate about responsibility. The RCN focused on the stress on staff created by a culture of fear and cutting jobs (see https://www.thcguardian.com/society/2013/sep/30/stress-nurses-patients-risk-rcn). This suggests that it is a false dichotomy to pit responsibility for care of patients/clients against responsibility for care of the RCN members. Both involve ethical value, and attention to care of professionals could have a major effect on the care of patients/clients. You can walk and chew ethical gum at the same time. The debate itself was raising questions about the nature of responsibility, how it is shared and negotiated. The Francis Report (2013) argued that the two roles should be clearly divided. However, the RCN argued that it was important to hold the two together. By 2017, 4 years after the second Francis Report, the RCN had determined that it would develop governance that would retain but separate the two roles (see https://www.nursingtimes.net/news/policies-and-guidance/rcn-to-begin-separating-oversight-of-union-and-college-roles/7016535.article). Partly as a response to the emerging challenge, the Chief Nursing officer for England, Pat Cummings, and Viv Bennett, Director of Nursing, Department of Health (DH) and Lead Nurse, Public Health England produced a document which refocuses the philosophy and practice of nursing (Cummings and Bennett 2012), and we will consider this in some detail below as part of a reflection on the nursing profession. First, however, we need to begin to consider what a profession as such is.

THE NATURE OF A PROFESSION

The case raises major questions about the nature of a profession. The Oxford Shorter Dictionary (Oxford Dictionary 2007) uses the term vocation to define the term profession: 'a vocation, a calling, one requiring advanced knowledge or training in some branch of learning or science'.

To be a member of a profession is therefore to:
- have specialised knowledge and skill;
- have power – the power of knowledge and the capacity to affect society;
- have autonomy of practice – this varies according to employment context, but focuses on the capacity of the professional to make decisions and judgements about practice;
- have a monopoly or near monopoly of a particular skill;
- have undergone an extensive period of training which includes not simply skills, but a strong intellectual element;
- be a member of a professional body which is responsible for regulating standards, protecting rights of practice and ensuring proper training (Fawkes 2017).

VALUES AND PROFESSION

Professional practitioners of all disciplines also require values. These focus on the core vision of the profession, the relationship and responsibilities to key stakeholders, including patients/clients, families, and professional colleagues. To ensure responsibilities are properly addressed these values include:
- Integrity, openness, and honesty, both with themselves and with others.
- Independence, to be free of secondary interests with other parties.
- Impartiality, to be free of bias and unbalanced interests.
- Responsibility, the recognition and acceptance of personal commitment, and accountability to others.
- Competence, a thorough knowledge of the work they undertake to do.
- Discretion, care with communications, trustworthiness (Robinson et al. 2012).

These values enable the professional to maintain principles and fulfil responsibilities in the best interest of the patient/client, and to do this in a context which is often complex and unclear. The professional works in a discipline with specialised knowledge that his/her patient/client may not have or fully understand. They therefore work outside the control of their patient/client and are trusted with their patient's/client's interests. Ethical meaning emerges then from the very nature of professions, built as they are on the imbalance of power between the professional and the patient/client. The values seek to protect the patient/client from any abuse, corruption, or coercion and to ensure that the interests of the patient/client take priority over the interests of the profession.

THE PURPOSE OF A PROFESSION

Airaksinen (1994) argues that in addition to the professional characteristics noted above, a key aspect of any profession is the underlying worth or the purpose of that profession. If the values above emerge from the professional–client relationship, then these values transcend that particular relationship and are focused on well-being and the common good. For the legal profession, for instance, the common good is justice and distribution of justice. It is hard for society to exist without such a good. The common good of the healthcare professions is the delivery of health and well-being. The professions are there to find ways of realising the common good. Of course, the concept of health or healthcare is not straightforward (Huber 2011) and is a matter of ongoing debate, across the health services and in each profession. But this is in itself part of any professional reflection. Hence, Tawney (1930) and others see professions as essentially serving society.

THE AMBIGUITY OF PROFESSIONS

Against this view of professions contributing to social development and wider ethical understanding, Fawkes (2017), in writing about all professions, echoes the concerns of Francis. In this view, professions are seen as using bureaucratic mechanisms to promote exclusivity and monopolistic practices. In Shaw's (1906) words, 'professions are a conspiracy against the laity'. Powerful bodies tend to protect their own interests, and focus on their power, prestige and wealth, built around a monopoly. Illich (2010) goes further, to argue that the very purpose of the professions has become to encourage the dependency of the patient/client. He suggests that the professions rose from the Middle Ages as soon as the definition of pastoral human need began to emerge. In this light, the priesthood became the key profession and acted 'arbiters' of the right way to live, taking away the responsibility from the individual. With the rise of the modern professions, far from this providing a disinterested service, power was simply transferred from the church to them. Illich (2010) argued that, in the medical profession, this led to the imposition of treatment and the over-prescription of drugs, leading to increases in iatrogenic illness, disorders inadvertently induced by a healthcare giver because of a surgical, medical, drug or vaccine treatment, or by a diagnostic procedure.

The picture of the professions as centres of power was also given credence by the focus on ethical codes. Fawkes (2017) notes that ethical codes have often been used as part of the defence of professions and their monopolistic power. They act as an attempted assurance of self-regulation; 'trust us, we have an ethical code'. Nonetheless, a formal professional body with accompanying bureaucracy is important if the core purpose of the profession is to be maintained. Without the professional structure it will be hard to sustain core values. The keys to the proper exercise of power, involving ethical judgement, is that the professional body should be transparent and critically reflective, and that the profession should be empowering not disabling the patient/client.

The Professional Body or Institution

The virtue of integrity is not simply an individual one but applies to the professional institution and management groups as well. The profession, as a whole, has to be consistent and be able to relate values to practice. Without this, the recognition of the profession as a body of experts concerned for public welfare will be eroded and with that will go the trust essential to the functioning of any professional relationship. The existence of an institution of professionals is essential for the development and maintenance of professional virtues. It enables the individual professional to reflect upon his own integrity and to learn from the experience of others, transmitting the culture from generation to generation. It provides an external perspective which enables proper reflection and responsibility. The Institution can:

- enable the professional development of moral awareness, skills, responsibility and identity, through codes, dialogues and training;
- ensure its processes and organisation are conducive to the development of moral responsibility;
- provide support and the opportunity for professionals to work through decision making and any conflicts of interest;
- regulate the practice of the individual professional;
- play a major role in communicating with the public;
- set standards for admissions to institutions and for initial and continuing professional training;
- act as a learned society, contributing to the advancement of the theoretical and practice skills central to the profession.

The Mid Staffs case suggests that professional bodies need to develop further roles: the appropriate support of the members (enabling them to do their job), and the wider role of communicating purpose and values beyond the professional body. In the first of these, this may involve addressing local conflicts of value, including critique of management decisions. In the second, the professions can be seen as contribution to focus on the common good; a role of social value leadership. The institution itself has to develop a means of reflecting on its own ethos and ethical culture – this is a prime responsibility of the Council of the Institution, requiring regular reviews of the professional code and ensuring sound practice by all members. Fawkes (2017) raises a critical question. How far does any professional body actually audit its values and practice? In other words, is the profession itself actually reflective? She views this from a Jungian perspective which argues that all individuals have a shadow side. This is not a 'bad' side necessarily but simply an aspect of the person that is not examined. Because it is not examined, this can lead to the person unconsciously projecting these underlying feelings and views on to relationships (Fawkes 2017). Fawkes argues that this dynamic is the same for any organisation, including professional bodies. The stress on self-regulation tends to be reactive rather than reflective; responding to crises such as Mid Staffs in healthcare. This reactive mode suggests a lack of ongoing reflective practice. Hence, there is an argument for developing on-going value audits at the level of the professional body, monitoring how the different concerns are held together.

Trust and the Professions

Crises surrounding professions are frequent; from clergy and child sex abuse and the leadership response (Lauer and Hoyer 2019), to the credit crises, to politicians, to police. Each time the cry goes up, 'how can we trust them anymore?' Trust is critical to the relationship between the profession and society; hence the need to maintain reputation. O'Neill (2002), in a major reflection on trust, argued that, in fact, trust in the main professions has been maintained. You still call an ambulance when you are in trouble is the gist of her argument. However, trust is a bit more complex than that, ranging from unconditional or naive trust (I trust you because you are a doctor), to trust which is focused not on the profession per se and more on the particular professional. Measurement of trust in professions has varied over the last decade according to the Edelman Trust Barometer (2019). Significantly, however, in 2019 the most recent report from Edelman noted a move away from trust in bodies to trust in particular CEOs or leaders: 'I trust my CEO'. This suggests that trust is focused on relationships, the embodiment of what is professed, in commitment and care over time. It also raises questions about the nature of the professional body. Is it an institution or is it a community, with members of the community responsible for that community? We will return throughout the book to explore trust.

The Professions as Empowering

In different ways Koehn (1994) and May (1985) suggest that the role of the professional is precisely to enable the development of autonomy. Many contrasts the image of the professional as adversary, fighting disease or fighting against the opposition in the courtroom, with the professional as teacher. This, they argue, involves a transformative process, with the client developing the capacity to make decisions, or the ability to make them in different contexts. May (1985) is careful to stress that such teaching would not be paternalistic but would involve a collaboration between one or more professionals and the patient/client around the project. Koehn (1994) takes this further, arguing that the professional does not simply seek to avoid harm but to develop the best for the patient/client. Developing the best can only be discovered in dialogue with the patient/client. In this light, Koehn stresses the importance of the professional enabling the patient/client to articulate his need through developing his particular narrative and the starting point for the professional is listening to the patient/client (Koehn 1994, p. 175).

Close to these is the view of Schön (1983), who argues for reflective practice as being central to professional development. This includes an understanding of the professional's own role in any context, noting both limitations and opportunities. Schön suggests also that a key part of the professional response is to treat the patient/client as a reflective practitioner. As a reflective practitioner, the patient/client would be empowered, learning, as well as using, knowledge, insight, and abilities in working out the particular problem. We will return to the definition of autonomy in the next chapter when we look at the ethical decision-making process.

The Nursing Profession

The nursing profession was founded in values of selfless, familial, care, focusing on the maternal role of nurturing. The very word nurse derives from the Latin verb *nutrio*, to nourish. The term *nutrix* was formed from this to denote a 'nurse' or 'foster mother'. This selfless narrative was reinforced in the 19th century with the story of Florence Nightingale (see Bivins et al. 2017). Here, nursing was associated with doing God's work through responding to those in need, highlighting a strong religious undercurrent of compassion. This in turn was reflected in the qualities said to be embodied by Nightingale, such as gentleness, kindness, and courtesy. As nursing in the mid-19th century began to evolve into a more regulated, professional activity, it continued to be associated culturally with this affect-led selfless vocation of caring. This led to a set of uncritical assumptions about nursing which have created tension for the identity of the profession, not least the underlying view focused on forms of labour that were gender specific, and to which women were uniquely adapted to by their family roles. On the one hand, this provided a view of nursing which underlined the worth of nurses, sanctioning their presence in homes and hospitals. This worked against the early Victorian stereotype of nursing as coarse, untrained, uncaring, and incompetent, exemplified by the character of Sarah Gamp depicted in the novel Martin Chuzzlewit (Dickens 1844). On the other hand, nursing became seen as largely affective, focused on altruism as motivation, and exemplified in the natural caring of women. This also became idealised with images such as nurses as angels (Campbell 1984). 'Nursing' and 'caring' remained largely synonymous and at the same time as 20th-century nurse training programmes began to stress accountability and competence, demanding an articulation of increasing levels of knowledge and specialised skills. These changes accelerated with the increasing use in hospital care of more complex technological interventions. In turn, this drove up training and educational needs set down by employers and regulatory bodies. This approach began to displace the paradigm of bedside compassion.

In the second half of the 20th century, nursing literature began to articulate concern with the apparent dichotomy between the affective image of nursing and the more scientific image of the professional expert. Part of this discussion was about sense of social worth, with the scientific view being more akin to the other professions' view of worth, especially the medical profession. At the same time, even in national healthcare context, there has been an increased focus on governance leadership and management. This is focused on sustaining organisations that deliver care. With that, professional advancement in nursing becomes more focused on specialisation and management roles, with less support for the affective role (Bivins et al. 2017).

The managerialism in the late 20th century, combined with a more scientific stance, fuelled a focus on quality and excellence in professional standards. To achieve such excellence demanded that quality be more tightly defined and more effectively measured, including the provision of compassionate care (Bivins et al. 2017). Attempts to measure compassionate care, however, have proved problematic, focused as it is on relationships which have a strong subjective element. Some influential models of nursing focus on care as holistic, focused on human interactions (Robinson et al. 2003; Watson 1985). This focus is in addition to a knowledge base and clinical competence (Sourial 1997).

Both models are based on the principle of equality (equal care). However, they have different understandings of that term. Watson (1985) sees equality as equal respect and therefore a concern for the particularity of the patient/client, including enabling particular needs to be answered. Sourial (1997) is more concerned with equitable provision of care – all receiving the same attention and provision.

Two things are important to note at this point. First, as the narrative of the nursing profession has unfolded, we have seen an ongoing dialogue and debate about the identity of nursing as a profession. In effect this has attempted to articulate the core purpose; the transcendent good at the heart of professional practice. Yes, it is health and healthcare, both focused on the common good of human well-being. The question then is, what does that look like in practice? Second, the debate can easily be seen as an either/or approach, with the more relational view of care as difficult to achieve, both in terms of time and of the emotional energy required. Two things work against this simplistic polarisation. Firstly, in some approaches, the idea of compassionate care as exhausting presupposes a view of care which focuses on the need for profound emotional engagement. Writers such as Campbell (1984), however, argue that care in a professional context has to be 'moderated' or mediated. In one sense, this sees the nurse (but also doctor) as akin to social workers or counsellors, professionally developing core psychological skills which enable patient/client empowerment. In effect, care is about an authentic concern for the other which also involves a distance which enables effective professional practice. Such a view of care also questions the idea of gender-focused innate care. The use of affective skills in a professional context requires training and development. The virtues of professional practice will be set out in more depth in Chapter 3, and meaning of care is developed in Chapters 4 and 11. The second argument against the polarisation of care models is that it focuses on the individual role of the nurse. Dutton et al. (2014) and others focus on the effect of culture in developing a compassionate response across the organisation. Compassion then becomes a function of the healthcare community not simply an aggregate of caring individuals. Hence, responsibility for care is shared across the organisation and between different professions and roles. The culture sets in place organisational and procedural architecture which mediates key aspects of the compassionate community including:

- Purpose and vision, with all engaged and committed to sustaining the practice of the vision. This means finding ways which refresh the core story;
- Training in skills and virtues that can develop congruent care;
- Provision of appropriate staffing levels;
- Training in leadership across all professions and roles.

The debate about the practice of compassion after the Mid Staffs crisis focuses on whether the cause was 'compassion deficit' or organisational culture that made it difficult to practise (Stenhouse et al. 2016; Paley 2014; Rolfe and Gardner 2014). The terms used in the debate, not least 'deficit', are limiting and other work has attempted to deepen the exploration of the meaning of compassion and related ideas such as empathy. Stenhouse et al. (2016) argue that the practice of both personal responsibility and organisational responsibility are necessary for the consistent practice of compassionate care. We will explore this in more detail in Chapter 3 and Part 3. At this stage, it is important to note that the compassionate care offered to the patient/client correlates to the creation of a compassionate workplace. It becomes difficult to practise compassion with patients/clients in a workplace that does not practise care in the workplace itself. These different elements of care have been part of an ongoing debate in the healthcare professions, and in the development in England of the six Cs, there is a systematic effort to hold them together in nursing and in all aspects of healthcare.

The Six Cs

In the middle of the Mid Staffs crisis, just before the Francis (2013) report, the core purpose of the nursing profession was revisited by the Department of Health in England with the introducing the '6Cs' as values for practice within a new nursing strategy (Cummings and Bennett 2012).

These were later included in the new framework for nursing (NHS England 2016). The six Cs grew out consultation with more than 9000 nurses, midwives, care staff, and patients/clients (Cummings and Bennett 2012). These represented the fundamental values of nursing practice:

- care,
- compassion,
- courage,
- communication,
- competence,
- commitment.

Cummings and Bennett (2012) aimed to embed the six Cs in all nursing as the unifying professional vision of the NHS and social care, and there is evidence of progress in this regard, both in professional identity and in the strategic development of the NHS (NHS England 2014, 2016). Cummings and Bennett (2012) acknowledged that the six Cs arose from ongoing debate and reflection, both with other organisations in the health service and with developing theoretical perspectives. The six Cs, for instance, echo the theories of care set out by Watson (1985) and Halldorsdottir (2013). Halldorsdottir (2013), for instance, suggests that compassion is a natural attribute of humanity but requires constant practice and reflection; 'compassionate competence, genuine concern for the patient/client as a person, undivided attention when the nurse is with the patient/client' (p. 44). The six Cs embody a view of care which is holistic (affective, cognitive, and somatic), integrated, focusing each of these in reflective practice, and thus stressing the importance of good judgement.

BOX 1.1 ■ Care

Care is our core business and that of our organisations, and the care we deliver helps the individual person and improves the health of the whole community. Caring defines us and our work. People receiving care expect it to be right for them, consistently, throughout every stage of their life (Cummings and Bennett 2012, p. 13).

Care is seen as a separate 'value' but is the core business, the raison d'etre, of the profession and the other five Cs can be seen as necessary elements in the practice of care. A conceptual analysis of care and nursing literature (Dalpezzo 2009) suggests the following definition: 'nursing care is a skilled, safe, high quality, holistic, ethical, collaborative, individualised, interpersonal caring process that is planned and designed based on best evidence available, and results in positive patient/client outcomes, optimisation of health, palliation of symptoms, or a peaceful death' (Dalpezzo 2009, p. 261).

BOX 1.2 ■ Compassion

Compassion is how care is given through relationships based on empathy, respect and dignity – it can also be described as intelligent kindness, and is central to how people perceive their care (Cummings and Bennett 2012, p. 13).

Compassion is a term which has a large literature base, and we will return to this in the final chapter on ethics of care. Its definition focuses on the quality of the relationship with the patient/client. This stresses a core ethical relationship involving awareness of the patient/client and their holistic needs (empathy), and respect for the dignity and autonomy of the patient/client. In a study of compassion in the care of chronic disease in older people, Van der Cingel (2011) suggested seven dimensions of compassion: attentiveness, listening, confronting, involvement, helping, presence, and understanding. This works against a simple instrumental view of care, that is a focus on technological means of caring. The term 'presence' links to the original Latin meaning of compassion 'suffering with', that is being with suffering, providing a human presence in the experience of pain. Cummings and Bennett (2012) suggest that all six concepts are of equal value, but if care provides the overall description of practice, compassion provides the key characteristic, reflected in the title, Compassion in Practice. This reflects the ontological nature of care, bringing humanity to the response to pain. This is close to Kohut's (1982) argument in the field of psychotherapy, that empathy per se has a therapeutic effect (see Chapter 11 for how this fits in with normative ethics).

This view of compassion is strongly integrative and holistic, not least in its reference to intelligent kindness (Campling 2015). Kindness is not focused on altruism or sacrifice, but rather on inclusion and solidarity, coming from the Old English *cynd* (kin; nature, family, lineage). Kindness, then, involves recognition of being of the same nature as others. The dynamic is one of respect and cooperation. The adjective 'intelligent' signals that this is not simply an emotional response, but also reflective, analytical, deliberative, and problem solving; focusing on the conditions and the means of kindness. Campling (2015, p. 4) refers to this as 'a binding, creative and problem-solving force that inspires and focuses the imagination and goodwill. It inspires and directs the attention and efforts of people and organisations towards building relationships with patients/clients, recognising their needs and treating them well. Kindness is not a "nice" side issue in the project of competitive progress. It is the "glue" of cooperation required for such progress to be of most benefit to most people'.

BOX 1.3 ■ Competence

'Competence means all those in caring roles must have the ability to understand an individual's health and social needs and the expertise, clinical and technical knowledge to deliver effective care and treatments based on research and evidence' (Cummings and Bennett 2012, p. 13).

Competence is commonly viewed as skilled performance (Bing-Jonsson et al. 2016; Garside and Nhemachena 2013). Bing-Johnsson et al. (2016) argue for a more holistic approach, involving knowledge, skills, and personal attributes, along with awareness of social, cultural, political, technical, and structural context. This view of competence takes in both technical excellence and the attitude of compassion. Whilst competence has a focus on technical practice, it has a strong ethical dimension in the sense knowing the limits of one's competence. It would be wrong to practise without competence.

BOX 1.4 ■ Communication

'Communication is central to successful caring relationships and to effective team working. Listening is as important as what we say and do, and essential for "no decision about me without me". Communication is the key to a good workplace with benefits for those in our care and staff alike' (Cummings and Bennett 2012, p. 13).

This description of communication returns the concept to relationships and away from the refinement of communication techniques and media. Effective communication communicates character and attitude, as well as ideas, both verbally and non-verbally. The stress on listening suggests that communication is both mutual and affective, as well as cognitive, and is thus critical both to the practice of the other Cs and the practice of accountability (articulating that gives an account to the self and others). Hence, Nyatanga (2014) argues that, in palliative care for instance, communication is the 'glue that makes the other Cs possible' (p. 463).

Many patients/clients, including those with intellectual/learning disability or affective disorders, have difficulty in communicating, reinforcing the need for clear communication. Similarly, the Mid Staffs case shows how many healthcare colleagues experience difficulty in communication in negative workplace conditions. Once more difficulty in communication involves both a technical and social element. One may have a clear idea about what has to be said but find difficulty in saying it, not least because of fear of personal consequences. Hence, communication is connected to character, and this includes courage.

> ### BOX 1.5 ■ Courage
>
> 'Courage enables us to do the right thing for the people we care for, to speak up when we have concerns and to have the personal strength and vision to innovate and to embrace new ways of working' (Cummings and Bennett 2012, p. 13).

Courage is a moral virtue (Aristotle 2004). It lies between the extremes of cowardice and foolhardiness. The practice of courage is central to all the other Cs. It is necessary, for instance, in addressing and defending safeguarding and standards of care or challenging accepted practices, and to implement change. This links directly to duty of candour and whistleblowing, which will be examined in more detail in Part 3. Courage (Lindh et al. 2010) is also needed in leadership and the workplace to lead innovation and change, face and respond to challenges, and motivate others through role modelling. Thorup et al. (2011) also suggests the need for courage in the act of compassionate care itself. They give the example of a nurse who remained with a patient/client who was struggling to breathe, noting that 'for a patient/client in that situation, it's really important that the people around them can bear to stay there and be present with the patient/client' (p. 432). Nurses in the same study also discussed the courage needed to challenge colleagues, 'daring to stick their neck out' (Thorup et al. 2011) in discussions. A slight critique of including courage in the six Cs is that, important though the virtue is, it is one of many which are demanded in care, and which form the basis of character. The virtues are examined more closely in Chapter 3.

> ### BOX 1.6 ■ Commitment
>
> 'A commitment to our patients/clients and populations is a cornerstone of what we do. We need to build on our commitment to improve the care and experience of our patients/clients, to take action to make this vision and strategy a reality for all and meet the health, care and support challenges ahead' (Cummings and Bennett 2012, p, 13).

The value of commitment is focused on patient/client-centred care; commitment to the patient/client over the time of treatment, and commitment to developing and sustaining care quality and improving the patient/client experience. Henderson et al. (2007) found that patients/clients were most dissatisfied when nurses showed what appeared to be a lack of commitment, such as forgetting tasks or not responding in a timely way to needs. As with all of the six Cs, there is a continuum of care. One extreme is care for patients/clients dying in the intensive care unit (ICU) where, for instance, Borhani et al. (2014) identified the quality of commitment to the patient/client as a dominant theme. Here commitment reinforces the direct and disciplined offering of compassion over time.

The Mid Staffs case showed that the nature of professional care cannot be assumed to be understood or practised. All the elements of care in this list need to be understood, articulated, and be a part of all decision making and practice. The power of narrative driven identity is critical to this kind of commitment. It was precisely, for instance, the powerful story of Florence Nightingale that strengthened the early views of nursing. There are, nonetheless, caveats:

- The practice of the six Cs is central to the profession of nursing. Mid Staffs showed us that metrics and the elements of practice they measure, such as waiting times, cannot be used as proxies for compassionate care. Compassionate care remains focused on relationships as well as outcomes and thus any audit must include this element (see Part 3).
- Though the Francis Reports and much subsequent work has noted the importance of an organisational framework for the practice of compassionate care, and its training and development, it has focused on nursing as the key example of compassionate care. Nursing, given the development of its professional identity and its understanding of the nature and practice of compassion, has an important leadership, advocacy, educational, and modelling role. Nonetheless, nursing cannot take the main responsibility for compassionate care, and, as we shall explore in Part 3, the whole service and related professions have to take responsibility for the culture and practice of care.
- The danger of the nursing profession taking too much responsibility in the provision of compassionate care is not simply the fragmentation of that care but also a return to the history of healthcare where 'care' was delegated to nurses as unpaid emotional labour, initially as women, then as subordinated professionals. Responsibility for care is now the whole organisations.

Nursing and Reflective Practice

The six Cs form the basis of common good, and thus worth or value of the profession, and the wider healthcare project. They also link to core ethical values. Alongside this, values are reinforced through the nature of professional reflective practice. Reflective practice is key to good nursing and good management (Howatson-Jones 2016; Freshwater et al. 2008). The process of reflective practice can be best seen as a recurring learning cycle involving several phases, summed up by Kolb's learning circle (Kolb 2014):

- Articulation of narrative in response to experience.
- Reflection on and testing of meaning.
- Development of meaning.
- Response, leading to new experience.

Donald Schön (1983) was instrumental in the development of reflection and, as noted earlier, there is an ethical basis to his view which focuses on the enabling role of the practitioner, respecting and enabling autonomy of the patient/client. Schön noted, through observation of a range of different professions, that in practice, there was a response which led not to an imposition of knowledge but rather a 'reflective conversation with the situation'. What emerged was a process involving:

- The analysis of the situation in order to work out what the problem might be and what issues are involved.
- The use of 'appreciative' or value systems that help to find significant meaning in the situation.
- Overarching theories that might provide further meaning.
- An understanding of the professional's own role in the situation, both its limits and opportunities.
- The ability to learn from 'talkback'. This involves reflective conversation about the situation.
- The professional treating clients as reflective practitioners, enabling them to better make decisions.

In a sense Schön is simply developing the idea of what it is to be a professional in any context. A professional in this sense is someone who knows what he or she is doing, develops meaning and learns in relation to practice, and understands how he or she affects patients/clients and the wider community, including the profession. Schön concludes that the technical skill of the professional couldn't and shouldn't be exercised without taking into account the relational context. Gibbs (1988) develops this further with a concern for understanding and engaging feelings and Oelofsen (2012) brings these elements together in terms of healthcare professional practice (https://www.evidence. nhs.uk/search?q=reflective+practice+in+nursing, see also Freshwater et al. 2008). It is important to note that reflective practice is not seen solely as a discrete activity. Schön (1983) views the first aspect of reflective practice as the capacity to reflect on action so as to engage in a process of continuous learning – pausing to reflect on practice. The second element of reflective practice Schön calls reflection in action, the capacity to reflect whilst practising; in effect thinking on your feet. This involves first developing awareness of patterns of thoughts, feelings, and physical responses as they happen, which involves metacognition, or the capacity to think about how we think (including the affective element of thought). This awareness is then engaged in choosing what to do from moment to moment. Hence, this focuses on taking responsibility for judgement in professional practice, and the core ethical practice of deliberation, careful decision making. We can usefully add a third stage, reflection for action, which combines insight with intention to apply learning in professional life. We will look more closely at this in Chapter 3 when we examine the nature of responsibility.

Emerging Values

Emerging from this chapter's reflection on professional purpose and practice, including practice in healthcare, is a series of connected ethical values:

- The common purpose of the profession – health and healthcare. This is played out through developing the meaning and practice of care and compassion. This is what it looks like to give professional care.
- This purpose gives the profession is worth in society, involves holding together different elements, not least technical and relational. This reminds us that the meaning and significance of such core value cannot be assumed. Boltanski and Thévenot (2006) suggested at least six views of worth and note that any of them has to be justified – their worth demonstrated.
- Core ethical values, principles, begin to emerge both from what it means to be a professional and from the nature of care itself. The first of these concerns a need to protect the patient/client, who is in a vulnerable power relationship with the professional. The second looks to respect the autonomy of the patient/client. We will examine these and other principles in the next chapter.
- The idea of reflective practice reinforces these values and deepens them, reinforcing the ethical dimension. Appreciative systems are precisely worldviews and perspectives on what is good which set out what is of worth. Attention to these apply both to the professional and the patient/client, not least because they say something about the identity of both parties. In turn, reflective practice focuses on the ethical principles such as respect for autonomy in both parties. Reflective practice also adds three other areas of value:
  - Concern for truth, and therefore clear evidence. What actually is happening or has happened? Truth becomes a key value and this will emerge in Part 2.
  - Concern for the consequences of actions. How might different decisions affect the different players, including the self and different institutions, in any situation?
  - Concern for careful planning that will take account of all of these aspects. This demonstrates the person or group has taken responsibility for learning and developing practice.

Paley (2014) suggests that the problems of cultures like Mid Staffs 'cannot be corrected or compensated for by teaching ethics, empathy and compassion to student nurses'. This is partly because he takes seriously organisational causes of such scandals. However, what is emerging from this chapter is a view that professional decision making is focused both on the culture and the individual professional; the two are intimately connected, and will inform any deliberations, careful decision making, and any decision-making framework. This suggests that ethics is a critical part of the professional culture and practice. Before moving into this, pause for thought and consider what this student nurse did next.

1.3 PAUSE FOR THOUGHT

What Happens Next?

As a trainee nurse I remember going to an elderly patient/client to do some brief observations. I had 5 minutes to go before the end of my shift and my boyfriend was waiting outside. We had seen the flat of our dreams and were going to meet the estate agent to nail it down; and had to be there in half an hour to make sure. Two minutes into my observations, as I was taking the patients/clients pulse, they began to shake and then cry. I was surprise by their reaction because my mind was focused on the flat. So it took me a minute to 'see' their distress. Now I had 2 minutes to decide what to do. Should I tell them not to worry, I would let my colleagues on the next shift know and they would come to see the patient/client? They would be here soon. Of course, I did not really have time to make the referral and in any case, it could be an hour or more before someone comes. Should I simply attempt to reassure the patient/client and then leave?

As I looked at this patient all I could see was fear. Perhaps then I could sit with him for another 5 minutes, help him calm down, and then ask a colleague to refer him to the next shift. I tried, swiftly texting my boyfriend to hang on. But as I sat with the patient all I could feel was my anxiety about the flat. I couldn't even make eye contact. What use was I to the patient if I couldn't focus? I decided I had to stay with the patient until he had properly calmed down, and to see if I could at least find what had triggered his anxiety.

I lost the flat and the boyfriend, but can't think he was up to much if he couldn't understand why I stayed.

Shared by a nurse on an MA course in medical ethics, and used anonymously with her permission.

This is a good example of ethical deliberation, which focuses on the practice of practical wisdom (see Chapter 3 for a detailed analysis). It involved:

- Reflection on and engagement with several different narratives, including: personal relationships; the needs of the patient; the practice of the ward and views of colleagues.
- Reflection on one's core purpose as nurse.
- Reflection on oneself, and in this case how the student nurse felt about the man she was caring for, and dialogue with herself about options and how they related to her practice.
- Deliberation that could be practised rapidly, but still remained true to core values and relationships. Practical wisdom does not necessarily require wearisome length, suggesting that the nurse was practised in such reflection, and thus able to do it as she practised care.

Taylor (1989) suggests that it is in this kind of dialogue in which we work out our ethical identity. In the process of doing this, the student was practising metacognition – reflecting on what they were thinking and the underlying feelings (Flavell 1976). The student could see herself and with that, begin to see the patient/client better. This involved all the three elements of reflective practice (reflection on, in, and for), in what was an exercise of ethical deliberation, and we will turn to that in the next chapter.

References

Airaksinen, T. (1994). Service and science in professional life. In R. F. Chadwick (Ed.), *Ethics and the professions* (pp. 1–13). Avebury: The University of Michigan.

Aristotle. (2004). *Nicomachean ethics*. London: Penguin.

Bandura, A., Barbaranelli, C., Caprara, G. V., & Pastorelli, C. (1996). Mechanisms of moral disengagement in the exercise of moral agency. *Journal of Personality and Social Psychology, 71*(2), 364–374.

Bauman, Z. (1989). *Modernity and the holocaust.* London: Polity.

Bing-Jonsson, P., Hofoss, D., Kirkevold, M., Bjørk, I., & Foss, C. (2016). Sufficient competence in community elderly care? Results from a competence measurement of nursing staff. *BMC Nursing, 15*(1), 5.

Bivins, R., Tierney, S., & Seers, K. (2017). Compassionate care: not easy, not free, not only nurses. *BMJ Quality & Safety, 26,* 1023–1026.

Boltanksi, L., & Thévenot, T. (2006). *On justification: economies of worth.* Princeton: Princeton University Press.

Borhani, F., Hosseini, S. H., & Abbaszadeh, A. (2014). Commitment to care: a qualitative study of intensive care nurses' perspectives of end-of-life care in an Islamic context. *International Nursing Review, 61*(1), 140–147.

Brand, B. L., Loewenstein, R. J., & Spiegel, D. (2014). Dispelling myths about dissociative identity disorder treatment: an empirically based approach. *Psychiatry, 77*(2), 169–189.

Campbell, A. V. (1984). *Moderated love: a theology of professional care.* London: The Society for Promoting Christian Knowledge – SPCK.

Campbell, D. (2013). Mid Staff Hospital Scandal Guide. London: The Guardian Newspaper, 06 February 2013. Online available: https://www.theguardian.com/society/2013/feb/06/mid-staffs-hospital-scandal-guide.

Campbell, D. (2018). Inquiry into deaths at NHS maternity unit widened. London: The Guardian Newspaper, 31 August 2018. Online available: https://www.theguardian.com/society/2018/aug/31/deaths-feared-shrewsbury-telford-nhs-trust-maternity-unit-investigation.

Campling, P. (2015). Reforming the culture of healthcare: the case for intelligent kindness. *BJPsych Bulletin, 39*(1), 1–5.

Cummings, J., & Bennett, V. (2012). *Compassion in practice: nursing, midwifery and care staff: our vision and strategy.* London: Department of Health.

Dalpezzo, N. (2009). Nursing care: a concept analysis. *Nursing Forum, 44*(4), 256–264.

Department of Health and Social Care. (2012). Winterbourne View Hospital: Department of Health review and response: Final report into the events at Winterbourne View hospital and a programme of action to transform services. Online available: https://www.gov.uk/government/publications/winterbourne-view-hospital-department-of-health-review-and-response.

Department of Health and Social Care. (2013). Independent Review of Liverpool Care Pathway for dying patients. Online available: https://www.gov.uk/government/publications/review-of-liverpool-care-pathway-for-dying-patients.

Dickens, C. (1844). *Martin Chuzzlewit.* The University of California: T.B. Peterson.

Dutton, J. E., Workman, K. M., & Hardin, A. E. (2014). Compassion at work. *Annual Review of Organizational Psychology and Organizational Behavior, 1*(1), 177–304.

Edelman Trust Barometer. (2019). 2019 Edelman Trust Barometer. Online available: https://www.edelman.com/research/2019-edelman-trust-barometer.

Fawkes, J. (2017). *Public relations ethics and professionalism: the shadow of excellence.* Abingdon, UK: Taylor and Francis Group.

Flavell, J. H. (1976). Metacognitive aspects of problem solving. In L. B. Resnick (Ed.), *The nature of intelligence* (pp. 231–236). Hillsdale, NJ: Lawrence Erlbaum Associates.

Francis, R. (2013). Report of the Mid Staffordshire NHS Foundation Trust Public Inquiry. London: The Stationery Office. Online available: https://www.gov.uk/government/publications/report-of-the-mid-staffordshire-nhs-foundation-trust-public-inquiry.

Francis, R. (2010). The Mid Staffordshire NHS Foundation Trust Inquiry. London: The Stationery Office. Online available: https://webarchive.nationalarchives.gov.uk/20130104234315/http://www.dh.gov.uk/en/Publicationsandstatistics/Publications/PublicationsPolicyAndGuidance/DH_113018.

Freshwater, D., Taylor, B., & Sherwood, G. (2008). *International textbook of reflective practice in nursing.* Oxford: Blackwell.

Garside, J., & Nhemachena, J. (2013). A concept analysis of competence and its transition in nursing. *Nurse Education Today, 33*(5), 541–545.

Gibbs, G. (1988). *Learning by doing: a guide to teaching and learning methods.* Oxford: Further Education Unit, Oxford Polytechnic.

Goodpaster, K. E. (2007). *Conscience and corporate culture*. Oxford: Blackwell.

Halldorsdottir, S. (2013). Five basic modes of being with another. In M. C. Smith, M. C. Turkel, & Z. R. Wolf (Eds.), *Caring in nursing classics: an essential resource* (pp. 201–210). New York: Springer Publishing Company.

Henderson, A., Van Eps, M. A., Pearson, K., James, C., Henderson, P., & Osborne, Y. (2007). 'Caring for' behaviors that indicate to patients that nurses 'care about' them. *Journal of Advanced Nursing, 60*(2), 146–153.

Howatson-Jones, L. (2016). *Reflective practice in nursing* (3rd ed.). London: Sage.

Huber, M. (2011). How should we define health? *British Medical Journal, 343*, d4163.

Illich, I. (2010). *Limits to medicine: medical nemesis, the expropriation of health*. London: Marion Boyars.

King's Fund. (2011). *The future of leadership and management in the NHS: No more heroes: Report from The King's Fund Commission on Leadership and Management in the NHS*. London: King's Fund.

King's Fund. (2016). *Improving quality in the English NHS: a strategy for action*. London: King's Fund.

Koehn, D. (1994). *The ground of professional ethics*. London: Routledge.

Kohut, H. (1982). Introspection, empathy and the semi-circle of mental health. *International Journal of Psychoanalysis, 63*(4), 395–407.

Kolb, D. A. (2014). *Experiential learning: experience as the source of learning and development* (2nd ed.). Upper Saddle River, NJ: Pearson Education.

Lauer, C. & Hoyer, M. (2019). Hundreds of accused clergy left off Church's sex abuse lists. New York: Associate Press News, 28 December 2019. Online available: https://apnews.com/f6238fe6724bdf-4f30a42ff7d11a327e.

Lindh, I. B., Barbosa da Silva, A., Berg, A., & Severinsson, E. (2010). Courage and nursing practice: a theoretical analysis. *Nursing Ethics, 17*(5), 551–565.

Markey, K., Tilki, M., & Taylor, G. (2019). Resigned indifference: an explanation of gaps in care for culturally and linguistically diverse patients. *Journal of Nursing Management, 27*(7), 1462–1470.

Mastracci, S. (2017). Beginning nurses' perceptions of ethical leadership in the shadow of Mid Staffs. *Public Integrity, 19*(3), 250–264.

May, W. (1985). Adversarialism in America and in the professions. In U. McLean (Ed.), *The end of professionalism?* (pp. 5–19). Edinburgh: CTPI.

McKenna, B., & Rooney, D. (2011). Wisdom in organizations. *Social Epistemology, 21*(2), 113–138.

National Health Service. (2015). NHS Constitution: the NHS belongs to us all. Online available: https://www.gov.uk/government/publications/the-nhs-constitution-for-england.

NHS England. (2014). *Five year forward view*. London: National Health Service. Online available: https://www.england.nhs.uk/wp-content/uploads/2014/10/5yfv-web.pdf.

NHS England. (2016). *Leading change, adding value*. London: National Health Service. Online available: https://www.england.nhs.uk/wp-content/uploads/2016/05/nursing-framework.pdf.

Nyatanga, B. (2014). Palliative care in the community using person-centred care. *British Journal of Community Nursing, 18*(11), 567.

O'Neill, O. (2002). *A question of trust: The BBC Reith lecturers*. Cambridge: Cambridge University Press.

Oelofsen, N. (2012). Using reflective practice in frontline nursing. *Nursing Times, 108*(24), 22–24.

Oxford English Dictionary. (2007). *The new shorter Oxford English dictionary* (6th ed.). Oxford: Oxford University Press.

Paley, J. (2014). Cognition and the compassion deficit: the social psychology of helping behaviour in nursing. *Nursing Philosophy, 15*(4), 274–287.

Robinson, S. (2013). Hearing voices: wisdom responsibility and leadership. In M. Thompson, & D. Bevan (Eds.), *Wise management in organisational complexity* (pp. 181–197). London: Palgrave.

Robinson, S., Dixon, R., Preece, C., & Moodley, K. (2012). *Engineering professional and business ethics*. London: Heinneman Butterworth.

Robinson, S., Kendrick, K., & Brown, A. (2003). *Spirituality and the practice of healthcare*. Basingstoke: Palgrave.

Rolfe, G., & Gardner, L. (2014). The compassion deficit and what to do about it: a response to Paley. *Nursing Philosophy, 15*(4), 288–297.

Rozuel, C. (2011). The moral threat of compartmentalization: self, roles and responsibility. *Journal of Business Ethics, 102*(4), 685–697.

Schön, D. (1983). *The reflective practitioner*. New York: Basic Books.

Shaw, B. (1906). *The doctor's dilemma.* Online available: http://www.gutenberg.org/ebooks/5070.

Sourial, S. (1997). An analysis of caring. *Journal of Advanced Nursing, 216*(6), 1189–1192.

Stenhouse, R., Ion, R., Roxburgh, M., & Smith, S. (2016). Exploring the compassion deficit debate. *Nurse Education Today, 39*, 12–15.

Tawney, R. H. (1930). *Equality.* London: Allen and Unwin.

Taylor, C. (1989). *Sources of the self.* Cambridge: Cambridge University Press.

The Insider Job. (2010). [DVD] Directed by Charles H. Ferguson. USA: Sony Pictures Home Entertainment.

Thorup, C., Rundqvist, E., Roberts, C., & Delmar, C. (2011). Care as a matter of courage: vulnerability, suffering and ethical formation in nursing care. *Scandinavian Journal of Caring Science, 26*(3), 427–435.

Van der Cingel, M. (2011). Compassion in care: a qualitative study of older people with a chronic disease and nurses. *Nursing Ethics, 18*(5), 672–685.

Watson, J. (1985). *Nursing: human science and human care.* Norwalk, CT: Appleton-Century-Crofts.

Making Decisions: The Ethical Dimension

LEARNING OUTCOMES

When you have read and worked through this chapter, you should be able to:
- Develop and practice an ethical decision-making framework
- Examine key ethical ideas within that framework
- Critically examine underlying theories about how we practice ethics
- Note key fallacies which affect ethical judgement
- Survey key ethical terminology

Introduction

This chapter will focus on professional decision making and its ethical dimension. It looks at how we do ethics, and argues that the professional decision making of the nurse and ethical decision making are not two separate practices, but rather two domains within professional practice – ethical value as part of professional competence. It begins with an extended framework for the ethical dimension of decision making. It then examines underlying descriptive theories about how we do ethics.

CASE 2.1	Older Patient and His Family

Tom was an 84-year-old man, who until 7 months prior to his hospital admission in January 2019, lived life fully, was self-caring, and the main carer to his wife, Sarah, who has hearing loss. Tom's symptoms included dyspnoea at rest and on exertion; anorexia; weight loss (clothes altered to fit); and heart working at 20% capacity. During this admission, Tom's wife and family were informed that, due to the condition of his heart, Tom could die 'tonight, in a day, a week, or a month'. Tom was discharged home with community support from the cardiac team. He was still judged to be self-caring. Over the next 2 weeks, there were increasing symptoms, with frequent contact/visits with the general practitioner (GP) and a deterioration in his general condition. Tom was sleeping/dozing most of the time but was reasonably comfortable. Tom developed diarrhoea, and was unable to manage the symptoms at home and thus unable to self-care. The GP visited and suggested that Tom may have diverticulitis, and Tom was readmitted to hospital. Tom was mobile but his voice was weak and barely audible due to dyspnoea.

Several different healthcare professions were involved in Tom's care. The dietician and the nursing team were encouraging, and at points pushing, Tom to eat, including taking build-up drinks. However, Tom could barely swallow, and it was a major effort to drink; he had been anorexic for months. The physiotherapists wanted Tom to walk 'aiming to rehabilitate for discharge home or to nursing home', despite the fact that he could not walk or stand without significant support. This action seemed to the family to contradict the judgement that Tom was close to death. The three doctors involved spoke with Tom's wife Sarah (also 84) without other family members present, leading to mixed messages and misinformation, with one mentioning a do not resuscitate (DNR), one discussing treatment, and one discussing possible investigation. Sarah often could not follow the speed of the delivery. Tom's daughter-in-law, Anne, a nurse, visited in early February and, after seeing him, requested the involvement of the Hospital Palliative Care team. This was arranged and the local hospice where Anne used to work agreed to transfer Tom to their care should the medical team consider this appropriate and that Tom required end-of-life care. Anne then met with Tom's consultant and discussed palliative care with her. The consultant had no difficulty with this. Anne expressed the family's concerns that Tom's condition was deteriorating and she believed the focus should now be on quality of life given that he was dying. Anne noted, 'the consultant expressed surprise that we had understood he was dying as she did not believe this was the case and that there may, as yet, be a reversible cause to his decline'. Tom had recently commenced a course of antibiotics. Anne noted the deterioration in her father-in-law since his original assessment, and the conversations with members of the team which suggested to them that Tom was dying, if not imminently then soon. Anne asked the consultant if, when the antibiotics were complete, she would review his future care with a view to not overburdening him with investigations, or treatments for an identified problem which would detract from his quality of life. Anne requested that when making her decision, she would look not just at the clinical picture but the holistic picture of Tom. He was now exhausted and he could only speak in a whisper, which was a huge effort, his throat was very sore which made drinking even more of an effort, and he was no longer able to stand/walk unaided. He was uncomfortable in the bed and had developed a pressure sore. The consultant agreed and also offered to review Tom's response to medical management the following week and discuss her plan of care with Tom's son after the ward round. Anne felt reassured that this would happen and returned to her home overseas.

Tom's son (Tony) took a day out of work on the Tuesday of the following week and was there to meet the consultant. It turned out that she was not there and not expected. A member of her team saw Tony and informed him that they planned to insert a line to help with his father's nutrition. From this Tony, who had no medical knowledge, understood an intravenous (IV) drip would be set up. Some days later a nasogastric tube (NG) was inserted. Tom later told his wife and grand-daughter, 'I've been through hell, it took three nurses – one held my head, one held my hand, and one put the tube down'. Tom was a man who never complained and had enormous respect for the medical and nursing profession.

Later that night Tom died. Tony was called in the early hours of the morning and informed of his death. He informed the nurse that he would contact his mother and brothers and they would be in to see dad as soon as possible. When they arrived to see him, he still had the NG tube in situ, taped to the end of his nose. Sarah is still haunted by this, 'it was horrible and it had stuff in it'. The family believed that Tom's symptoms reflected those outlined in National Institute for Health and Care Excellence (NICE) guidelines (https://www.nice.org.uk/guidance/qs144) as appropriate for palliative care. They believed that the burden of investigating and treating Tom unto death significantly detracted from the quality of his life in his last days. Although they knew and understood that Tom had a limited life expectancy, they believed that the strain imposed on Tom in inserting the NG tube may have contributed to the timing of his death, a death that came sooner than they were given to expect during this admission.

2.1 PAUSE FOR THOUGHT

Consider the Case Study

Consider for a moment what you would have done as a nurse in this case.

What questions would you have of your colleagues across the professions in reflecting on this event?

If you were a member of the family, what questions would you have of the different professions?

With a colleague, consider what you feel the key issues and problems were in this case, i.e. what were the most important values involved?

This case is not a simple ethical dilemma, where you have to choose between stipulated options, focused on a crisis. It is, rather, an example of everyday professional and inter-professional practice where the underlying ethical dynamic is evident, involving different values. The 'ethics' are not neatly parcelled but are part of the professional judgment, and involve relationships with family and colleagues.

2.2 PAUSE FOR THOUGHT

Unpacking Ethical Decision Making

When was the last time you made an ethical decision in your training and professional practice? Take a little time with your colleagues and share with them how you believe you make ethical decisions in nursing. Is the process a long one? Do you find it 'instinctive' or 'intuitive', so you feel the right decision quickly? Is it an easy or difficult experience? Do you have a decision-making framework?

ETHICAL DECISION-MAKING FRAMEWORK

There are different approaches to ethical decision making. One strong approach focused on nursing focuses on consequences and assessing the consequences (Table 2.1).

Analysis of Tom's case reveals further stress on the core principles and values and on the shared nature of ethical decision making, involving: data gathering and problem definition; value clarification and management; option examination and planning; and audit. The case study is precisely one where there is no discrete ethical dilemma, for example whether to end life support or not. The point about the key ethical issues is they are often just below the surface, and need shared reflection to focus on them more clearly.

TABLE 2:1 ■ The Steps of the Ethical Decision-Making Process

Problem definition	Define the problem in a clear description of the ethical issue and the circumstances intertwining with it.
Data collection	The data collection phase involves reviewing professional ethics codes, published evidence (peer reviewed, professional statements/position papers/literature).
Data analysis	Organisation and analysis of the data.
The identification, exploration, and generation of possible solutions to the problem and the implications of each	All options and solutions to solve the ethical issue are explored and evaluated.
Selecting the best possible solution	All options and solutions are considered to decide upon the most appropriate ethical action to be taken.
Performing the selected desired course of action to resolve the ethical issue	Implementing the chosen most appropriate ethical action.
Evaluating the results of the action	Similar to the nursing process, the actions taken to solve the ethical issues are evaluated and measured in terms of their effectiveness to resolve the ethical issue.

From Burke (2020)

DATA GATHERING: UNDERSTANDING THE SITUATION

The starting place of ethics is reflection on the situation. The term 'data gathering' sounds formal and scientific but Tom's case shows that understanding the situation involves clarity about the situation and how we perceive it. This means identifying:

- The purpose of being involved—What is the core value and how is it being embodied?
- The key stakeholders—The term stakeholder simply means anyone who had a significant relationship with the patient/client. How did they see the situation and how were they involved?
- The main needs that required response—Was there one or many? If many, what was the priority and how do you decide that? Some are identified and others not. Anne is the one who begins to take control, partly because of her health background and what coordination there was came from her.
- The technical issues surrounding those needs.
- The ethical issues around identifying and responding to the needs.
- Whose responsibility was it to address these needs.

Clearly the core purpose in this case was to provide care. However, what that purpose actually means in practice is determined by the situation. In this case, the purpose of care could have involved rehabilitation or palliative care. None of the different professions critically questioned which of these was most appropriate. Hence, there was an unresolved tension, with the family left with the view that Tom was close to death, with one junior doctor suggesting that it might be best to sign a DNR, only to hear from the consultant that she did not think that Tom had reached that stage. Core to all data gathering is clarity about the expectations of stakeholders, which means that it is important to work with stakeholders at this stage. This requires communication and with that, how each of them perceives the patient/client and how they perceive the treatment. Dialogue with all the stakeholders in this case seemed at a minimum, which made it hard for the different stakeholders to see what was happening. In the case of the family, this meant that it became hard for them to become involved.

Stakeholders in this situation are not just Tom and his family, but the different healthcare professions. Even within the family there are very different perspectives. Anne has clear view of the need for palliative care. Tony is less clear about treatment and more hopeful of keeping hold of his father. It is hard to find the voice of Sarah or Tom, and neither seems to be involved in the developing situation. The arc of Tom's experience has been rapid. From being a carer, he quickly moves to being an exhausted patient. Making sense of that for him would require him to develop his story, not least the loss of his major purpose and his feelings about his situation now. This requires dialogue. There was some stakeholder push back from the family, not least from Anne about setting palliative care into place, and this was heard and acted upon. There was no push back from the professionals. This was partly because there had been no professional dialogue about the core purpose. Hence, purpose for the dietician and physiotherapist was not defined in terms of the patient/client but in terms of their professional identity and what they had been told to do. There was no attempt to push back on their part. Clearly no one had asked them how they perceived the response of Tom. The nurses' response was chequered, with some finding time to be with Tom and others giving him little attention whilst still caring.

A key part of nursing purpose is advocacy, which could have included raising palliative referral and interventions. Yet it was the family who raised this issue, focusing on the NICE guidelines for palliative care. Hence, there was no push back from the healthcare professionals. There was a suggestion that some of the professionals did not see push back as a part of their role. They felt they had to follow the direction of care in good faith, and in this they were doing what they thought was best for the patient/client. There may be a further indication that they were uneasy about pushing back because they saw this as raising conflict. Or it may be that they thought any such push back would take time and thus take away from the care. Much of this suggests unreflective practice, with the dominance of task-orientation. The job has to be done and there is no time to reflect. The result is a lack of awareness about the situation. The professional ends up with a narrow perception of the situation. This also might be because decision making was based on a narrow few. Were the nurses, for instance, involved in the decision making about inserting an NG tube? With three nurses involved, this was clearly a deeply affecting experience for Tom. He deeply respected the staff but this experience clearly felt abusive. As the family reflected on their experience, they believed that the burden of investigating and treating Tom until death significantly detracted from the quality of his life in his last days. Although the family knew and understood that Tom had a limited life expectancy, they believe that the strain imposed on Tom by inserting the NG tube may have contributed to the timing of his death, a death that came sooner than they were given to expect as active treatment was still underway.

Lederach (2005) argues that finding out about the situation requires 'web-watching', taking time to see how all the different elements of the situation connect to each other. He argues that this demands care because the social web does not exist apart from the observer – we are connected to it. It is easy from a purely scientific perspective to feel that the situation exists apart from us, and thus that the professional is not one of the stakeholders. But as Lederach suggests, where we place our foot affects the web. He also argues for the need to exercise aesthetic imagination. The term aesthetic is used in the arts, and means a 'sharpening of the senses'. Great paintings, for instance, draw you into their perspective. When a family comes to visit their deceased father, this is especially a moment requiring a sharpening of the senses. The body becomes the existential focus of myriad feelings of loss, guilt, pain, and care, and draws the family members into the significance of the person they mourn. The question then is why the NG tube was still in place when they arrived?

Lederach also suggests that a key part of this awareness is the capacity to learn as we travel (cf. Schön 1983), and the development of a systematic scepticism. The first of these brings us back to reflective practice, and the importance of reflecting as we practice. This reflection is not a separate function bolted on to practice but a key part of the practice. Hence, there is no question of not having time to think these issues through. Thus systemic scepticism enables critical reflection on purpose and what we really think. As a core to professional ethical practice, we will return to this. Again, it is easy to see these as simply a function of the professional. But it is a key part to the ongoing dialogue with patient/client, enabling the patient/client and the family to be fully aware of the situation, to learn as they proceed, and to respond with questions. The questions from the family about the NG tube were left until the end because at the time Tony was simply not aware of what this process meant. He was thus not empowered to give voice to any concerns or scepticism.

VALUE CLARIFICATION AND MANAGEMENT

The second stage of ethical decision making is the clarification and working through of ethical principles involved. In this case, there are clearly several different kinds of principle that the nurse may need to be aware of such as personal and professional ethical principles, public ethical values, and managing value conflict.

Personal Ethical Principles

Most of us assume that we have personal ethical principles, derived often from the families we grew up in or the different groups that we have been a part of, not least religious communities. However, it is worth noting just what these might be. What are the core moral principles which guide you in your life? How would you prioritise these? How do these principles relate to the principles of your profession? For some, personal principles relate directly to the professional principles. Indeed, awareness of the ethical identity of healthcare might be a key reason for joining the profession in the first place. Nonetheless, a healthcare professional may bring personal principles to the situation which begin to reinforce or clash with professional ethical principles. Equally importantly are the principles of other stakeholders. In the case presented, there was no attention paid to the family's principles, as a whole, or as members. Learning about these is part of any dialogue which helps them to find a voice, and enables a coherent value narrative of the case to emerge. In this, the family was primarily concerned about how they could express their love and care for Tom.

Professional Ethical Principles

These can be seen as fundamental and procedural principles. It is generally accepted that the fundamental principles of healthcare professions are respect for autonomy, justice, and non-maleficence and beneficence (Beauchamp and Childress 2019). *Respect for autonomy* (self-governance) can be seen in two ways. Firstly, in a negative sense it involves not interfering with the freedom of the patient/client or colleague to decide for themselves (Berlin 1969). Secondly, in a positive sense it refers to enabling the person to make his or her own decision. Each of these requires dialogue with the patient/client. The first involves making clear the limitations of the nurse and the importance the patient/client taking responsibility. The second involves actively enabling the other to develop autonomy, encouraging reflection, articulation and justification of felt needs, and articulation of values and hopes. In the first, autonomy is largely about respecting choice and leaving the other to determine what will happen to them. The second focuses not on the action of choice but the capacity to make a choice. For many patients/clients, the first of these is sufficient. Choosing how to deal with a compound leg fracture is fairly straightforward (unless you are a professional footballer). Choice for Tom was much more complex. He came to treatment having been recently the key carer of his wife, thus losing an important part of his identity, and he was faced by the possibility of imminent death. Hence, if Tom is to make a choice about his treatment, he would have to think through two existential challenges (challenges to his identity and to his very existence). There is no evidence in the case that this happened. It is not clear that either sense of autonomy was respected. Some members of staff were keen to get Tom involved. There was real communication effort by all members of the medical team; they were attentive, courteous, and kind to Tom and appeared anxious to deliver the best possible care to improve his condition and rehabilitate him. All practitioners responded to requests for meetings and/or instigated meetings.

However, there seemed to be an overall lack of team focus and working. Each member of the multidisciplinary team (MDT) went in and carried out their own individual role, but it was not joined up. The focus was on discrete task-oriented interventions. No one seemed to be looking at the whole patient/client and seeing what was happening to him. During one of Anne's visits, the dietician came in and advised Tom over his diet, encouraging food and supplement drinks. She told Tom he must eat, even though Anne had told the dietician that Tom even found drinking difficult. This visibly upset Tom and when the dietician had left, he turned to Anne and said 'but I can't eat. I am trying. I haven't felt like eating for months'. Similarly, the physiotherapists had been told Tom was for 'rehab' and so were focused on getting him up and out even though Tom was very weak and dyspnoeic. The lack of attention to detail in this case led to a lack of 'basic' nursing care:

- Mouth care: Anne cleaned Tom's dentures, which had clearly not been cleaned for several days.
- Pressure area care: Tom was left sitting for long periods (3 hours) on a chair and he had developed a pressure sore.
- Tom also complained of a crick in his neck because as he slept so much his head fell forward.
- The call bell was frequently on the floor when family or other visitors arrived.

At points, there were behaviours which disrespected Tom:

- One nurse was seen shouting in Tom's ear, despite the family being able to communicate effectively without doing this. As one of the family said, 'Just because Tom did not have the voice to speak didn't mean he was deaf or stupid'.
- Tom reported to his family about the embarrassment of two nurses arguing above his head in the bathroom, 'I was undressed....I was really embarrassed, I think they were arguing about me'.
- On another occasion, when Tom told a nurse that he needed to go to the bathroom, the nurse told him in front of his granddaughter, 'you've got a pad on, you can do it in that'.

For the most part, however, staff were friendly, kind, attentive, and 'respectful'. It could be that the staff for the most part thought they were being respectful. It is perfectly possible to think you are practicing respect. It raises the question as to what respect looks like. What constitutes respect? Kant (1964) offers one of the most convincing views on this principle. Respect is when you treat the other as an end in themselves, not as a means to an end. If the other is simply a means to your end, then you cannot actually see them or understand what their hopes are in any clinical situation. Often, then, respect is seen as the same as unconditional care or love (Robinson 2008), or unconditional positive regard (Rogers 1983). The unconditionality of this means that respect does not depend on any condition, such as an attractive quality, in the other. This in turn assumes mutuality in the relationship. Campbell (1984) writes about care as developing genuine partnership. Such mutuality would assume genuine dialogue (Buber 1937), where both parties learn something about the other not simply about the treatment. Bakhtin (1993) argues that dialogue is more than dialectic (debate about a proposition or a practice). It reveals something about the nature of each party. Dialogue then becomes a key evidence of respect and moves to mutual respect rather than a one-way dynamic.

Respect. *Respect* in this case then focuses on the particularity of the other – the particular voice of Tom, the particular voice of the carer. At its heart is the practice of listening and questioning. It is, of course, communicated not just by dialogue but by body language, and evidence of commitment and continuity. There was little evidence of the practice of this respect. Tom espoused great respect for nurses but this was built on generality – the nursing profession as a whole not the particularity of his carers. The carers espoused great respect for Tom, but again without any knowledge of his particular concerns. Such respect would demand evidence of autonomy, and there was little. Whilst Tom was included in some discussions, the case suggests that he did not see much hope of getting home, and that treatment was rather done to him, with the assumption that he knew, and had bought into, the way ahead, that he was capable of rehabilitation, and that the role of the professional was to motivate him to that end. There was little evidence of listening even to Tom's physical concerns. Hence, in this case, respect for the patient had become secondary. The primary concern was to fulfil a care agenda determined elsewhere, and respect was really the positive support offered to Tom to get him through the treatment.

The principle of respect cannot be solely about respect for autonomy. Later in the book we will examine ethics and intellectual/learning disability and dementia. In these areas, respect for persons requires something broader than respect for autonomy, that is respect for the particular humanity of the other, regardless of apparent limitations. Hence, the concept of autonomy will be further addressed. Rosen (2012) extends this to respect for the dignity, the humanness, of the other even when characteristics of human life are gone, that is respect for the dead body. In the case discussed here, it is natural to feel concern for the family when they saw Tom's body. In effect, his body was not an object of respect. This begins to show how the decision-making framework should not be treated as a series of discrete stages – follow these and ethical practice will be fulfilled. On the contrary, even in the initial practice of engaging in the situation, the practice of respect is demanded. Without this and the related skills of listening to the patient/client and the others involved in the situation, the full data about key relationships will not emerge. Moreover, purpose and principle are interconnected. A narrow view of purpose, focused on task per se, runs the danger of a weak view and practice of respect. A broad view of purpose (person centred) leads to a deeper practice of respect and shared autonomy. Reflective practice demands reflection on the practice of respect.

Justice. *Justice* illustrates well the nature of principles. Principles are general, and if used without care, can result in shaping any data to a narrow end. However, principles do give some idea of values which can be shared across different areas. At the same time, the particular meaning of the principle emerges as one engages with the situation. The principle of justice is quite complex. Rawls (1987) argues that it means fairness. But what does fairness mean? Perhaps a form of equal respect. Others argue that it involves different forms of equality, such as equality of access or opportunity (Tawney 1930), and Nozick (1972) argues that it involves desert, that is making the punishment fit the crime or rewarding good behaviour – as in, why should we give new livers to an alcoholic, their practice does not deserve it. Lambourne (2004) goes further offering:
- Retributive justice, about settling accounts.
- Restitutive justice, involving recovery of losses, compensations for pain.
- Restorative justice, restoring or healing relationships between conflicting parties.
- Social justice, in which parties are given what they need to achieve social equality or resolution.
- Distributive justice, involving fair distribution of goods according to need.
- Environmental justice, which looks to take into account the future of the environment.

Any of these meanings might surface in different healthcare contexts. How, for instance, can we enable every dying patient/client to experience a good death? The NICE guidelines (https://www.nice.org.uk/guidance/qs144) are meant to ensure this kind of equality of experience. Hence, these would have supported any advocacy for Tom. However, three key points emerge around justice. First, it sounds like a portentous principle which we have to learn to apply to situations. But as noted in the introduction, we are brought up thinking and arguing about justice. In fact, because of the many meanings of this principle, it can only be understood and embodied through dialogue with those who make up the situation. This kind of dialogue helps us to test what we think we mean. We will look at this kind of dialogue in detail in the case study in Chapter 3 which looks at a dilemma about conjoined twins. Second, it becomes clear that justice is not just about metrics, a means of calculating, but is also relational. How the nurse practices justice signals to the patient/client and colleagues a sense of concern for the other and so a sense of worth. When you do not get the treatment you had hoped for, that may seem to be against you as a person. Hence, the process of justice is not simply rational but also affective. Third, justice infuses organisational meaning, from how remuneration is calculated in any organisation, to how patients/clients and family are treated, to how the nurse frames their identity. As noted above, advocacy is based on justice and putting/making the case on behalf of others – seeking justice for the patient/client. Justice is also there in the foundation of the UK health service, offering equal care, not based on capacity to pay, and we will return to this in Part 3. The concern for justice is, then, there at every point of professional practice, and the task of working with that principle demands a continual reflection on it, and how it relates to professional practice with the different stakeholders in any situation. This is as much a part of professional practice as any technical skills.

Beneficence and non-maleficence. *Beneficence* and *non-maleficence* are very broad principles, meaning seek the best possible outcome and do no harm. Interpreting these in the situation then becomes important. It is hard to see the same weight in these principles as respect or justice. However, these principles focus on consequences and how any action will affect the parties involved. Again, this would have to be worked through with the other interested parties to see how these principles actually work out in practice. Because it is hard to estimate exact consequences, then these principles, like justice and respect, demand continual reflection on outcomes.

Veracity. *Veracity,* along with fidelity and accountability, emerge from respect and justice. It involves communicating the truth to patients/clients and colleagues (see communication in Chapters 1 and 9). This principle is complex, not least because the communication of truth can lead to difficult, even painful outcomes, setting up possible conflict with the principles of beneficence and non-maleficence. These tensions will be explored in more detail in Parts 2 and 3, leading up to such issues as the duty of candour. In Tom's case, it is hard to find where the truth is addressed, with different views of his condition and of treatment emerging. It is striking that the seriousness of Tom's condition when originally stated, whilst painful to the family, was not something that led to a bad consequence (sometimes used as a reason for not telling patient/clients or family about bad news). On the contrary, they simply focused on their commitment to Tom and how to support appropriate care.

Fidelity. *Fidelity* connects to veracity – it is about being there for the patient/client (see commitment in Chapter 1) whatever the outcome, being true to the patient/client. For the professional, it is also about being true to the professional body, to the healthcare organisation, to the core purpose of healthcare. In Tom's case, the staff remained true to him, that is they stayed with him. However, without honesty, such commitment loses a key part of the relationship that you are true to. This becomes important for a sense of ongoing trust. We will look in more detail at veracity and fidelity in the next chapter when we consider the virtues.

Accountability. *Accountability* is a key ethical principle focused on responsibility and we will examine it in detail in the next chapter. It is about 'owning' one's practice and the worth of that practice, and being able to give an account of this. Consider the stakeholders (those involved in the care) in Tom's case. Who was responsible for his care and how far did they fulfil their responsibilities?

Procedural Principles. *Procedural principles* are the values which inform the professional's engagement with the situation, and are really instruments of the basic principles (Beauchamp and Childress 2019): confidentiality; informed consent or decision making; cost–benefit analysis; and risk–benefit analysis.

    Confidentiality. *Confidentiality* is often essential for respecting the autonomy of the patient/client. Such confidentiality needs to be formally established. How would that work through the case above?

    Informed Consent. *Informed consent* is also essential to respect for autonomy. This involves sharing the technical details of the treatment and what probable consequences may be. Again, the proper context for this is dialogue, giving space to the patient/client and family to explore what this means. In Tom's case, there was little of this involved, with professionals not taking account of Sarah's hearing problems, and lack of clarity about the nature of the NG tube.

TABLE 2.2 ■ **Summary of Professional Ethical Principles**

Fundamental Principles	Procedural Principles
• Respect for autonomy of the patient/client • Justice • Beneficence • Non-maleficence • Veracity • Fidelity • Accountability	• Confidentiality • Informed consent or decision making • Cost–benefit analysis • Risk–benefit analysis

Cost–benefit and risk–benefit analysis. Cost–benefit analysis and *risk–benefit analysis* are both focused on consequences and how the different stakeholders are affected. In the first, the resources of the healthcare organisation are taken into account, whereas the second connects directly to risk management. In the light of the different scandals, risk management has become increasingly important. Table 2.2 provides a summary of the fundamental and procedural professional ethical principles.

Public Ethical Values

Public ethical values focus on social ethics, not least around the distribution of healthcare. As such, the classic social principles include freedom, equality, and community (Tawney 1930). For the UK, these principles were central to the creation of the Welfare State and the National Health Service, and we will look at them in more detail in Part 3 of the book, when we compare different approaches. At this stage, three points will suffice. First, these principles are distinct from the professional principles but relate directly to them. Equality relates directly to justice (Rawls 1971) and freedom to autonomy. Second, these principles are also complex and need to be thought through in relation to practice. The term equality, for instance, has over 100 logically distinct meanings (Rae 1981). The main candidates are equality of treatment, equality of opportunity, and equality of respect. Of course, as Tawney (1930) suggests, equality may not mean that all get the same treatment. On the contrary, equality of respect will lead to different treatments based on the needs of the patient/client. All healthcare professionals operate in a system which is focused on such principles and increasingly have to manage local distribution of healthcare. In all this, equality demands dialogue and negotiation, working through the needs with the patient/client. The principle of freedom is often expressed in terms of rights. The idea of right brings with it a sense of negative freedom and a defence of what is seen as a right. In Parts 2 and 3 we will look at how these principles are worked through, and in particular how ideas like rights can radically affect how we view distribution.

Managing Value Conflict

Once values are clearly articulated, there may be value conflict or value congruence. Value conflict may emerge in terms of a dilemma, as noted above, involving no simple solution. Conflicts may be between values of different areas such as personal, professional, or public, or between different professional values. This requires first some attempt at prioritising them. Core principles may be equally important and have to be held together. The professional principles of justice and equal respect for autonomy have to be held together. The core principles of healthcare have to be held together with the principle of organisational sustainability, that is it is the healthcare organisation which ensures the practice of care. Values conflicts can be addressed in several ways:
■ Recognise that there is a value conflict. The default position is to deny or ignore such a conflict, partly because recognising and managing value conflict is not an academic exercise. Values connect to identity and relationships and can lead to relational conflict if those

involved feel they have to defend them – something most of us want to avoid (see Haidt below). In Tom's case, there were different views of care amongst the stakeholders, leading to task conflicts, but none of these were addressed.

- Value clarification, which is not a conceptual exercise. Values come alive in practice and therefore reflecting on practice helps focus in on the values expressed in that practice. Value clarification, then, demands mutual dialogue, helping all parties to look at their practice and see if that practice reflects the values they think they hold.
- Value congruence. As value reflection progresses, some form of value congruence should be aimed for, in order to establish a sense of shared value. This can form the basis of shared trust.
- Genuine reflection on values, and especially core principles, enables their meaning to be established in context. This is what justice or respect look like in this situation. In Tom's case, the core principles seem to have been assumed, without any attempt to see how they were instantiated. Hence, there was never any sense of dissonance about values and practice amongst the healthcare teams, and thus no learning that might involve addressing any dissonance.
- Involving the wider community in the value reflection. This may be simply a wider dialogue, hearing the views of different professions, the healthcare organisation (including any account of principles, such as codes), and members of the family. Dialogue in this way has a mediating effect, taking away from possible relational conflict. It may also involve more formal mediation.
- Where dialogue fails to establish any sense of shared value, this may demand a more formal process of testing the values and the associated practice. This may involve whistleblowing. We look at this in detail in the third part of the book. It is worth noting here that whistleblowing involves careful deliberation with all parties about values and practice (see Chapter 9).

Identifying Options and Planning

As noted above, ethical decision making has grown from the simple rational practice of deciding between two options into an exercise which explores the different possibilities. At one level this is about examining possible consequences and ensuring there is a risk–benefit analysis, that is practicing the principle of non-maleficence. However, it is, by definition, hard to know exactly what might happen in the future, especially if you aim not to simply avoid possible dangers but seek to find the best possible embodiment of principles. Such possibilities are precisely not evident unless the different agents in the situation are consulted and become part of the deliberation. In our case perhaps most importantly, Tom and Sarah were not given a real voice because they were not part of exploring the possibilities. Exploring the possibilities would have involved working through their relationship. How would Tom feel going home to die? Did he want to protect his wife Sarah from the experience of this? In this he may have still seen himself as her carer. How did Sarah feel about what was happening – the impending loss of her husband and thus of her carer? Both in turn could not begin to explore possibilities fully until there was clarity about Tom's condition, something not there in the team as a whole.

Possibilities, of course, will be dependent upon limitations and resources. These can only be identified through analysing, first the capacities of individual 'actors', and then the resources in relation to the potential partnerships. Options will increase in relation to the different partnerships. At the base of this will also be exploration of responsibility, owned by individuals, or shared with others. Without negotiation of that responsibility, the options could not be put into practice. The key ethical category of responsibility will be explored in detail in the next chapter. How far were possibilities examined in the medical team in Tom's case? If not far, what was getting in the way? There might have been reluctance to send Tom home because of 'risk'. Could risk management actually obscure possibilities? Examining possibilities relates directly to the core principles. In one perspective, this looks to how far different possibilities and their consequences fulfil these principles. Equally, those possibilities would not emerge without the practice of those principles enabling all those involved to become part of the deliberation.

Audit

In a sense the decision-making process ends with the decision about how the core ethical principles are to be embodied. However, some form of audit is important in the reflective process. The term audit is often associated with formal processes, and with measurement of practice. However, its key meaning is to do with giving an account of value and practice (from the term *audire*, to hear). In Chapter 10 we note the importance of ethical audit in clinical governance. The simple process of hearing principles as part of reflective practice links meaning to practice, encouraging responsibility for both. Gregory and Willis (2013), in work with hospital Trust boards, ran a simple audit, asking board members what they thought the key principles of the Trust were. The boards could identify these fairly easily. However, in a follow-up question they could not identify any decision made over the previous 12 months which was explicitly informed by these principles. This suggested that decision making is often tied to targets rather than values or principles.

Ethical audits do not have to be formal but should be part of the discipline of reflective practice and professional development, in healthcare teams, with critical friends or mentors, and so on. They usually involve identifying practice: the key ethical principles that guide the different professions; the key ethical principles that guide the wider healthcare organisation; recent practice where these principles have been consciously used in deliberation (Gregory and Willis 2013). Given the holistic nature of the ethical decision-making framework, this would not simply be a cognitive process. Reflection on feelings about a case can unearth dissonance which leads to learning, as much as reflection on principles. It is important to underline that any ethical decision-making process is not discrete, that is not separate from any professional decision making per se.

Making a decision about the delivery of healthcare is not a separate process from ethical decision making. As we shall see in Part 3, any aspect of delivering healthcare involves core principles and perceptions of purpose, not least questions about justice and responsibility. This applies to all healthcare professions, including management. The ethical dimension of deliberation is at the heart of professional practice. Hence, ethical decision-making frameworks have the same shape as reflective practice, and are premised in the same dynamic of learning. We shall see in the next chapter how the core skills and attributes of ethics, the virtues, also interrelate with all the professional skills – intellectual, psychological, scientific, and practical.

Reflecting Practice and Ethical Decision Making

Of course, the deadlines of work mean that embodiment of values cannot be 'perfect', and the fitting of values to practice will be a matter of ongoing reflection. Indeed, given such constraints any ethical response may involve choosing the best of several difficult options; there is no absolute ethically right 'solution'. Nonetheless, the use of a framework that is understood and accepted by colleagues can enable rapid critical reflection for the immediate situation. Clearly, such a framework may not be used in detail for every situation. Moreover, the experienced reflective practitioner may well use the framework without consciously working through it in a serial way. However, it provides a means of making ethical sense of any situation. It embodies and reinforces a view of ethics that is dialogic, participative, collaborative, and transformative. Hence, ethical practice involves several things:

- Dialogue is key to ethics at every point. It cannot be about hands-off problem solving. Dialogue engages not simply issues and techniques but the people involved. It communicates something about the patient/client and the carer and this relationship enables the development of autonomy and trust (see Chapter 9 for a more detailed analysis of trust).

- The ethical process is essentially a learning process, learning more about the situation, stakeholders (including the self), values, and possibilities.
- Ethical decision making involves both the individual and the wider community of practice. It is essentially social. Ethical judgement needs others (Hoffmaster and Hooker 2018; Taylor 1989). Without different perspectives we get locked into uncritical acceptance of values.
- A key part to the learning process is the challenging of perceptions. Perceptions matter, perceptions about principles and values and perceptions of the world, how it functions and what is important in it. One of the key reasons for the credit crisis of 2007/8 was perception that the marketplace was self-regulating, despite indications to the contrary. The challenge of perception is part of dialogue, because dialogue involves different perspectives and enables reflection on one's own narrative. Hence, contradictions begin to emerge. Whitehead (1989) argues that only once we experience such contradiction is there real learning and motivation to change. In his learning theory, he argues that absolute ethical fit is not possible. On the contrary, each individual, and by extension every group, is a 'living contradiction', a mismatch of values and practice. Historically, this is exemplified in the way that often very morally upright people in the industrial revolution had little problem with child labour (Gallop 2010). Such figures only began to learn when campaigners such as Shaftesbury faced them with their actions and they saw that these were at odds with beliefs and values, including beliefs about children. Prior to this point children were not seen as fully human.
- If ethical decision making involves this kind of reflection, then it must also involve feelings as well as cognitive reflection. Seeing values and beliefs at odds with action creates an affective (emotional) as well as cognitive dissonance. All values are related to feeling precisely because we form some commitment to them and they are important to identity (Cowan 2005). It is this feeling that motivates change.
- Identity, a sense of the self, is key to ethical deliberation, both of the professional and the patient/client. Such identity is developed implicitly or explicitly through self-narrative, hearing the self (Ricoeur 2000). The practice of deliberation/decision making further establishes identity (Taylor 1989), not least when decisions are compared to those of others in any situation. This also establishes responsibility, and we look at that in more detail in the next chapter.

It is important to underline two points, about purpose and everyday ethics.

PURPOSE

As noted in the analysis of the case, the purpose of care underlies all the ethical reflection. All parties were trying to find the care that was right for Tom. This perspective is critical to the decision-making process, because it brings the nurse and all involved back into the relationship with the patient: how he/she sees what he/she is doing in that relationship, how he/she justifies to his/herself what he/she is doing, how he/she justifies to others what he/she is doing, and how he/she justifies to her patient what he/she is doing. We use the term justify in a positive sense here, of simply giving an account, something the principle of accountability suggests is reasonably owed to others as a part of professional practice. All professionals involved believed they were caring, and the analysis suggests that this belief was not properly tested. This also suggests that the reflection care cannot be purely individual. We need others to help us reflect.

EVERYDAY ETHICS

The case reinforces the importance of starting professional practice with ethical reflection focused on care. Raising the ethical questions, and issues about respect and dignity, after Tom's death were too late. Ethical meaning was there from the word go, and by not addressing it, the consequences were care for Tom that was not truly responsive to his needs. This demands making time for reflecting on principles from the word go – ensuring that ethics are an everyday focus.

Descriptive Theories: Making Sense of Ethical Practice

An ethical decision-making framework then is basically the framework of reflective practice which enables the professional to address ethical issues as an ongoing part of reflective practice. It enables careful deliberation and judgment. *Descriptive theories* of ethics help us to understand what we might need to make such judgements. These are distinguished from *normative ethical theories* which try to establish the foundations of ethics. Historically, this has emerged from philosophical and theological studies which often seek to justify one theory over others, and thus establish normative practice, that is how we ought to behave. We will examine these theories more closely in the final chapters. Descriptive ethical theories are focused on how we actually make ethical decisions; the domain of social sciences, especially psychology. The distinction between the different theoretical areas are useful, though, as we will argue, they are interconnected. Rest (1994), for instance, argues for a complex, multiple-stage decision-making process, which requires:

- moral awareness (taking in the situation and the key ethical issues);
- moral judgment (deciding that a specific action is morally justifiable);
- moral motivation (the commitment or intention to take the moral action);
- moral character (persistence or follow-through to take the action despite challenges). Note that, in this book, we use the term 'moral' as interchangeable with 'ethical' (see the list of terms at the end of this chapter).

POPULIST DESCRIPTIVE THEORIES

'It's easy to be ethical!' was part of the headline in *Star Tribune Minneapolis-Saint Paul* (28 June 2002, quoted in Trevino and Brown 2004). The litmus test is 'if something stinks, don't do it.' Such thinking advocates other approaches, including the well known the *light of day test*. The best form of this is, when faced by a problem that seems to be ethical, imagine what your parent, spouse, or your children would say if you were part of this practice and if this practice were headlined in today's papers. This can be intensified in the *consequence test*, namely what would the consequences be for me or my organisation, if I got involved. Such tests are useful tools to bear in mind but they do not get us very far. First, they are not really tests at all but rather precautionary perspectives that remind us that we might be found out. Second, all they tell us to do is not to get involved. But what if not getting involved leads to making the unethical practice even worse? And what if my mother or partner were to read the headlines about the subsequent enquiry and saw that I had not done anything about the practice when I could have? A warning does not help us to make judgement. Third, what if my ethical 'sense of smell' is not very good? I might be aware of a practice and consider that it is strange but note that the practice seems to have been accepted by colleagues and line managers. Fourth, and connected, the way in which the 'smell test' is set out assumes that ethics is about an immediate ethical dilemma, and that it involves responding to that dilemma. But the dilemma may not be obvious, not least if the culture in which one operates discourages critical reflection. Hence, in the Mid Staffs case, many professionals simply did not see a dilemma in their practice. Fifth, it assumes that ethical decision making is individualistic. It simply involves the individual making up his or her mind. But even the reflection up to this point in the chapter indicates that ethical decision making cannot simply be about one person. By definition there are many people whose judgement is involved, who radically affect both the ethical meaning and practice. Nonetheless, such popular theories have a real strength focused on the concern for how people will think about what we have done, linking to a sense of shame.

RATIONALITY BASED THEORIES

Such theories argue that ethical decision making is a function of rationality. The best-known is the stage theory of moral development from Kohlberg (1969). A stage is a period in a person's development where they exhibit typical behaviour and establish particular capacities. Kohlberg argued for six stages in moral development. Building on Piaget's (1965) work, Kohlberg's theory suggests that the key to moral development is the development of cognitive capacities stages. Kohlberg based his stage theory upon research and interviews with groups of young children. A series of moral dilemmas were presented to children, who were then interviewed to determine the reasoning behind their judgments of each scenarios. These involved decisions made for the good of, for instance, the family which involved breaking the law. Kohlberg was not interested so much in the answer to the question of wrong or right, as in the *reasoning* for the participant's decision. From this work, Kohlberg identified six stages of moral reasoning grouped into three major levels, each divided into two stages (Table 2.3). Each level represented a fundamental shift in the social-moral perspective of the individual.

The stages move from a simple acceptance of authority through to a reasoning about the nature of authority and the underlying ethical principles of society. The stages according to Kohlberg form an invariant sequence, with moral development never skipping stages, and occur across all cultures. Cross-cultural research shows that individuals in 'technologically advanced' societies move rapidly through the stages of moral development, whilst in isolated communities, few go beyond stage three (Kohlberg 1984). This seems to indicate that greater awareness of different ethical perspectives assists moral development.

TABLE 2.3 ■ **Kohlberg's Stages of Moral Development**

Level I Preconventional Morality	*Stage 1. Obedience and Punishment Orientation* – In this the child assumes that powerful authorities hand down a fixed set of rules which he or she must obey without question. Kohlberg calls this thinking 'preconventional' because children do not yet see themselves as members of society. Morality is seen as something external to themselves, something adults impose upon them.
	Stage 2. Individualism and Exchange – At this stage children recognise that there is not just one right view that is handed down by the authorities. At stage two, punishment is a risk that one naturally wants to avoid.
Level II Conventional Morality	*Stage 3. Good Interpersonal Relationships* – This marks the beginning of the teenage years, when the children see ethics as more complex. They believe that people should live up to the expectations of the family and community and behave in 'good' ways. This is conventional thinking because it assumes that the attitude expressed would be shared by the entire community.
	Stage 4. Maintaining the Social Order – This focuses on society as a whole. The emphasis is on obeying laws, respecting authority, and performing one's duties so that the social order is maintained.
Level III Postconventional Morality	*Stage 5. Social Contract and Individual Rights* – A core motivation in stage four is to keep society functioning. However, a totalitarian society might be well-organised, but has little moral content. At stage five, people begin to ask the underlying question about what makes a good society. Critical questioning is introduced, and one's own and other societies are tested. Rights and democracy dominate this thinking.
	Stage 6. Universal Principles – Stage six respondents also saw themselves as working out a conception of the good society. Laws are evaluated in terms of their coherence with basic principles of fairness rather than upheld simply on the basis of their place within an existing social order.

However, there are several criticisms of Kohlberg's theory; Gilligan (1982) argues that it is incomplete, not least because it devalues the morality of care and community. Kohlberg, as a member of the educated, elite, white, male, Western culture, viewed individual autonomy and justice as the premier moral values. In effect, he equated ethics with justice, ignoring other possible core principles, such as equality of respect and compassion and care. Gilligan views this as partly a gender issue. Feminist ethics (Nussbaum 2000) argues that care is at the centre of ethics and that this looks to work through ethical issues not in an individualistic way but through members of the community sharing responsibility. Gilligan argued there was a difference between male and female respondents, with the latter stressing shared responsiveness. This involves more affiliative ways of living, tying ethics to real, ongoing relationships rather than abstract solutions to hypothetical dilemmas. Non-Western and tribal societies, and historically the lower classes in the West, also frequently see the community as more important than the individual. According to Kohlberg's Western view of moral reasoning, communitarian morality is doomed to rest forever at a lower stage of development. This view disregards the possibility that communitarian morality may be as advanced as individualistic morality, if not more so, and makes little room for cross-cultural inclusion.

From an empirical methodology, some critics claim that the use of hypothetical situations skews the results because it measures abstract rather than concrete reasoning. When children (and some adults) are presented with situations out of their immediate experience, they turn to rules they have learned from external authorities for answers, rather than to their own internal voice. Therefore, young children base their answers on rules of 'right' and 'wrong' they have learned from parents and teachers (stages 1 and 2). Gilligan (1982) noted that if young children are presented with situations familiar to them, on the other hand, they often show care and concern for others, basing their moral choices on the desire to share the good and maintain harmonious relations, placing them in stage 3 or 4 (which Kohlberg claimed was impossible at their age). It is difficult then to see how the idea of invariant sequence can be sustained. It may be that individuals and groups locate themselves in different stages depending on the context, with major crises causing access to higher or lower stages. Furthermore, it is not clear that making a moral decision can be confined to a narrow view of rationality. Feelings are a critical part of any ethical decision making. The very idea of values indicates that we feel strongly about certain principles. Such positive feelings can inform any decision making (Solomon 2007). Feelings also reflect something about significant relationships. Hence, feelings have to be involved in decision making. The case of Tom shows that feelings were intentionally avoided, perhaps for fear how to engage them. Kohlberg's stage theory then has important elements. However, it does not take full account of the complexity of moral decision making. To do that requires greater understanding of the effects of aspects such as culture and gender on the decision taken. It also demands closer attention to the role of feeling in ethics.

Non-Rational Theories

In response to the stress in Kohlberg on individual rationality, non-rational theories stress the role of feeling. One of the best examples focuses on social intuitionism. Haidt (2001; 2012) argues that our ethical decision making is based more on feelings and, in particular, intuitions. There is a long history of this view in the study of ethics (see Hume 1975 on intuitions and Smith 2016 on moral sentiments). There is considerable neuro-scientific evidence that many evaluations, including moral judgments, take place automatically without rational reflection, and these initial intuitions anchor subsequent judgments (Haidt 2001). Such moral reasoning is further influenced by two psychological pressures which motivate any response. The first involves 'relatedness', how we manage impressions and ensure smooth interactions with others. The second involves 'coherence', and how we maintain a coherent identity, including an underlying worldview.

If ethical decision making is based on these affective intuitions, then the ethical reasoning process is secondary. Haidt's (2001) research suggests the reasoning process is generally used to create convincing post hoc justifications for the intuition and for the associated behaviour. Such justifications are often arrived at despite the person involved being unable to accurately describe the reason underlying his or her judgement. Given this dynamic it is perhaps not surprising that when the person seeks to convince others of this moral reasoning, it involves a focus on the affective dimension. Such judgements are in turn significantly influenced by others who hold similar views or practice similar behaviours. Hence, we turn to like-minded people to reinforce our views.

Haidt (2001) does suggest that logical reasoning may override the person's intuition but that this is rare. He also suggests that later individual reflection may alter or refine the initial intuition, but not radically change it. The implication of this is that life becomes fixed in certain 'tribal' ethical positions. Haidt (2012) later develops this to argue that ethical and political views are dominated by these intuitive perspectives on principles, such that partisan groups find it difficult to appreciate the different perspectives of other groups. Focusing on the Democratic and Republican parties in the US, he notes how they hold key values and principles such as freedom and equality but have very different views of what these mean. For Republicans, for instance, freedom is about not being constrained by others (freedom from) (Berlin 1969), including government regulators, and about the individual taking responsibility for their lives (economically or in terms of health and well-being). This view of humanity has major consequences for the provision of healthcare as we shall note in Part 3. Democrats tend to see freedom as more an enabling concept (freedom to) (Berlin 1969) and thus to stress human rights as empowering people. Here freedom is given rather than taken. Ethical partisanship tends to focus on defending the value against the threats of other group values. Not surprisingly, it becomes hard to understand the other group – to see them as part of a coherent or rational association – and this is part of the problem with social intuitionism. As Corporal Willis, whilst on duty outside Parliament, puts it, '…every boy and every gal, that's born into the world alive, is either a little Liberal or else a little Conservative!' (Gilbert and Sullivan's *Iolanthe* Act 2).

CRITIQUES OF INTUITIONISM

There are significant problems with Haidt's position. First, if our moral intuitions are predetermined then the theory can give no adequate account of agency, of the person taking responsibility for making up his or her own mind about an ethical issue. It is this kind of agency that Kohlberg does show us in his later stages. In the earlier stages, ethical views are indeed pre-determined, and reinforced by groups, but in the final two, there is agency that enables the person to take a view that is different from the community, but also to stay with the community. This is the basis of *autonomy*, which literally means the capacity to govern oneself. Second, evidence suggests that effective challenges of initial intuitions are not simply a rational activity but are also affective, based either on the challenge of relationships with others or on reflection on core values that transcend partisan positions. Research into what led sports drugs users to change their mind (Backhouse et al. 2006) points to reflection on family relationships, and their associated feelings about what was of worth, causing individuals to reflect on their practice and the underlying rationalisation that held this in place. Third, Haidt's model of social learning is inadequate. How would anyone learn and thus develop different views about value and practice if their value world is pre-determined? This also does not take into account plural identity, allegiance to several different groups that may have different perspectives. It is precisely when such allegiances are part of one's identity that they will, as a matter of course, challenge values held.

Haidt's theory nonetheless reminds us that ethics cannot be simply based on rational reflection. It involves the interplay of feeling and rationality (Solomon 2007) based on perspective, how we see the world, personal, professional, or political, and how we appreciate that world; that is how we value that world and our interaction in that world. If feelings have a positive role in ethical judgement, they need to be expressed. If they are negative or are holding back an awareness of the situation, then they need to be critically examined. Hence, in Tom's case there needed to be more dialogue: self-dialogue and dialogue amongst the different stakeholders. This means that how we talk about ethics should evidence rational thinking, coherent thought, and emotional engagement. Problems with ethical decision making often involve an absence of logical coherence, or emotional engagement. This is often revealed in ethical fallacies.

2.3 PAUSE FOR THOUGHT

Ethical Arguments and Fallacy Alert

Food campaigner: *I think people should eat fewer fatty hamburgers as part of developing public health.*

    Burger customer: *What? Are you trying to put farmers out of work? Trying to disrespect ordinary people who see this a part of their social gatherings? You posh protesters and your moralising, all part of the nanny state, robbing us of our freedom!*

    This neatly combines two fallacies: the straw man and the *ad personam* or *ad hominem*. In the first, the argument is misrepresented as an extreme one and then attacked. By exaggerating the campaigner's argument, the customer had created a straw man (i.e. an argument with no substance, and this is easier to attack than the actual argument). This original argument is ignored and thus not actually addressed. *Ad hominem* arguments address the person, not the issue. Here the focus is on do-gooders who want to take away my freedom. The exclamation mark reveals strong feelings and a determination not to deliberate about public health and diet.

ETHICAL ARGUMENTS AND FALLACIES

Knowing what the major fallacies are can help you strengthen ethical dialogue. Other fallacies commonly used include:

The *slippery slope argument* asserts bad consequences that will happen in the future if some action is allowed to happen. The classic versions of this are applied to ethical issues across the board, including change in drug legislation or euthanasia. If you allow cannabis to be legalised then this will lead to a breakdown of society. If you allow euthanasia, this will lead to the indiscriminate killing of elderly people who feel they are a nuisance. The problem with such logic is that the conclusions simply do not follow. It is possible, for instance, to put in place safeguards that ensure euthanasia is properly practised. The dire end that the slippery slope argument predicts may or may not happen. However, the fear that it might can give the argument a (false) sense of authority. The slippery slope fallacy is one version of the *non-sequitur* (it does not follow) fallacy. This involves the argument trying to bring two or more logically unrelated ideas as if they were related.

Many arguments rely on an *analogy* (strong similarity) between two or more objects, ideas, or situations. The argument goes that if A is like B and B is wrong then A also must be wrong. Everything then hangs on the analogy, which may or may not be valid. One version of weak analogy is *moral equivalence* in which minor problems are compared to much more serious issues (or vice versa). For instance, mandatory seatbelt laws might be compared to the coercion of Nazi Germany. The analogy in this case tries to compare regulation which systematically saves lives and regulation which systematically tried to destroy whole peoples. The underlying emotion is apparent, belief in the value of freedom and fear of regulation as a loss of freedom. However, once the logic is challenged it becomes apparent that regulation can have value and that is dependent on its end. In this case, the end is a common good.

We often try to strengthen arguments by referring to respected sources who support them – *appeal to authority (ad verecundiam)*. For example, we may refer to the writings of Ghandi to support the idea of equality. However, simple appeal to Ghandi is irrelevant unless he can provide clear argument or empirical support for the importance of an argument or a moral idea. A different form of appeal fallacy is the appeal to the practice of others – *ad populam*. In the Mid Staffs case, some senior staff tried to persuade junior colleagues not to be concerned because it was claimed that this is how every Hospital Trust operated these days. This fallacy is common across all organisations and at all levels. Junior professionals in accountancy research told researchers that they are happy about systemically failing to carry out important checks, because 'everybody else did it' (Gill 2013). The Vice Chancellor of Nottingham University said that one of the reasons why his university accepted several million pounds from British American Tobacco for a Centre for Corporate Social Responsibility was because 'if they had not accepted it, others would have' (Campbell 2001) – everybody else does it. None of these arguments were coherent justifications for what they did.

The *tu quoque* fallacy ('you too') is a variation on 'everybody else does it'. Faced by the accusation, for instance, that, as a leader, you give favours to your family, you might respond to the accuser that he also does this. The aim is to discredit the accuser by pointing out their hypocrisy. However, someone else's guilt does not excuse your own.

A *false dichotomy* is where one tries to dominate the argument by arguing that there are only two options to be followed, for example if you have discovered questionable behaviour at work, you can either make it public or do nothing. This fallacy is often used as a tool to manipulate an audience and is designed to polarise thinking often focused on ties of loyalty – 'you are either with me or against me'.

Causal fallacies suggest causal connections which are not in fact established. One of the main ones is *post hoc ergo propter hoc* (after this, therefore because of this). A manager might suggest, for instance, that poor performance in one part of the hospital only began after the leader of that area was appointed. However, because something happens after something else does not necessarily mean this was the cause.

Appeal to ignorance suggests that ignorance has evidential power. For instance, faced by lack of evidence about UFOs, the retort is often, 'ah, but no-one has definitely proved they don't exist!' Again, feeling predominates in this case as well as the desire to believe in the argument.

A *red herring* derives from prison escapees who would drag fish across their trails to put dogs off the scent. In the same way, an arguer might introduce another issue to take away from the central debate in the hope that we will follow it. A student caught cheating, for instance, might accept they made a mistake and argue, 'but think how this will affect my professional future', hoping that this becomes the focus.

It is important to know that fallacious arguments are common and can be powerful and persuasive if you are not watching out for them. Many of these fallacies reveal underlying feelings that actually dominate the argument. *Ad personam*, for instance, show feelings, such as vulnerability and fear about opponents. Slippery slope arguments, applied, for instance, to abortion, are dominated by fear for the fetus and a desire to protect it.

In fact, this kind of thinking is common. In politics, fallacies are used constantly. When the 2009 UK Members of Parliament expenses scandal hit the headlines (Grice 2009), the favoured response was 'I did nothing wrong, I was simply doing what everyone else did'. At this point, we see that fallacies are commonly used to avoid responsibility and excuse behaviour, as in much of the dynamics of the Mid Staffs case. We will return to this question of responsibility in the next chapter. It is important to be alert to the use of fallacies and to focus on the dynamics that are underlying them. This requires careful challenge. First, the underlying feeling should be acknowledged; 'I hear your concern', 'I hear you feel strongly about this'. This is an expression of respect and concern. In some cases, this can help the person to recognise their own feelings, and how they have arisen. Second, the focus should then become the issue itself. In focusing on the issues, this begins to address responsibility and take the argument into the possibilities of how the core issue might be addressed. The important point is that ethical decision making and conversations never take place in a rational bubble. This leads to a more dialogic approach to ethics.

A Third Way: Dialogue and Narrative

Kohlberg stressed the act of ethical decision making as a rational individual activity, with stipulated choices, either A or B. Haidt focused on ethical decision making as based on social intuitionism (affective), with the decision made before any rational reflection. The first of these saw moral deliberation as objective, the second more subjective, reinforced socially. Between those two poles have sat many different views of how we do ethics which involve rationality and feeling working together. These have focused on the good person and good community rather than the good act. Virtue theories argue that it is these strengths that are most important and they should be cultivated by the community (MacIntyre 2013). The community shows what are the most important virtues through its narratives. They show what good character looks like – what attributes are needed to be good and do good. These theories focus on the act of decision making and how individuals and communities work together to achieve this.

Feminist ethical theory is part of this approach, based on empathy and compassion, and showing, for example, how ethical decisions are best arrived at through dialogue which stimulates the imagination and leads to shared responsibility. Gilligan's (1982) research argues that this builds on women's voices which have worked against conventional, individualistic, and patriarchal constraints. Key to this affiliative way of thinking is that it shows people working together to find a solution. Autonomy then takes the shape more of individual and shared governance. Gilligan argues that women's conceptions of care and affiliation are embedded in real-life situations, and rather than imposing an ethical judgement, enabling judgement to emerge from immersion in the situation. This approach to ethics is focused on identity, dialogue, and narrative, and we will develop it in more detail in the next chapter. Identity reflects the complexity of the personal, professional, social (a member of an organisation or wider society), and ecological (part of the wider physical environment). Dialogue reflects ongoing dialogue with the self (Burkitt 2008) and personal values, with the profession and individual members of the profession (who bring guidance on ethical meaning and practice through codes), with wider stakeholders (who bring different values or different perceptions of values), with organisations who enable practice (such as Healthcare Trusts and their publicly stated vision and values), and with wider society. Each of these dialogues enable a firmer focus on principles in practice, a greater mutuality (including an affirmation of the different perspectives) and a concern for shared action that will bring principles to life.

THE MORAL IMAGINATION

Narrative development enables individuals and organisations to develop a clearer, practice-based ethical voice. This is my story; this is our story. The two are never quite the same, and should not be so, because it is the slight differences which emerge though the questions brought by new challenges, which ensure that the belief that we are always 'the good guys' is tested. Hence, as noted in the decision-making framework, ethics is about continuous learning, and practice of the imagination. The moral imagination in applied ethics is most strikingly associated with the work of Patricia Werhane (1999) who focuses on moral deliberation. Moral imagination is seen as 'the ability to understand a context or set of activities from a number of different perspectives, the actualising of new possibilities which are not context dependent, and the instigation of the process of evaluating these possibilities from a moral point of view' (Werhane 1999, p. 5). Biss (2014) deepens this analysis, suggesting four aspects of the moral imagination: perception; judgement; radical perspective; and moral possibilities:

- Perception. Nussbaum (2000) and Murdoch (2001) both see perception as preceding any theoretical or abstract moral ideas (Levinas 1991; Bauman 1989 – pre-rational primacy of responsibility). It is how I *see* the world that really determines my ethical response. This demands that I take responsibility for testing my perception. Nussbaum argues that this requires use of the moral imagination, an effort to see the other and the social and professional network I am involved in. This means working out my identity and how I relate to the world. Nussbaum often focuses on literature to illustrate this. One example by Nussbaum (1990) is Henry James's *Golden Bow*. The central relationship in this book is between father and daughter, and Nussbaum shows how the imagination enables them to see each other and allows both to let go. Imagination becomes the means of 'apprehending morally serious features' (Biss 2014).

- The practice of deliberation (judgement). Dewey (2007), for instance, sees imagination as being used in rehearsing the rational decision-making process, partly a result of self-dialogue and partly dialogue with others.

- Radical perspective/moral imagination. Babbit (1996) focuses on the imagined self and the imagined society, based on core moral values, and how these proceed into deliberation. This focuses on the self as socially constructed, and responsibility as involving the working through of this identity in relationships. In the light of those different relationships, there is discovery of new moral possibilities.

- Moral possibilities. This focuses on moral imagination in action. It is about creativity, seeing what is possible, with the suggestion that the moral choice demands that possibilities be seen (in projects and people). Ethics in this sense cannot be abstract. The use of the imagination can lead to possibilities well beyond such stipulated choices, partly because involving others increases possibilities. Of course, this takes us into the aspects of the debate between Kohlberg (1984) and Gilligan (1982) on moral development. The developed feminist perspective in that debate (e.g. Robinson 2008; Koehn 1998) was able to see possibilities that were not apparent in individual rational decision making precisely because it focused on people and the relationships of the people involved in any situation as well as ethical values and principles. The focus on relationships involves reflection on identity, how the person or organisation relates to the other, what the significance of that relationship is (worth in society), and with that, the awareness of possibilities that reside not just in plan or project but people. The person (self or other) or organisation (own or other) may not know if they are capable of making a project possible. To be aware of that requires the exercise of imagination about oneself and others, to see moral context, connections, capacities, and so on. Diamond (1991), building on Nussbaum's view of Aristotle, takes this further into the possibility of improvisation. The ethical improviser can see the possibilities and respond with appropriate timing. This idea takes us back to reflective practice, underlining moral deliberation as part of practice, rather than always having to enter a formal decision-making process. Nonetheless, the framework is important in keeping the imagination focused on core principles.

As Tom's case has shown, this involves good communication at all times with all stakeholders, building up awareness and trust. The 'solution' in the case above demanded good communication amongst all the team members in order to clarify not just diagnosis but what each of them meant by care; remember they were all focused on the desire to care. Communication was also critical with Tom and Sarah. At all costs Tom wanted to avoid being a nuisance, and so did not give any cues about how he was feeling. Good communication demanded much more active listening from the team, empowering Tom to direct his care. Wider communication with all the family was also lacking and it meant that the moral imagination could not be practised. Can you imagine your end, and how you would want it to be? The real question may be 'but if it was so easy why did it not happen?' Perhaps the most important question, going back to Mid Staffs, is what stops it from happening. We will look at this in the next chapter and in the development of an ethical culture (see Chapter 10). For some professionals there is the feeling that all the dialogue and narrative is too complicated, another skill to be practised and added to the great list of things to do. This is to mistake ethics as a discrete skill not fundamentally part of professional practice. It might also be a hangover from the time when ethics was thought to be purely about the exercise of the intellect. In fact, ethics is involved and ongoing in everyday practice and ethical judgement often takes place on the hoof.

2.4 PAUSE FOR THOUGHT

Analogies of Ethical Practice

The ethical practice outlined above can be thought of as like driving a car. You are in the car, and so want to get from A to B. How you get there is not just a matter of choosing the quickest route, you have to make a number of ongoing reflections and judgements about how you will respond to:

- National guidelines about speed;
- Motorists and pedestrians;
- Immediate issues, from areas of risk, such as schools, to limited visibility and so on;
- The constraints of your own situation, such as deadlines;
- Consideration of the consequences of one's actions for all involved or potentially involved.

The Motivations to be Ethical

Traditionally, the different reasons that support attention to ethics involve self-interest, mutual interest, and the common good.

SELF-INTEREST

- Management of reputation. Effective professions depend upon trust. Trust is built through the perception of good reputation and the practice of integrity.
- Effective internal regulation can minimise external regulation.
- Ethical focus can actually enable greater awareness and more effective decision making, leading to clearer strategy and more effective enterprise.
- Attention to purpose, justice, and values can enable a more motivated and creative workforce (see Chapter 10).
- 'Be sure your sin will find you out!' (Numbers 32:23). This comes from the book of Numbers in the Old Testament and is part of the Jewish wisdom tradition. In other words, it is based on practical wisdom. It is easy to imagine that we are invisible and that we cannot be seen. Hence, Plato's story of the ring of Gyges (Plato, 2007). Gyges is a shepherd who discovers a ring that makes him invisible. If you are invisible, do you have to be good? The answer is twofold. First, you are not invisible to yourself. This is about living with yourself and thus integrity (see Chapter 3). Second, the truth is that we operate in a world where we are seen by somebody, if not now then later. This is true most of all in relation to our information technology (IT) dominated environment. If it is likely that bad things will come to light, then it is in our interest to get things right in the first place.
- Stakeholders can cause negative pressure that could affect individual or organisational reputation.

MUTUAL INTEREST

- Healthcare is part of a complex network of stakeholders with mutual interests, account-ability, and values. It is the interest of all to develop ethics and responsibility together. There is an argument that developing ethical meaning and practice across any shared project or with wider stakeholders improves ethics and the effectiveness of the profession or organisation.

COMMON GOOD

- The common good recognises a good which is of value to all. Classic examples of the com-mon good are a sustainable environment and society, and health for all. Hence, healthcare is founded in the common good, with the healthcare professions and society in general together responsible for it.

Ethical Terminology

- **Ethics**: The philosophical study of what is right or wrong in human conduct and what rules, or principles, should govern it. Hence the term is singular. This is often subdivided into meta-ethics, and applied and professional ethics.
- **Meta-ethics**: The systematic study of the nature of ethics. This looks to the issues such as how an ethical judgment can be justified and the theoretical underpinning of ethical deci-sion making, that is what values should inform ethical practice. We will look at the different kinds of theory below and in the final chapters.
- **Applied ethics**: The application of ethics in a particular area of practice, for example busi-ness or bio-ethics.
- **Professional ethics**: The ethical identity, codes, and practices of particular professions, such as nurses, doctors, lawyers, or engineers.
- **Morality**: Morality often refers to standards of moral conduct – right behaviour. In the his-tory of philosophy there have been many attempts to differentiate the concept from ethics. Nietzsche (2008), for instance, argues that morality involves 'mores' (social norms and obli-gations), whilst ethics involves the freedom to determine for oneself what is right or wrong. However, the term morality is most often used interchangeably with the term ethics, which is how we will use it.
- **Principles** (from *principium*, source or beginning): These are fundamental concepts which are the source of inspiration or direction for ethical action. Principles form a basis for moral reasoning which is worked though in response to the situation. Kant (1964) distinguishes constitutive and regulative principles. The first involves something about the nature of an enterprise. Sport, for instance, is about individuals or teams competing to win. Sport, how-ever, has to be regulated, hence rules must ensure fairness, that is the practice of the prin-ciple of justice. Kant suggests that the human person, bearer of rights and responsibilities, is a constitutive principle (telling us something about human beings and relationships), and *respect* for the person (as free to determine and practice responsibilities) is the regulative principle.
- **Rules** (from *regulare*, rule or govern): These involve public statements which prescribe prac-tice or define duties. Hence, rules are often procedural – about how we go about a social practice. Despite their prescriptive nature, rules still have to be interpreted.
- **Attitudes and opinions**: Unexamined and conditioned views of reality leading to knee jerk responses. Opinions, as in the legal profession, are focused on good deliberation. However, it is common to justify opinions simply on the basis of freedom to hold them: 'I am entitled

to my opinion!'. However, even if we accept your entitlement, it does not mean that your opinion can be effectively justified. Note the old saying, 'opinions are like "anal sphincters", everybody has one, and they need regular and rigorous examination'.

- **Beliefs**: Trusted worldviews based on a range of foundations, from science to religion, which form the basis of actions. Beliefs, like opinions, are always contestable, in terms of logical coherence or empirical foundation. Such beliefs are often a key part of appreciative systems. They inform in different ways what we think is of significant worth. We will note below how beliefs can dominate ethical debate.

- **Ethos**: The characteristic spirit of a community or organisation which reveals values, attitudes, and aspirations. Ethos tells us something about the character and identity of a group. As the Mid Staffs case shows, identity is not always what we think it is, and the character of an organisation cannot be assumed. Hence, in Part 3 we will look at the role of different professions in the healthcare project in developing and maintaining ethos.

- **Values**: This a general term about things that are valued to practice and relationships. Ethical principles, for instance, are ethical values. Virtues are dispositions that have value.

- **Right and wrong**: These are terms that refer to the moral principles underlying the duties. We judge something to be right or wrong according to whether it has fulfilled a principle.

- **Good and bad**: Refers to goals or outcomes that are either beneficial or detrimental.

- **Virtue and vice**: Refers to the moral competence of the person. Virtues are the moral muscles (*virtus* meaning man, focused on strength). They are key to any ethical action – the qualities or dispositions that enable it to happen. The term vice is not often used these days but has real utility in professional ethics. These are dispositions which cause the person to avoid ethical practice. We will examine virtues and vices in more detail as part of professional competence in the next chapter.

- **Conscience**: This is often seen as 'personal', a feeling that makes one uneasy at the prospect of doing the wrong thing, or after doing the wrong thing. It is even referred to as 'a voice'. Aquinas (1981) defines 'conscience' as the 'application of knowledge to activity'. This involves the exercise of reason and the natural disposition of the human mind to apprehend general principles of behaviour. Goodpaster (2007) argues that conscience was originally a cultural or community attribute, not simply personal. In this case, ethical reflection would focus on organisational decision making. We will return to this in Part 3 and the development of ethos.

- **Deliberation**: Deliberation, careful consideration (in decision making) is at the heart of ethics because it involves the individual owning both critical reflection and making a judgement. Deliberation is often thought to be slow, but if the elements of deliberation are well-practiced, it does not have to be (see the example of judgement in nursing practice in Chapter 1).

- **Ethical problem**: A difficult ethical challenge which can be resolved with effort.

- **Ethical dilemma** (*di-lemma*, a double argument with conflicting assumptions): This involves a choice to be made between two or more alternatives, all of which are problematic. This may involve conflicts between core principles or duties, with no guidance about how to resolve the conflicts.

- **Ethical quandary**: The simply perplexed state, involving uncertainty about ethical choices.

Conclusion

This chapter has examined ethical decision making through some descriptive theories of ethics. Stage theories show the importance of personal development, moving from a view of the person as influenced by the social context to more autonomous decision making, based on rational reflection. Gilligan and others argue that this focuses on two extremes, the person who simply follows rules and the person who thinks for themselves. Between those, argues Gilligan, is a social approach to ethics that is not just about individual decision making but about people working together for an ethical response. The conclusion of that debate is that ethics is *both* about thinking for oneself and working out the response with others. The decision-making framework confirms, for instance, that data gathering is more effective if it includes all stakeholders. All this suggests that ethical thinking is focused on personal maturity. This also suggests that ethics is both about responding to difficult dilemmas often faced by the individual, and also about how values are handled in day to day decision making and planning. In turn, this stresses the importance of developing professional practice which enables dialogue, and the development of a culture that makes ethical values and thinking explicit, as part of any vision and value statement. Many of these values are rooted in the six Cs. Commitment involves fidelity. Compassion involves both respect and justice. Communication involves veracity. Competence includes concern for patient's/client's safety (non-maleficence). Care connects to all of the core principles. The final C is courage, often needed to fulfil responsibilities for care, and part of a wider concern for character, the virtues needed to develop ethical practice. We turn to these in the next chapter.

References

Aquinas, T. (1981). *Summa theologica*. New York: Resources for Christian Living.

Babbit, S. (1996). *Impossible dreams: rationality, integrity and moral imagination*. Boulder, CO: Westview Press.

Backhouse, S., Mckenna, J., & Robinson, S. (2006). *International literature review: attitudes, behaviours, knowledge and education – drugs in sport: past, present and future*. Montreal: World Anti-Doping Agency – WADA.

Bakhtin, M. (1993). *The Dialogic Imagination*. Austin: University of Texas.

Bauman, Z. (1989). *Modernity and the holocaust*. London: Polity.

Beauchamp, T. L., & Childress, J. F. (2019). *Principles of biomedical ethics* (8th ed.). Oxford: Oxford University Press.

Berlin, I. (1969). Two concepts of liberty. In A. Quinton (Ed.), *Political philosophy* (pp. 141–155). London: Penguin.

Biss, M. (2014). Moral imagination, perception, and judgment. *The Southern Journal of Philosophy*, *52*(1), 1–21.

Buber, M. (1937). *I and thou*. Edinburgh: T and T Clark.

Burke, A. (2020). *Ethical Practice: NCLEX-RN*. RegisteredNursing.Org. Online available: https://www.registerednursing.org/nclex/ethical-practice/.

Burkitt, I. (2008). *Social selves: theories of self and society*. London: Sage.

Campbell, A. V. (1984). *Moderated love: a theology of professional care*. London: The Society for Promoting Christian Knowledge – SPCK.

Campbell, C. (2001). Should Nottingham University give back its tobacco money? *British Medical Journal*, 20, 1118–1119.

Cowan, J. (2005). The atrophy of the affect. In S. Robinson, & C. Katulushsi (Eds.), *Values in higher education*. Cardiff: Aureus.

Dewey, J. (2007). *Human nature and conduct*. New York: Cosimo.

Diamond, C. (1991). *The realistic spirit*. Cambridge, MA: Massachusetts Institute of Technology – MIT Press.

Gallop, A. (2010). *Victoria's children of the dark*. London: History Press.

Gill, M. (2013). *Accountants' Truth*. Oxford: Oxford University Press.

Gilligan, C. (1982). *In a different voice: psychological theory and women's development*. Cambridge: Harvard University Press.

Goodpaster, K. E. (2007). *Conscience and corporate culture*. Oxford: Blackwell.

Gregory, A., & Willis, P. (2013). *Strategic public relations leadership*. London: Routledge.

Grice, A. (2009). *Review of the year 2009: expenses scandal*. The Independent, 23 December 2009. Online available: https://www.independent.co.uk/voices/commentators/andrew-grice/review-of-the-year-2009-expenses-scandal-1847865.html.

Haidt, J. (2001). The emotional dog and its rational tail: a social intuitionist approach to moral judgment. *Psychological Review*, *108*(4), 814.

Haidt, J. (2012). Moral psychology and the law: how intuitions drive reasoning, judgment, and the search for evidence. *Alabama Law Review*, *64*, 867.

Hoffmaster, B., & Hooker, C. (2018). *Re-reasoning ethics: the rationality of deliberation and judgment in ethics.* Cambridge, MA: MIT Press.

Hume, D. (1975). *Enquiries concerning human understanding and concerning the principles of moral.* Oxford: Oxford University Press.

Kant, I. (1964). *Groundwork of the metaphysics of morals* (translated by Paton, J.). New York: Harper and Row.

Koehn, D. (1998). *Rethinking feminist ethics.* London: Routledge.

Kohlberg, L. (1969). Stage and sequence: the cognitive developmental approach to socialisation. In D. A. Goslin (Ed.), *Handbook of socialization, theory and research.* Chicago: Rand McNally.

Kohlberg, L. (1984). *Essays in moral development.* San Francisco: Harper and Row.

Lambourne, W. (2004). Post-conflict peace building. *Peace, Conflict and Development, 4,* 1–24.

Lederach, J. P. (2005). *The moral imagination.* Oxford: Oxford University Press.

Levinas, E. (1991). *Entre nous; the thinking of the other.* New York: Columbia University Press.

MacIntyre, A. (2013). *After virtue: a study in moral theory.* London: Bloomsbury.

Murdoch, I. (2001). *Sovereignty of the good.* New York: Routledge.

Nietzsche, F. (2008). *Thus spoke Zarathustra: a book for everyone and nobody.* Oxford: Oxford University Press.

Nozick, R. (1972). *Anarchy, state and utopia.* New York: Basic Books.

Nussbaum, M. (1990). *Love's Knowledge: Essays on philosophy and literature.* New York: Oxford University Press.

Nussbaum, M. (2000). *Love's knowledge: essays on philosophy and literature.* New York: Oxford University Press.

Piaget, J. (1965). *The moral judgment of the child.* New York: The Free Press.

Plato (2007). *The Republic.* Penguin: London.

Rae, M. (1981). *Equalities.* Cambridge, MA: Harvard University Press.

Rawls, J. (1971). *Justice as fairness.* Oxford: Clarendon.

Rawls, J. (1987). *Justice as Fairness.* Oxford: Clarendon.

Ricoeur, P. (2000). The concept of responsibility. In P. Ricoeur (Ed.), *The just* (pp. 11–35). Chicago: Chicago University Press.

Rest, J. (1994). Background: theory and research. In J. Rest, and D Narvaez (Eds.). *Moral development in the professions: Psychology and applied ethics* (pp. 1–26). Hillsdale, NJ: Erlbaum.

Robinson, S. (2008). *Spirituality, ethics and care.* London: Jessica Kingsley.

Rogers, C. (1983). *Freedom to learn.* Columbus: Merrill.

Rosen, M. (2012). *Dignity.* Cambridge, MA: Harvard University Press.

Schön, D. (1983). *The Reflective Practitioner.* New York: Basic Books.

Smith, A. (2016). *The theory of moral sentiments.* Oxford: Oxford University Press.

Solomon, R. (2007). *True to our feelings.* Oxford: Oxford University Press.

Tawney, R. H. (1930). *Equality.* Crows Nest, NSW: Allen and Unwin.

Taylor, C. (1989). *Sources of the self.* Cambridge: Cambridge University Press.

Trevino, L., & Brown, M. (2004). Managing to be ethical: debunking five business ethics myths. *Academy of Management Executive, 18,* 69–81.

Werhane, P. (1999). *Moral imagination and management decision making.* Oxford: Oxford University Press.

Whitehead, J. (1989). Creating a living educational theory from questions of the kind: How do I improve my practice. *Cambridge Journal of Education, 19*(1), 41–52.

CHAPTER 3

Whose Responsibility Is It?

'Ven the rockets go up I don't care vere they come down, that's not my department'
says Wernher Von Braun.

Tom Lehrer (Wernher Von Braun)

LEARNING OUTCOMES

When you have read and worked through this chapter, you should be able to:

- Examine a case study which focuses on the interpretation of principles and responsibility in ethical practice
- Set out a three-fold definition of responsibility and the dynamics of responsibility in professional practice
- Examine the function of ethical codes
- Introduce and examine the virtues and how they relate to professional practice

Introduction

In this chapter, we will begin with a very different kind of ethical case, one that focuses on an explicit ethical dilemma. We will analyse the case in terms of the last chapter's ethical decision-making framework, noting especially the importance of dialogue in and beyond the healthcare organisation. It also demonstrates a broader view of rationality in ethics. This case further reinforces the importance of the concept and practice of responsibility in ethics at all levels of the organisation. The chapter will then focus on three modes of responsibility in individual, professional and organisational practice. We will then examine professional codes of practice in general, their critiques and how they might best be used to develop responsibility. We will end this by analysing and critiquing the latest iteration of the Nursing and Midwifery Council Code (NMC 2018), comparing it briefly with other codes. Ways of anchoring such codes in an ethical culture will be developed further in the third part of the book. In addition to the guidance of codes, ethical deliberation requires the practice of ethical capacities, that is virtues. We will analyse the key virtues, noting how they connect to intellectual and practical virtues. This holistic view of the virtues will then focus on integrity (personal, professional and project integrity) and the practice of practical wisdom (*phronesis*).

CASE STUDY 3.1   **Conjoined Twins**

In 2000, conjoined twin babies, referred to as Jodie and Mary (pseudonyms), were born in Gozo and taken to a Manchester hospital (see Lee 2003). Jodie was a bright, alert baby, sparkling, sucking on her dummy and moving her arms. She had a functioning heart and lungs. Her legs are set wide apart, but that could be rectified by surgery. The probability was that, separated from Mary, Jodie would be able to lead a relatively normal life, probably walking unaided, attending school, and being able to have children. For Mary, things were very different. Her face was deformed but, more importantly, she had no effective heart or lung function. It became clear that both could not survive together and that if the two were separated, then the weaker one, Mary, would die, partly because she depended upon Jodie's respiratory system. Three options existed:

- Continue as before, until the death of both twins probably within 3–6 months or at best in a few years.
- Elective separation. In the hospital's view this would lead to Mary's death, but would give Jodie the opportunity of a 'separate good quality life'. There was a 5%–6% chance of death at separation. Jodie would subsequently require several operations for bladder and genital repairs. She had musculoskeletal abnormalities, which would require future surgical intervention. Separation would allow Jodie 'to participate in normal life activities appropriate to her age and development'.
- Urgent (emergency) separation. In this case, mortality was projected at 60% for Jodie and 100% for Mary.

The hospital argued that the two should be separated. The parents did not want to agree to a procedure that would lead to the death of one of their children, arguing that God should ultimately determine what would happen, and they should leave it to God. This led to the issue going to the courts, which upheld the hospital decision. The parents, supported by the Roman Catholic Church, appealed against this. What followed was a very public ethical debate, largely between the appeal court and the Roman Catholic Church. The former dealt in case law and attempted to find cases analogous to this one. The latter dealt in broad principles. Neither approach was wholly adequate. The Church, through the submission of the cardinal archbishop of London, set out the following principles as central their argument:

1. Human life is sacred. This was seen as an inviolable principle that one should never intend to end an innocent person's life by omission or commission.
2. A person's 'bodily integrity' should not be invaded when the consequences to that person involve either no benefit or harm.
3. There is no duty to preserve life if the preservation of that life involves a grave injustice to another. Hence, it was argued that the grave injustice of taking life away from Mary made the preservation of Jodie's life unacceptable.
4. There is no duty to preserve life if extraordinary means have to be used.
5. The natural authority of the parents should be accepted and their rights only overridden if there is clear evidence that they are acting contrary to what is owed to their children.

The judges accepted the first four principles but came to exactly the opposite conclusion. The sacredness of human life, they argued, required that the twin who had the chance to survive should be given that chance. The weakest twin would be likely to die whatever decision was taken. As a result, the twins were divided. The judges also argued by analogy and precedent, offering several comparable cases. One in the United States involved conjoined twins, and the parents agreed to have a similar operation within a few minutes. Deeply religious Jews, they refused to make a decision without the guidance of their rabbi. Some of the hospital staff also refused to be involved until advice from Christian priests had been sought. Rabbis and priests were all agreed that it was permissible and based their own judgement on analogies. One, for instance, involved the scenario of two men jumping from a plane. The parachute of one does not open and he clings on to the first man. His parachute cannot support both of them. The rabbis agreed that it was permissible for the first man to kick the other away, as the man whose parachute did not open was already 'designated' for death. However, none of the analogies exactly fit the situation.

One supporting argument against the operation was that if this was allowed to happen, it would lead to a slippery slope. The argument ran something like, 'we must maintain a moral standard now or this will lead to a desensitisation of practitioners, such that in the future they will allow this to happen without genuine reflection'. As noted in the last chapter, slippery slope arguments are a form of logical fallacy. First, the argument simply assumes that the decision involved a lack of care and sensitivity to the issues. Far from that, the evidence shows that the hospital, the professionals involved, and the different legal practitioners took great care. Second, the argument presumes there will be many such cases in the future, and there is no evidence to back this up. Third, the assertion that a decision to separate the two will lead to desensitisation is simply speculation.

Making the Decision

We suggested in the last chapter that ethical decision making involved principally: careful reflection on the situation, including all the stakeholders; critical reflection on the principles and values and consideration of the options, including all possible outcomes. The key stakeholders in this case were the children, the family, the Church and related interest groups, the healthcare professionals, whose judgement was taken up by the hospital and the courts. The parents, not surprisingly, found it hard to make a decision. They did not want to be directly responsible for the death of one or both of their children. Responsibility was therefore literally given to God. Of course, the proxy for God was the Christian Church, in this case the Roman Catholic Church, to which the parents belonged. The Church saw it as their role to defend the rights of the parents, hence the fifth principle above, and to defend the twins. Critical to working through such a situation is not simply looking at the different aspects of the tragedy but also the psychological process of coming to terms with the tragic situation. For the parents, this involved moving through the process of coming to terms with loss. In effect, this involved anticipatory grief. Anticipatory grief involves deep pain experienced before loss (Al-Gamal and Long 2010). It can be similar to grief after death but is also unique in many ways. Grief before death often involves more anger, more loss of emotional control and atypical grief responses. These may be related to the limbo experienced by family, involving a delicate balance between trying to let go and trying to maintain some form of hope. This in turn fuels feelings of guilt and shame, that the carer can do nothing about the problem or even may feel responsible for the problem.

For the parents of Jodie and Mary, this was further exacerbated by the fear that their decision would directly lead to the loss of one or both of the children. Working through such anticipatory grief is essential to the stakeholders developing their sense of agency in the process of deliberation. Critical to this case is the question of who supports the parents in developing that agency, so that they can begin to determine what would happen (Bouchall et al. 2015). At one level, this might have been the role of the nurse, acting as supporter and empowering the parents, as part of the team response to the situation. We do not know if this did happen, not least because most of the reporting of the incident focused on a narrow view of ethics: the rightness or wrongness of the of the action of dividing the children, or even, as we shall see, the definition of personhood. The dangers of this approach are, first, it fails to include key stakeholders in either working through the situation, in the reflection on principles or in the exploration of consequences. Second, it can lead to polarisation based on defending some stakeholders or certain key principles. In this case, it could be argued that the Church had decided to take responsibility for the deliberation rather than give it to the parents. Elements of this polarisation are in the statements of The Guild of Catholic Doctors (2000) who questioned the legal rulings. These included the argument that the parents had the right to follow their faith in this matter. There are several problems with such an argument:

- The simple asserting of rights is not sufficient without a critical examination of the ethical situation. In this case, the tragic nature of the situation suggests that no answer is without tragedy, and this demands dialogue about the beliefs expressed by the parents.
- Connected to this is the assumption that the faith argument had only one clear articulation. However, the reference to two other cases showed that different religions could see other possible outcomes based on their reflection on the same principles. This takes away any temptation to defend a narrow faith position.

Clearly, without attention to how the different stakeholders view the world and the situation, it would be hard to see the principles in a dispassionate way.

BELIEFS AND PRINCIPLES

Lee (2003) suggests that the conflict was not so much between different principles, as differences found *within* such broad principles. When faced by a case such as this, the broad principles can point to different and conflicting outcomes. Respect for life, for instance, can precisely underpin any of the choices. Lee notes that several doctrines seemed to underlay the principles set out in this case. In particular, there was a theological anthropology that sets out human beings as both uniquely valuable and also interdependent. Once again, however, this does not begin to point to a solution. The doctrine and principles rather provide a framework of meaning in which the tragic experience could be worked through. Bouchall et al. (2015) point out 'the strong need to offer protection was part of the anticipatory mourning experience of striving to be within the present'. Once protection is a primary motivation, this radically affects how the different ethical principles are viewed, and this in turn can prevent a deep reflection on the tragic situation. The self-identity of defender becomes primary, the basis for doing one's job both as parent and as a Church.

The polarisation can then be reflected in the way that different aspects of the situation were spoken of. In terms of ending Mary's life, for instance, some argued that it involved consciously killing her, in effect murder (cf. Paris and Elias-Jones 2001). The second and third principles led to language involving defence against the aggressor (Paris and Elias-Jones 2001). Even when principles are examined dispassionately, things are not straightforward. The Kantian principle of respect for persons depends upon the use of other criteria to define person, not least the view of the person as a rational agent. Also at play is the intent of the agent. Did the hospital intend primarily to save the life of Jodie or to end the life of Mary? The Roman Catholic Church has recognised this distinction through their principle of 'double-effect' (Cavanaugh 2006). For instance, if the intent of the action of abortion is to save a pregnant woman's life, then the loss of the child cannot be blameworthy. Strictly speaking, it remains wrong to be involved in the taking of a life, but the primary good intent makes this acceptable. Hence, it could be argued that the primary intent of the hospital was to save the life of Jodie. Other reflections on the case have questioned what it means to be a person. Bratton and Chetwynd (2004), for instance, argue that the view of person-hood informing the decision was limited; both individualistic and adversarial. We assume that a person must have one centre of consciousness in one body; why not two centres of consciousness in one physical entity? It is not clear, however, how this would help in deliberation on the case.

WORKING THROUGH THE POSSIBILITIES

In one respect, the options available were very constrained. However, it became clear that the significance of the options depended on worldviews and how principles are interpreted. What was critical to this was the way in which dialogue was developed across the stakeholders. Firstly, the debate was handled sensitively, working against the polarisation into secular or spiritual/religious views. At the heart of this was a strong sense of commitment from all parties and to all parties. There was no sense of a divide between law and ethics, but all parties explored belief and values, brought together in the need to respond to tragedy. Secondly, as all parties tried to work through the truth about the situation, this was the basis of a critical hermeneutical (interpretive) approach. Spirituality and values were articulated and illustrated by all participants, and their meaning was tested in the situation. Precisely because of this underlying concern about the family, there was no attempt to make this a knock down philosophical argument. In this light, spirituality and values were not seen as exclusively owned by any one group. Hence, it was acceptable for judges and the Church to test and challenge each other's interpretation of the values and principles. In that light, it was a good example of wrestling with something that went beyond boundaries, be that religious, spiritual or philosophical.

Thirdly, as Lee notes, this was a learning experience for all involved. Because the different perspectives were taken into account, this enabled a change in the understanding of the moral imperatives (Lee 2003, p. 47). The very idea of the Common Good, underlying much of the religious input, gives space for such change, precisely because it does not aim to impose some worked out view of the good but looks to give men and women 'the freedom to assume responsibility for their own lives' (Lee 2003, p. 47). Lee sums up the dynamic in this way, that it is possible to argue:

- That it was right for the parents to stake out their position.
- That the doctors were entitled to challenge their decision.
- That it was right, given some public criticism of the parents' standpoint, the challenge from the doctors and the decision by the first instance judge (who was deciding against the parents without the benefit of all the arguments which the Court of Appeal heard), for the archbishop to articulate the overarching moral considerations.
- That it was permissible nonetheless for the judges to apply this framework, or their own variation on its themes, to reach a different conclusion.
- That the best reasoning to defend such a decision has yet to be formulated.
- That we are all, therefore, learning from this 'uneasy case'.

Fourthly, the case underscores the importance of all key stakeholders being involved in the deliberation process. Hoffmaster and Hooker (2018, p. 192) argue that deliberation is 'most reliable and productive when it is a collective and social enterprise'. Models of physician-patient/client acknowledge the idea of joint decision making but tend to focus on the person who is entitled to make the decision; patient/client choice trumps everything. This case shows that the process of deliberation is more critical, enabling all parties to test out not simply their principles and values but also their perspectives. This also works against simplistic ideas of health and healing, which generate the belief that all medical problems can be solved.

Finally, the case shows how central to the process of deliberation is the development of responsibility in all the parties. For the parents, there was the danger of letting go of their responsibilities. This is not to underestimate their tragic experience. Nonetheless, by handing over responsibility to God, and his proxy the Church, this runs the danger of not facing the tragedy of the situation, and thus not beginning to come to terms with the situation. The Church in this case accepted responsibility for both the parents and the children. Inevitably, this led to the taking of the identity of the protector of the children and defender, more widely, of key moral ideas and rights. The question at this point is did the Church take too much responsibility? The hospital had to take over the responsibility from doctors and nurses for working through what had become an impasse. In turn, the courts took over responsibility for developing the arguments and reaching a decision. The question here is could the deliberation have been better handled had the medical and nursing staff been able to focus on enabling a deliberative process, such that the parents could begin to come to terms with the situation and trust the doctors and nurses? Again, the questions raised here are not meant as a criticism of those involved in the case. They are rather intended as a reflection on how the different stakeholders might face the issue now.

In the other two similar cases noted above, the parents and staff retained responsibility for deliberation and religious or philosophical leaders acted as consultants, further enabling the process. The legal framework enabled a shared responsibility for working through the principles and consequences, and for publicly articulating the reasoning behind the deliberation. In all that, the emotional burden of the process was shared, and different perspectives were developed. The twin who lost her life can then be seen as less a victim and more someone who gave her life for her sister. This importantly, then, albeit by proxy, begins to include the two central stakeholders, the twins themselves, as an exercise of the moral and compassionate imagination. In that light, working through the principle of respect becomes central. All this takes the process of deliberation beyond a simple idea of stages and more into the development of learning cycles that gradually help responsibility of all parties to be developed, including the negotiation of responsibility.

Responsibility

The term responsibility tends to be focused on areas of responsibility. You have been given responsibility for a particular task and have to give an account of how you have fulfilled this. However, this simple view of responsibility is not as straightforward as it seems. Not everyone might agree on how the responsibility should be fulfilled or what the objectives of the task actually are; hence the problems of Mid Staffs. There is the problem of what do you do when faced by something that demands your attention and is not part of your immediate professional responsibility.

3.1 PAUSE FOR THOUGHT

What Would You Do?

You are a nurse going off duty and you see a young woman limping badly, making slow progress towards A&E. Would you take responsibility for getting a wheelchair?

You are a student nurse who sees a senior shouting at a patient. Would you take responsibility for raising this with the senior or is that someone else's responsibility?

You are a physiotherapist who sees a senior doctor verbally abusing a ward cleaner. Would you take responsibility for stepping into this situation?

Writers such as Levinas (1998) and Bauman (1989) argue that responsibility is the starting point of ethics (see also Jonas 1984). It is about our commitment to the good and to the 'other', in whatever situation. Hence, Levinas suggests that ethics begins with 'the face of the other', and associated need; not with an abstract principle but with a concern for the other. Precisely how that responsibility can best be fulfilled requires deliberation, and may involve many different players sharing responsibility. Schweiker (2010) and Robinson (2008) suggest three interrelated modes of responsibility, the first two of which originate in Aristotle's thinking: agency, accountability and positive responsibility.

AGENCY

This attributes agency to the person (hence sometimes referred to as attributability or imputability). There are strong and weak views of agency. The weak views (McKenny 2005) simply refer to the causal connection between the person and any action. Person A has caused, or was responsible for, action B. Such a view does not help in determining just how much the person is actually involved in and therefore fully responsible for the action. A stronger view, then, suggests that to be fully responsible for something necessitates a rational decision-making process. Taylor (1989) argues that this decision making constitutes a strong valuation that connects values and action. This owning of the thoughts and related decision and action is what constitutes the moral agency and identity of the person or group. This empowers persons and organisations to take responsibility for their thoughts, including purpose, values and principles and practice, in effect developing rational agency. In the context of professional practice, this involves knowing about ideas, overall purpose, values (including ethical principles) and practice.

In relation to thoughts, this demands clarity about the concepts that are used and the capacity to justify them rationally. We can hardly be said to be responsible for our thoughts if we cannot provide some account of and justification for them. Any account and justification of thoughts and actions also demands openness to critical intellectual challenge. Purpose takes us back to the purpose of the nursing or related professions, that which gives them social and personal worth. The individual nurse is responsible for their own view of purpose. Values demand the capacity to appreciate values, including the principles noted in the last chapter, underlying thoughts and action. This is not just that they are coherent, it is also that they have distinct meaning and value, such that one prefers one practice to others. Even at this stage, responsibility involves a comparison with other practices and their values. Hence, deciding upon one's own values or the values of the organisation does not take place in social isolation or apart form the core relationships to the social and physical environment.

Purpose and values are both focused on feeling (Cowan 2005; Goleman 2005), not least because they associate with what we believe to be of worth and also with our identity. This demands responsibility be taken for feelings. It might be thought that, by definition, one cannot control feelings. When you feel afraid, for instance, this feeling can dominate and erode personal agency. However, Ricoeur (2000) argues that whilst feelings may arise spontaneously, we nonetheless are responsible for what we do with them. This also demands responsibility for critically examining those feelings and the underlying world views that may be responsible for keeping those feelings in place. Practice includes developing and 'owning' technical and scientific competency. It also includes social awareness, not least of the effects of one's actions, and thus the connection between oneself and the other, patients/clients, colleagues and so on. None of this prescribes a particular response. What it does demand is awareness of what one is doing, how that fits into the purpose of the organisation and how that effects the internal and external environment. In other words, there is a relational context to agency that goes beyond the individual self and that demands awareness and responsiveness.

Critically then, this first mode of responsibility includes responsibility for meaning. Taylor (1989) argues that self-interpretation is key to a sense of identity. All this is developed in critical dialogue and thus engages plurality inside and outside the group. Only in that context is meaning articulated, defended and developed. By extension, this also involves responsibility for how we perceive the world. Mustakova-Possardt (2004, p. 245) sums up this responsibility for both world views and awareness of the social and physical environment in the idea of 'critical moral consciousness', and this involves:

- A moral sense of identity;
- A sense of responsibility and agency;
- A deep sense of relatedness on all levels of living;
- A sense of 'life meaning or purpose', linking to underlying beliefs.

These connect:

- Core intellectual values, not least the development of rational agency.
- Moral values. These include core principles such as justice and respect.

- Spiritual values. Spirituality here is used as a generic term pointing to underlying beliefs about the world, sometimes expressed in terms of worldviews.
- Competency values, not least professional and technical skills and values – from communication, to teamwork, to concern for excellence.

3.2 PAUSE FOR THOUGHT

I'm Free

Responsibility as agency is often associated with freedom, in particular, free will. Put simply, the argument is that we cannot be free if we are unable to make a decision, and the capacity to make a decision depends upon knowing what we are thinking and doing and the effects of this upon our environment. This extends ideas of freedom beyond the negative freedom and positive freedom (freedom from coercion and freedom to practise (Berlin 1969)). Such a freedom is tied to learning and development, relationships and so to the autonomy noted in the last chapter. The person is always learning more about how to respond to his/her social and physical environment.

As a nurse or healthcare worker, are you free to determine how you respond, focus on your values and practice? Or does someone, or something, else determine what you do or how you do it?

Philosophers continue to argue whether humanity is free or determined (see Callender 2010). In fact, our agency, our freedom, emerges from the many forces which determine or seek to determine our thinking: behavioural, social, psychological, neurological, political and organisational. It is determined (in terms of autonomy, self-governance) through individuals and organisations challenging and engaging these forces.

In the Mid Staffs case, it was precisely the powerful forces which sought to determine the action of staff which blocked effective agency for a significant period.

ACCOUNTABILITY

Accountability is, in one sense, another aspect of moral agency. A lot of the stress in moral agency is about making sense to oneself, that is self-justification. Accountability is about making sense to others, a wider sense of justification. Accountability is about being answerable to another about what one is responsible for, hence ongoing opening oneself to judgement. It presumes a relationship of some significance which might be embodied in formal or informal contracts of some kind. Contracts can be empowering if they include rights as well as responsibilities of the participants, setting out the nature (meaning) of the relationship and what is expected, from function and role to ways of relating. The danger of professional relationships is when accountability becomes focused on one direction. Accountability in the Mid Staffs Trust was from professionals to management. The line of accountability, then, goes back to the government and, in particular, to the Treasury. For nursing, this runs the danger of obscuring mutual and plural accountability, in which leadership is not questioned and compliance around narrow targets dominates. This leads to isomorphism, and the polarising and defensive attitudes found in the Mid Staffs case. Accountability to central government encourages communication aimed at giving the best possible view of data, in effect self-promotion (Francis 2013, p. 44), not a critical reflection and deliberation on the case in hand. However, in the light of the inert-connected relationships in healthcare, accountability is both plural and mutual.

Plural Accountability

Plural accountability reflects the different relationships and their associated narratives which go to make up the social interactions of personal and professional life. Our accountability to family, for instance, is expressed for many in the formal contract of marriage, for others in different expressions of commitment. The associated narratives are both about the nature of that commitment, and, in the case of marriage documents, the commitment of society to such relationships. Accountability extends and deepens with the growth of family, to the children, to other members of the family, and to associated institutions such as schools. The plurality of accountability suggests that our identities are plural, and that making sense of our identity demands plural dialogues – the dialogic self (Burkitt 2008). The nursing dialogues involved include accountability to:

Oneself, this includes developing and maintaining personal development throughout working life and ensuring a proper balance between work and personal life. This also involves awareness of limitations and the need for self-care.

To *the profession* which is essentially accountability for one's own professional performance, including ongoing learning and supporting the values of the professional body. However, the accountability of the professional goes beyond these elements of professional practice. The nurse is accountable to the profession for maintaining the very meaning and purpose of the profession and for maintaining the relationship of the profession with wider society. When a nurse does not maintain standards and values, this brings the whole profession into question. Hence, it is possible to speak of the professional as being responsible for the integrity of that profession.

The employer/organisation, which involves being accountable to one's immediate employer and responsible for the performance of duties, so long as they are consistent with the professional code. The relationship between the nurse and employer seems to be qualitatively different from that of the nurse and profession, not least because the former is based on a financial contract. Nonetheless, the purpose of a healthcare institution remains the same as the profession within that project. The key question, as the Mid Staffs case showed, is when the purpose and aims of the two different organisations seem to conflict. In this case, accountability demands that the nurse questions the nature of the conflict. This will be examined in more detail in Part 3.

Finally, to *the patient* which includes giving impartial and competent advice and reporting any conflicting areas of interest. The key aspect of this accountability is enabling the patient/client to take responsibility for decisions about treatment and lifestyle. As noted above, this may involve a number of different responses from the nurse or doctor, from simply setting out to the patient/client the different options and their consequences, to enabling the patient/client to develop critical autonomy in coming to terms with the situation. As the case above shows, this may also involve the family. Importantly, this begins to focus on the nature of patient/client-centred care. Patient/client-centred care reflects the accountability of the nurse to the patient/client, but it also reflects a broader responsibility for the nature of care itself. As noted above, appropriate care has to be worked out in the situation, with all its limitations, and this might conflict with a narrow view of consumer care. Such accountability is not straightforward, partly because it includes the core ethical values of justice, care, beneficence and non maleficence.

3.3 PAUSE FOR THOUGHT

What Does Patient/Client-Centred Care Look Like?

As a nurse, are you accountable to a patient/client for what they want or need?

Does the patient/client have the identity of a consumer or customer, with your job to keep them happy?

How do you feel when patients/clients complain?

How do you respond when patients/clients complain?

This includes awareness of the overall social and physical context of healthcare, and the impact of the project on society and the environment. There is a concern for the sustainability of healthcare delivery systems, including an awareness of their limitations and awareness of their effect on society. Again, this means that accountability is not straightforward, with a concern for just distribution of healthcare. With respect to other groups or professions, the nursing profession shares with other professions responsibility for the project of healthcare, and as such, is also accountable to those professions. It is important to note both the shared values of these other professions, focused on the healthcare project but also the different narratives, based on a sense of professional identity, that each brings to the table.

Mutual Accountability

Mutual accountability is both vertical and horizontal. It does not require absolute equality, recognising that all relationships are asymmetrical, involving differences not least in power (Buber 1937). Key to such accountability is the capacity to communicate with, to give an account to, people and groups who are of different power levels. If the professional has accountability to the profession as a whole and to the professional body, who represents the profession, the professional body is accountable to the profession and its members. Despite the criticism of the Francis Inquiry (2013) the Royal College of Nursing, for instance, is responsible not simply for establishing standards but also for supporting and even defending members of the profession. Hence, the professional body acts as an advocate standing up for justice and respect for its members. If members of the health service have accountability to the organisations which employ them, then the leaders of those organisations have accountability to them. We will develop this further in looking at leadership and leadership ethics in Chapter 8. At this point, it is sufficient to note, for instance, that leadership is accountable to staff for ensuring that their directions and the culture they establish do not cause them harm, either psychological or physical. The leadership in the Mid Staffs case created a workplace environment that was unsafe for the staff, primarily because of the dominance of a narrow set of objectives. These included cutting over a hundred nursing posts, thus putting greater stress on the nursing workforce.

The UK government was a significant part of that failure in mutual accountability. The broad assumption is that the government is accountable to the electorate. However, in the Mid Staffs case, they were precisely accountable to the patients/clients and staff for instituting a focus on narrow targets, and for allowing a system of regulation that did not focus on mutual accountability for the shared project. The government was also responsible over time for instituting too many major changes in practice and process, with the effect of focusing professional attention further on process and targets, rather than on the overall shared purpose of care (Francis 2013). This had the effect of a form of teleopathy generated by the government. In healthcare in general, this has involved a focus on saving costs rather than on best care practice (Seddon 2014). Critically, there was no articulation of the narrative of the overall project, and the related purpose and worth at any level. The narrative was assumed, and not therefore part of the ongoing professional reflection.

Unfocused leadership can attempt to avoid accountability, as we note in Chapter 8, not least through ambiguous communication (Eisenberg 1984). This demands dialogue that will test that communication, and require clearer accountability from leadership for communication. Importantly, this suggests that mutual accountability is not confined to reporting processes but is a function of ongoing professional interaction. The same dynamic is there for the relationship of the nurse to the doctor, or the nurse or doctor to the patient/client, or the nurse or doctor to the institutional management team. All this adds to the accountability of the leader, because the questions cannot be asked if there is no way of hearing them, or hearing underlying feelings.

There was a lack of mutual accountability in the Mid Staffs case, extending to the different professions, different institutions (including the government), the patients/clients, volunteers, families and different regulators. All these groups were responsible for what might be termed the project of health. Hence, all were accountable to each other for the project. The mutuality was supposed to be expressed in different ways. Regulators were accountable to the government, professions, and others, to give an account of their findings. Ultimately, they were accountable with others to the patients/clients and to the wider community, to ensure that the right level of care was maintained. Key regulatory bodies, however, raised the alarm without ensuring that a practical response occurred (Francis 2013, p. 45). They assumed that other bodies would take responsibility for this. Some regulatory bodies were focused on finance, and financial and institutional responsibilities, others on care, with little sense of how they all connected or how different narratives had to be critically sustained. Audits had no sense of holistic or responsibility connection.

The dynamic here was essentially one which lacked mutuality. Reports go one way rather than leading to dialogue and action. Mutual accountability demands that value narratives of all parties be shared. It is precisely the appreciation of different perspectives and values (Bauman 1989) that guards against a totalising perspective, simply one way of looking at values and practice, and with that a loss of truth. The truth in the Mid Staffs case should have been focused on the overall narrative of care, which was meant to sustain the core purpose, with all parties accountable to each other for that purpose. As noted in the first chapter, one of the key responses by the nursing profession was the re-articulation of the core purpose and value of nursing – giving a public account. The Mid Staffs case and the case above suggest that value, purpose and worth are not engaged unless there is a regular account given of these, reinforcing mutual accountability. Mutual accountability, as suggested above, is also there in the nurse-patient/client relationship. If the nurse is accountable to the patient/client, then equally, the patient/client is accountable to the nurse and all other members of the care team. This is partly based on the directions the patient/client chooses to take, and responsibility the patient/client takes for their own care. Choosing not to take diet or exercise seriously is to ignore patient/client accountability to carers. This will be explored further in Chapter 10 and the attempts of the NHS Constitution to specify the responsibilities of the patient/client.

POSITIVE RESPONSIBILITY

The third mode of responsibility goes beyond accountability and looks to moral liability (as distinct from legal liability), which is a concern for others, a sense of wider liability for projects, people or place. Some ethical thinkers view this in terms of universal responsibility. This suggests that the foundation of ethics is a sense of responsibility for everything, whatever the context. Levinas (1998) and Bauman (1989) argue that this stance always challenges the individual to find ways of responding to the needs of others. The danger of this view of responsibility is that it is interpreted as always being responsible for the other, leading to taking too much responsibility. The danger limiting a sense of responsibility is that the consciousness of the situation becomes limited, that is it is always somebody else's job.

This is exemplified much in religious ethics. The classical focus of Christian ethics is in the parable of the rich man Dives (Luke 16: 19–31). Dives sees no responsibility for his community, and as a result, can literally not see Lazarus, the poor man at his gate. This suggests that perception of the social context is based on a sense of moral responsibility. Cohen (2001) develops this point about responsibility in the context of responses to atrocities. He argues that a State's, denial of responsibility emerges in one or more of four paths: obedience to authority; conformity with social norms; necessity and splitting of the personality. The first two place responsibility on others. The thirds denies that the individual or group had a choice – I had to do it. The fourth denies what the person can see before them, choosing to focus on a dominant narrative to justify the action. This is confirmed in a wider context by Burleigh (2011). In examining the testimony of SS troopers involved in mass killings, he notes how they refer to their murder of children through reference to the dominant narrative that Jews and others were a threat to Germany and beyond, and principles dictated that they should defend against this threat.

The way around the default of denial is to see responsibility as never exclusively individual, but rather social and shared (May 1992). Each person or group has to work this responsibility out in context. This demands an awareness of the limitations of the person or organisation, avoiding taking too much responsibility and a capacity to work together with others and to negotiate and share responsibility. Finch and Mason (1993), in the context of single parent family care, note the way in which negotiation of responsibility was more powerful than simply following principles, not least because it led to the development of ethical identity. It is precisely when creative dialogue around shared responsibility is practised that the possibilities in any situation are maximised. This includes developing a creative way of seeing any situation, always looking for the possibilities (see the moral imagination in Chapter 2). This works against the narrowing of responsibility. As noted above, the nurse is responsible for their own actions, and also for the whole project of healthcare, something they share with all colleagues. This search for the best is, of course, central to the practice of *beneficence,* and takes the healthcare professional beyond a narrow contract to a broader covenant, a commitment to what is best for the patient/client.

Interactive Modes of Responsibility

The three modes of responsibility have to be practised together. Without, for instance, the practice of critical agency, including regular reflection on value, purpose and practice, the practice of accountability runs the danger of losing focus. This can involve first denying accountability beyond the immediate task, that is it was not my job to check the patient/client. The second danger is simply to avoid giving an account – the leader, CEO or professional, focuses on the demands of the task. The third danger is of hyper-accountability, the multiplication of forms and checks so that the process of account becomes more important than the practice of care. This is exacerbated by systems of compliance which further stress guilt and fear associated with non-compliance. Ricoeur (2000) refers to this, an embodying negative responsibility, a form of moral responsibility which focuses on the individual, their guilt and the negative consequences for the individual. Ricoeur argues that the focus on negative responsibility leads to a lack of support in the workplace and avoidance of practising positive responsibility. The fear involved is fear of retribution if the individual gets things wrong. Hence, negative and positive responsibility mirror two of the different views of justice: justice as merit (you get what you deserve) and restorative justice. Restorative justice recognises that we get things wrong and looks to learn from this and restore the person to contribute to positive responsibility. Both have their place and need to be fostered. In Chapter 9, we look at this in relation to the duty of candour and the danger that healthcare professionals might be discouraged from being open about crises if there is the possibility of this leading to legal or professional retribution. The question then emerges as to how we might begin to anchor such responsibility in practice. Three elements emerge; codes, character and culture. We will deal with the first two here and the third in Part three.

Codes

Codes, as noted in the first chapter, are often seen as a critical part of the identity of a profession. Expressed either as Codes of Ethics or Codes of Conduct, they provide guidance about ethical practice. However, not all philosophers agree with the idea of codes. One of the most important arguments against them comes from Ladd (1980). Ladd (1980, p. 154) argues that codes go against the very nature of ethics. If ethics is about developing practical decision making around principles, consequences and the situation, then it cannot be imposed by authority or rule. Rules are prescriptive, and this leads to a diminution of autonomy and responsibility. Hence, Ladd refers to professional codes as 'an absurdity – moral and intellectual'. Ladd (1980) highlights two further harms of codes. First, they place the responsibility for ethical response on the code or on the committee which polices the code. Second, if conduct is summed up solely in terms of the code, then anything not explicitly covered in the code might be thought to be acceptable.

Ladd (1980) goes on to argue that there are no ethics specific to any profession. On the contrary, all ethics espouses concern and respect for patients/clients, customers, family members and so on. Moreover, all of us understand cheating, lying, deceit or injustice to be wrong. Nothing extra then needs to be said about the context of nursing or the healthcare professions as a whole. There is no doubt that codes run the danger of being used legalistically, which can obscure the principles or spirit of the code. Arguments against Ladd's ideas include:

- The idea that ethics is simply about autonomy is unrealistic. Descriptive theories (see Chapter 2) suggest that autonomy has to develop, and that part of the development has to involve a sense of shared practice focused on community. Codes help to express meaning and values in and of the community.
- The idea that at least explicit guidelines are not necessary is confounded by Milgram (2005) and Gill (2013). They suggest that without articulation of ethical ideas, a majority of people will opt not to take responsibility for ethical reflection and response. Codes are important precisely because they articulate ethical ideas. The question then becomes how does the culture and practice of the organisation enable the continued articulation of ethical ideas. The argument here is that if ethics is not talked about, then it is not practised.
- There are ethical issues specific to a work place or profession. In the medical and nursing professions, for instance, there is the constant tension between two core principles, the autonomy of the patient/client and best interest of the patient/client, which historically have been thought best articulated by the doctor. Clearly, both are important and require the doctor and nurse to develop the capacity to hold together both.
- Ladd's argument depends upon the view that ethical deliberation is a purely individual activity. However, the decision-making framework of the last chapter shows that ethical deliberation is essentially social. Dialogue enables critical thinking about ideas, values and practice and ongoing learning about how to embody the ethical dimension of practice.
- Ladd also fails to recognise the importance of particular reflection to the practice of ethical principles. Yes, ethical principles are general but they do not take practical embodiment without reflection on particular practice.

The danger of codes is that they become the total focus of ethical thinking and they ossify to an unthinking system. Any code should be rather a part of a total culture that precisely aims to enable the members of the organisation to take responsibility for practising the good; in Bader's words, 'rules are for the guidance of wise men and obedience of fools' (cited in Brickhill 1954, p. 69).

CODES OF ETHICS

Clearly then codes can have an important function, but must not be used to take away responsibility from the individual or group. To get this right, the purpose of the code needs to be established. Initially, it will be a function of the professional body to identify this in consultation with experts and stakeholders. The purpose of a code should be linked to the history, identity and culture of the profession or institution. A code may be intended either primarily to prevent unethical behaviour (with a prescriptive stress), or primarily to promote and encourage ethical behaviour (focusing on ethical aspirations). Professions tend to combine elements of both types, providing clear guidelines around common ethical issues and dilemmas, and broader values and principles to frame responsibilities to stakeholders. The first tends to focus on typical ethical issues of dilemmas in that area, such as how to deal with conflicts of interest, respectful treatment of stakeholders or the profession's judgement on receiving gifts. The second focuses on broad responsibilities, encouraging thought about how they will be managed.

The code may have several focuses. It may be intended primarily for leaders, managers and employees, or may include external stakeholders, such as in a supply chain, or any partnerships. The code may also have wider target audiences. Professional codes are core to the identity of professions, tied to foundation values, not least health (its administration and distribution), and aim to demonstrate the integrity of the profession. They aim to establish and maintain trust in the profession as a whole, and as such are often tied to compliance procedures, not least the withdrawal of the right to practise. Codes then can include any or all of the following:

- Define accepted standards of behaviour for the group.
- Promote high standards of practice.
- Provide benchmarks by which members can measure and develop their personal standards.
- Define the ethical aspirations and identity of the group both internally and in relation to the public and communities around them.
- Exhibit a level of maturity and integrity to the outside world.
- Pre-empt calls for government regulation of professional practice.
- Act as the basis for ethical training.

Codes are used across a wide spectrum of institutions and professions, and these include:

- Professional codes, as noted above.
- Industry codes. These are adopted by entire sectors, such as insurance, banking and healthcare organisations.
- Issue codes. These codes may focus on narrow areas of practice, such as the World Health Organisations (WHO 1981) International Code of Marketing of Breast-milk Substitutes (https://www.who.int/nutrition/publications/code_english.pdf), Codes of Governance noted in Chapter 10, or codes to do with advertising, such as the Advertising Standards Authority (ASA) (https://www.asa.org.uk/codes-and-rulings/advertising-codes.html).
- International codes such as that of the United Nations Global Compact (https://www.unglobal-compact.org/).

NURSING AND MIDWIFERY COUNCIL CODE (NMC) 2018

The first thing to note is that the Code is not referred to as an ethical code, not even as a code of conduct. It is simply, the Code. The meaning of it is summed up as 'Professional standards of practice and behaviour for nurses, midwives and nursing associates'. This tells us that ethics is part of the wider identity of this professional body, not a bolt on extra. The introduction begins to fill out this identity, noting that care is at the heart of the practice but that the Code applies to a range of roles which inform or develop care, including leadership, education and research. We will look at these in greater detail in the third part of this book. For the time being, it is simply worth noting that all three areas have the same relational dynamic as the nursing profession, involving asymmetrical power relationships (and therefore vulnerability) and a learning process. The standards identified within the Code:

- express the nature of the professional body.
- are expected not just by patients/clients but by the wider public. This reinforces the underlying worth of health and healthcare. Health is critical to the human experience, and all experience vulnerability and the limitations that can compromise that.
- are expressed in the whole Code, and the Code aims to show what these standards 'look like'. By definition then, the Code is focused on embodied practice not abstract ideas.
- reinforce professionalism and continued professional development.
- act as a focus for ongoing dialogue with employer organisations, educators, safety regulators, and patients/clients.

Already at this stage there are two questions. First, how will that dialogue, the basis of transparency, be achieved? Is this the responsibility of the professional body, the employer or organisation or of the wider national service? Part 3 of this book develops ideas around this. Second, and connected, how will professional responsibility actually be practised? In the introduction, some markers are set down. First, whilst different groups may have different *responsibilities*, for example nurses and associate nurses, all professions share the same *responsibility* for the overall project.

Second, the professional must work within their own level of competence. This is about understanding the limits of professional competence. Hence, though a nurse or midwife is deemed responsible for the whole service, they cannot in practice be responsible for every detail of practice. Awareness of limitations is a critical part of shared responsibility. Third, it is suggested that the Code can be of help to other groups, and that other groups, not least employer organisations, should be responsible for supporting the standards set out.

The Code then moves into four areas:

- Prioritise people.
- Practise effectively.
- Practise safety.
- Promote professionalism and trust.

Prioritise People

This section is suffused with core ethical principles. It does not explicitly set out the ethical principles noted above, but the stress is on equal respect. As noted in the last chapter, this involves the Kantian principle of respecting people as an end in themselves. This is developed in two ways. The first is upholding the dignity of all involved. Dignity involves the worth of the other, including the person's sense of worth (Rosen 2012). Hence, upholding dignity involves supporting and developing that sense of worth. This is connected to rights language, not least in respecting the right to privacy and confidentiality. The second picks up on the responsibility of the nurse to provide this respect. Responsibility is also mentioned in relation to the patient/client. Listening to the patient/client and responding to their needs involves enabling them to take appropriate responsibility for their health and care: enabling decision making; respecting involvement in decision making; respecting the right not to receive care and so on.

Practise Effectively

Core to this section are the values of professional excellence, safety and accountability. Professional excellence is based on evidence-based practice and therefore requires that the practitioner maintains knowledge and skills. This requires good communication, cooperative working and sharing skill, knowledge and experience for the good of the patient/client and colleagues. Concern for safety (*non-maleficence*) runs throughout the code. Accountability is expressed in giving an account, through the keeping of records.

Preserve Safety

The stress on safety is underlined with a separate section. At the heart of this is the importance of the professional working within the limits of competence. Again, this is focused on not taking on too much responsibility. It is also about a realistic assessment of one's professional identity. This includes responsibility to the self. This is further stressed in a section where the professional is charged to offer help in an emergency but to act with care, for the self and other, and to look for all options in responding to the emergency. Candour is an important principle in this section, both in being open about mistakes made and prompt in reporting the need for extra support or for response to emergencies. We will examine this in more detail in Part 3. The final two paragraphs of this section reinforce the potential for harm associated with care, not least in the administration of drugs, and thus the need to be aware of the possible consequences of all actions.

Promote Professionalism and Trust

This is anchored in the individual practitioner's responsibility for the integrity and reputation of the profession as a whole. This partly involves the leadership role of modelling good behaviour, and stresses the professional relationship involves caring people who are vulnerable to open exploitation, and the dangers of conflicts of interest. The basis of trust is the integrity of the professional, which involves both competence and character. Hence, when faced by investigation, audits or complaints, the practitioner should respond in an open and constructive way.

The Code's strength is its focus on safety and responsibility, both in terms of the agency of the practitioner (knowing what one is doing) and his or her accountability. Pattison (2001) has questioned other versions of the code. His critique includes:

- Lack of attention to core ethical principles and their meaning. There is no listing of the key principles and what they mean. Understanding these elements involves an interpretation of the Code.
- Lack of attention to related ethical ideas such as integrity, kindness and trust, and how the professional competence relates to ethics.

In addition to these points, the Code's stress on the first two modes of responsibility and the issue of safety means issues of justice are not fully articulated. In reflecting on the NMC Code, it is worthwhile contrasting it with other related codes. The National Association of Social Workers (NASW 2017) Code of Ethics explicitly uses the term ethics. It takes time to set out key values and principles and how these relate to the profession of social work. It then drills down, to examine in the standards section, to six key areas of social work responsibility. The Nursing and Midwifery Board of Ireland (NMBI 2014) Code is also explicit about the term ethics, distinguishing it from conduct and stresses the key principles and works through each of those. Codes are an important part of practising ethics and to be effective they require:

- Regular reflection, to ensure that ethical value and practice remain part of reflective practice. This also requires dialogue.
- Regular development, which ties into the development of an ethical culture.
- Regular reflection with other professions about key issues.

The Codes themselves also indicate the need to develop key ethical strengths or capacities that enable the practice of professional ethics and virtues.

3.4 PAUSE FOR THOUGHT

Codes

Why do all healthcare and social care professions have to have their own code?

Are not the core elements of the different codes actually the same?

In which case, the difference would be largely in how the different principles and responsibilities are worked through in practice. Compare the three codes above in terms of the core principles and how responsibilities are worked through. If there is an opportunity, compare the codes with a member of another care profession.

How do they view your code?

Reflect on how you use your professional code in practice, and how important it is to know the core principles of other professional codes and organisational codes.

Different codes can act as the basis for interprofessional dialogue, and also for awareness of shared principles. A good example of the latter is the joint guidance of the General Medical Council (GMC) and NMC on the duty of candour (see Chapter 10).

Character

Character involves the mental and moral qualities distinctive to an individual. As we shall see in Part 3, this can also apply to an organisation, in terms of its culture. The qualities in question are virtues (strengths). It is the virtues that show ethics in operation, that is what ethics looks like. There are many different perspectives on virtues, and we shall focus on the generally accepted ones where virtues:

- are of the 'mean', that is middle, between extremes (Aristotle 2004).
- enable rational deliberation. The person or group are not drawn into narrow defensive reactions but can actually work through meaning and practice.

- demand reiteration of the core narrative of the organisation (MacIntyre 2013). Narrative enables reflection on identity and thus reflection on core purpose.
- are only learned through practice (Aristotle 2004). Conversely, when they are not practised, the virtue is lost, the ethical analogue of muscle strength to physical activity. Hence, any organisation has to find space for and enable the practice of the virtues.
- enable the practice of responsibility as set out above.
- are not exclusively moral. They can be characterised as intellectual, moral and psychological. The practice of each kind of virtue strengthens the others.

INTELLECTUAL VIRTUES

Practical Wisdom. This is Aristotle's virtue of *phronesis* (see Curzer 2014), the capacity for rational deliberation that enables the wise person to reflect on their conception of the good and to embody this in practice. This virtue is often the one most tested when targets have to be met, precisely because it is about reflecting on purpose. *Phronesis* is a virtue that is brought into play whenever there is a value conflict, or an uncertainty about ends. Hence, there was little evidence of the practice of this virtue in the Mid Staffs case. Practical wisdom (Latin *prudentia*) for Aquinas (1981) had at its heart several elements, including: openness to the past (*memoria*), openness to the present, involving the capacity to be still and listen actively (*docilitas*) and openness to the future (*solertia*). This openness stresses care before any hasty judgement or decision. It also presumes a critical, testing stance on our perceptions. This means that other intellectual virtues are essential to any ethical deliberation, and to any view of professional competence, including (in Aristotelian terms, as noted in the introduction):

- *Sophia* – wisdom (rational intuition and scientific knowledge directed toward the highest and most valuable objects).
- *Episteme* – scientific knowledge of objects that are necessary and unchanging.
- *Nous* – rational intuition of first principles or self-evident truths.
- *Techne* – craft knowledge, art, skill. This includes knowledge of possibilities.

This works against a primarily target-centred approach to leadership and management. This relates closely to the practice of responsibility, especially ethical agency. *Phronesis* is often characterised as an individual virtue. However, as noted in the first two chapters, deliberation is most effective in a social context focused on open dialogue.

MORAL VIRTUES

Additional to the deliberative virtues, the practice of ethics needs virtues, which will make a difference and lead to action.

Courage

In the conjoined twin case, it took courage for the hospital authorities to test the case in law. For individuals, it is less easy to practise courage. As the Mid Staffs case showed, ethical challenges occur in situations where there is strong pressure not to get involved, including fear of management and loss of job. The psychological pressures on the parents of the twins were too great for them to be involved directly in the deliberation.

Aristotle (2004) sees courage as resilience and the capacity to withstand a variety of pressures. Courage is one of the clearest examples of virtues as involving the mean. In this case, the mean is between the extremes of foolhardiness and cowardice. Foolhardiness involves knee-jerk reactions, without taking account of context. Cowardice involves giving in to pressures, and not addressing the issues. Courage enables the person to stand up for the good in a thoughtful and determined way. Hence, courage for Plato includes a capacity to persevere with an aim, whilst also holding a critical relationship to that aim, enabling one to modify it as and when it is right to do so (Reid 2002). Again, there is tension in this virtue, between the courage to stick something out, literally going the extra mile, surviving perhaps great suffering and knowing when to stop. Any healthcare professional will need courage to articulate, test and stay with or alter a moral purpose, faced by competing purposes. In this sense, courage is also tied to relationship and how we deal with different narratives. A key aspect of the abuse of power in the workplace is the way in which the narrative of power is accepted by the workforce. Courage is required even simply to ask questions about meaning and practice in oneself and others, challenging the narrative and unexamined assumptions. It is worth adding that the Alcoholics Anonymous prayer refers to the virtue of courage, as well as wisdom and serenity (Harle 2005).

Patience

In the conjoined twin case, we see a good illustration of patience. For Aristotle, this is partly about good temper. At one extreme is irascibility and at the other is lack of spirit. This has clear implications for how we see and handle time. The irascible person will tend to try to do this quickly. The person without spirit will have little sense of the need to make a timely decision. This suggests that patience is important for making a timely decision. In the Mid Staffs case, one of the pressures caused by management and some nursing leaders was to prevent this kind of patience. There was never enough time to consider the different options; deadlines had to be met. Moreover, there was never enough time for people, especially concerned families. In this, the virtue of patience is focused on deliberation and relationships. Avoiding both was critical to the failures in Mid Staffs.

Temperance

Temperance does not involve abstinence from drink or anything else but rather moderation, balance and self-control, hence a virtue of the mean, between abstinence and incontinence (in a general sense). This is important for effective judgement, self-reliance and the acceptance of responsibility. Plato's *sophrosunê*, temperance or self-control, Reid (2002) suggests, corresponds to discipline. Discipline, for the nurse, involves continued good practice for decision making, including regular meetings that focus on core objectives.

Justice

If *phronesis* enables clarity about and awareness of the social and physical environment, justice enables fair and disinterested practice in those relationships. As noted in relation to professional principles, justice can involve several different meanings, from fairness as equal distribution to receiving just deserts. Perhaps the key point about justice is concern for the other, for fair treatment that applies to all. This demands both rationality, with attention to desert, and awareness of the needs of the other. This connects justice directly to accountability and applies both to relationships within the organisation and outside. In all this, justice is focused on relationships and is in turn closely related to the care or respect for the other and for a sense of self-esteem. Justice in this sense, as a virtue, is a capacity for fairness, both inside and outside the organisation. This relates directly to the care of colleagues and patients/clients and to the development of meaning in the sense of self and organisational value. Once again, this virtue was often absent in the Mid Staffs case.

PSYCHOLOGICAL VIRTUES

The focus on psychological virtues has been reinforced by the work of positive psychology (Miller 2003), which has focused on the virtues that enable individuals and communities to thrive, including empathy, humility, hope, veracity and faith or trust.

Empathy

Empathy is closely connected to the virtue of benevolence, and enables the carer to identify with the other. If wisdom is an intellectual virtue, then empathy is an affective (to do with feelings) virtue. It is the capacity to hear and understand the underlying identity and feelings of the other, and respond to them. This involves an awareness of others and their needs, regardless of who they are. It does not involve total identification (sympathy), but rather enables an appropriate distance between the self and the other. Such a distance is necessary if the other is to be understood, and if the nurse is to operate impartially and effectively. Hence, any professional cannot do their job if too close to a situation. As such, empathy can form the basis of the professional's perception, data collection and judgement. Similarly, empathy enables the professional to be aware of and accept their own limitations, and to avoid the kind of self-conscious caring that wants to impose the manager's own needs on the relationship.

There has been much criticism of the concept of empathy, not least because it seems patronising to assume that one can know what the other person feels (Bloom 2017; Verducci 2000), a sort of affective imperialism. Hence, many argue that the dynamic of empathy is one of mutuality (Swinton 2001). Augsburger (2014) extends the term to interpathy, to include cultural awareness. Epley (2014) argues that the associated idea that empathy can understand what the other is feeling without any account offered is false. The 'inner' feeling can only be discovered through the articulation of some language, of the body or the word. Empathy then involves awareness of the emotional meaning so expressed, or any conflict in that meaning. Empathy is closely connected to the capacity for humour. Aristotle sees wit (*eutrapelia*) as one of the virtues. There are, of course, negative aspects to humour, not least the danger of using humour to put down the other (Bakhtin 1981). At its best, however, humour is a vehicle of empathy. It enables a distance and perspective such that the self and the other can be seen and accepted in all their incongruity (Pattison 1988, p. 186). Hence, Shakespeare and Bakhtin (1981) stress the importance of comedy, often expressed in the carnival, enabling us to see different perspectives more clearly. Many of Shakespeare's plays include the fool, the institutional jester who is able to help leaders see perspectives they have lost (such as Feste in *Twelfth Night*).

Empathy does not of itself involve concern for the good of the other (see Chapter 11). A figure such as Iago in Shakespeare's Othello shows acute understanding of all the characters in the play. Hence, he is perhaps the most trusted figure. However, he uses this virtue to a bad end. Therefore, there is the additional need for compassionate care. The Australian aboriginal term *dadirri* includes a sense of deep listening, such that one is open to all the different elements of the other and of the situation. This enables the carer to see just what the issues are and help to take the bull by the horns. In the case of the conjoined twins, this meant being open to all the psychological, ethical and treatment issues.

Humility

The virtue of humility involves an awareness and realistic appreciation of the limitations and strengths of the self or the organisation. Humility is often seen as a nervous doubting of competence, self-deprecation, quite the opposite of the leadership image. Tangney (2000), however, summarises a very different view of humility, reminding us that all virtues rest between extremes. It involves:

- Accurate assessment of one's ability and achievements.
- Ability to acknowledge one's mistakes, imperfections, gaps in knowledge and limitations.
- Openness to new ideas, contradictory information and advice.
- Keeping one's abilities and accomplishments – one's place in the world – in perspective.
- Relatively low self-focus, 'a forgetting of the self', while recognising that one is but part of a larger project.
- Appreciation of the value of all things, as well as the many different ways that people can contribute to our world (Tangney 2000).

In other words, humility is directly related to meaning making and practice and awareness of the nature of the social and physical environment. Vera and Rodriguez-Lopez (2004) sum up the importance of humility for learning and resilience, both individual and organisational. In learning, it enables openness to new paradigms; eagerness to learn from others; acknowledgement of limitations; pragmatic acceptance of failure and the ability to consult and ask for advice. In resilience, it involves acceptance of simplicity; avoidance of narcissism and avoidance of self-complacency. This virtue is central to the practice of moral agency and accountability, and was well summed up in the conjoined twins case, not least in the way that all parties became involved in the deliberation, claiming no privilege.

Hope

Hope has often been associated most closely with the so-called theological virtues, faith and love. However, any organisation needs hope if it is to flourish, not least because it is necessary in empowerment for change. Hope is about the capacity to envision and take responsibility for a significant and meaningful future. As such, it is distinct from a generalised attitude of optimism. Snyder (2000) suggests that the development of hope as a real virtue depends upon three factors: goals; pathways and agency. The capacity to hope is generated through a sense of morally significant purpose or goals. Such good hope provides meaning, which affirms the worth of the person or group. In the light of such purposes, realistic goals need to be set out. Hopefulness develops on goals which can be achieved. Hope may be a major virtue but it needs specific aims for it to be meaningful and aims worked through in dialogue. Hopeful thinking looks to find pathways to the goals. This involves a development of the creative imagination to be able to see what ways forward there are. This is enabled through the development of method and through practice, not least the development of multiple possibilities through negotiation of responsibilities (Snyder 2000).

Hope centres on the experience of the person as subject, capable of determining and achieving the goals they look to through agency. This applies once more to the person and to the organisation. If such hope is to be realistic, it cannot be built on deceit or untruth. Hope also has a psychological dimension, based on the presence of the other (Robinson 2008). The continued presence of the other, the carer, signals the worth of the patient/client, whatever their condition. The term 'hopeless' is often used as a putdown: 'there is no hope for you'. All of these elements can be the focus of hope, even for a terminally ill patient/client; finding, for instance, pathways to communicating with family or friends in the future, through letters and gifts for significant events.

Veracity

The virtue of truthfulness or veracity is professional, relational and personal. Some truth is based on medical knowledge, truth that the patient/client has a right to hear. Truth is also about revealing the authentic self. Hence, Aristotle (2004) writes about truthfulness (*alētheia*) as the truthful and reliable re-presentation of the self across different contexts. In the case of the conjoined twins, it could be said that the different parties remained true to themselves across the different contexts but also true to different possibilities. Veracity is not simply about telling the truth to the patient/client. It is rather about sharing the truth in such a way that he or she can begin to take responsibility for it. In a sense the practitioner takes on a pedagogical role, enabling the patient/client to reflect and to explore. Genuine reflection and exploration will not only begin to handle the truth about the situation, it will also explore the different possibilities for the future.

Faith

Fowler (1996, p. 394) defines faith as 'the foundational dynamic of trust and loyalty underlying selfhood and relationships; in this sense faith is a human universal, a generic quality of human beings'. Such faith will vary from complete trust in the other to partial or working trust. Trust can be seen as an essential prerequisite to relationships and therefore key to health. Trust involves a personal dimension; the authenticity of the person (connected to truthfulness); being true to the other. It also involves the practice of professional competency, that is the nurse knowing what they are doing and about the social and physical environment within which they operate (the first mode of responsibility), able to give a credible account of her practice and be open to question (the second mode) and able to share in responsible practice (mode three).

Integrity

In different ways, integrity is often seen as the capacity to stand up for one's principles or vision of the good or ethical identity (Williams 2005; Calhoun 1995; Halfon 1989; Rawls 1971). In different ways, these suffer from the problem that whilst one may intend to follow an ethical path, the overall ethical vision may be flawed or questionable. The film *In Bruges* (McDonagh 2009) is a good example of this.

3.5 PAUSE FOR THOUGHT

In Bruges (DVD Universal Pictures)

The leader of a criminal gang has a strong belief about the wrongness of killing children. To allow one of his 'hit-men' to live after he has killed a child, albeit by mistake, would go against this belief, which he takes to be part of his integrity and that of his organisation. This is ultimately tested for him when he believes that he too has killed a child.

What should he do to remain a man of integrity?

Ultimately, his integrity is only within a narrow moral boundary. Outside that boundary, it is permissible to kill, and the very purpose of the business is murder.

Integrity is not one virtue but a collection of several virtues, brought together to help form a coherent character and identity (Solomon 2007). It is precisely this character that forms the basis of trust, and from all this we can sum up integrity in the following ways.

Integration of Identity

Integrity involves integration of the different parts of the person: emotional, psychological and intellectual. This leads to holistic thinking, and an awareness of the self, alongside awareness and appreciation of external data. Taylor (1985) takes self-integration further, to involve acknowledging the 'plural person', the different cultural aspects of the person (ethnic, civic, professional, family identity and so on) and how these can operate together.

Consistency between: the self, values and practice; past, present and future and different relationships, situations and contexts. Integrity is tested most of all in the relationship with stakeholders, who may have very different claims and perceived needs. This demands a consistency of approach, with a clarity about core values and capacity to develop dialogue. The response may not be exactly the same in every context but will remain consistent to the identity and purpose of the person of the organisation. Central to this is the idea of being true to purpose and identity, requiring the practice of *phronesis* or continued critical reflection.

Honesty and Transparency

This involves an openness to the self and others whilst remaining focused on the truth of a narrative. Such a truth, of course, is not a simple objective truth, found apart from the network of relationships. As Smail (1984) notes, much of 'truth' about ourselves and others is illusional, built on social myths and often avoiding genuine reflection on the self or one's group. Hence, honesty is very much about how one is able to examine the self and others in a way which both understands and tests such illusions. Key to this is accountability and the capacity to give a public account of principles and practice.

Independence

This is a key element of integrity. It ensures distance, such that the professional can stand apart from competing interests, and more effectively focus on the core purpose, enabling professional autonomy.

Responsibility

Responsibility for values and practice. Without accepting responsibility for ethical values and for response, neither the individual nor the profession can develop a genuine moral identity or agency.

Learning Process

Given the limitations of human beings, it is impossible to have complete integrity. Hence, practising integrity can involve genuine struggle (Cottingham 2010) and is best viewed in terms of a continual learning process, with the person discovering more about the different aspects of the self and others and how these connect. Central to this is the capacity to reflect critically, to evaluate practice, to be able to cope with criticism and to maintain, develop or alter practice appropriately. Here, integrity connects to humility and the acceptance of limitations. In this light, integrity can be seen as a continuous struggle (Cottingham 2010; Robinson 2016), to deal with conflicting values and principles.

Several things should be noted about virtues as a whole:

- All the virtues above are focused both on individuals and organizations. The organization or community, as MacIntyre (2013) argues, develops its culture through the development of narrative, critical reflection on that and other means. A culture can enable the development of the virtues at individual and organisational levels (Brown 2005).
- Virtues are connected to and deepen the idea of skill. Traits tend to be utility- and skills-centred. Virtues look more to the depth of value and purpose. Skills and virtues enhance each other. Hence, the practice of virtues will both maintain ethical meaning and positively affect core competencies (Robinson 2005). Empathy, for instance, is central to data gathering in depth. Several skills, such as listening, teamwork and communication skills, require empathy. Empathy and practical wisdom enable appreciation and care of the other and support imagination, creativity and openness, key to the creative process and making effective decisions. Practical wisdom reinforces the skills of intellectual reflection, analysis and synthesis. Empathy also enables better awareness and appreciation of stakeholders.
- The virtues reinforce each other, but it is difficult for one person to embody all the virtues. This would look to the development of virtues through dispersed leadership, with leadership teams collectively developing the virtues.
- Virtues are never 'complete', and indeed might diminish if not practised. A one-off training in the practice of virtues is as useless as a one-off training about professional skills. The practice of the virtues requires regular reflection as part of ongoing professional development. This means that there has to be an appropriate discipline and culture, something we will examine in Chapter 9.

3.6 PAUSE FOR THOUGHT

Integrity

Think of a colleague who embodies integrity. How would you describe them?
   What are the virtues that you practise in your professional life?

Conclusions

This chapter has argued that the practice of the three modes of responsibility is central to professional ethics. Principles provide a compass, giving ethical direction. Codes provide a map that outlines ethics in professional practice. Virtues provide the moral muscle for the ethical journey, enabling balanced judgement about direction in practice and capacity to sustain the journey. Ethical judgement does not attempt to impose an ethical perspective, claim the moral high ground or polarise ethical positions. Rather, it involves staying focused on the situation and ethical issues. This involves critical engagement with ethical plurality inside and outside the organisation, building dialogue and shared narrative over time, that is working with others to find an ethical response focused on the practice of care. Care, of course, is not simply the purpose of nursing and healthcare more widely. It is also the key virtue, the capacity to care. The background of care is critical to the practice of the other virtues. As purpose, it is central to the practice of *phronesis*. As virtue, it is important in any critical engagement of values, without which this can become simply criticism rather than creative reflection. Without care, empathy can lose its positive concern for the other. These connections will be explored in more detail in the final chapter when we set out an ethics of care as a normative stance.

References

Al-Gamal, E., & Long, T. (2010). Anticipatory grieving among parents living with a child with cancer. *Journal of Advanced Nursing, 66*(9), 1980–1990.

Aquinas, T. (1981). *Summa theologica*. New York: Resources for Christian Living.

Aristotle. (2004). *Nicomachean ethics*. London: Penguin.

Augsburger, D. (2014). Interpathy re-envisioned: reflecting on observed practice of mutuality by counselors who muddle along cultural boundaries or are thrown into a wholly strange location. *Reflective practice: Formation and Supervision in Ministry, 1*, 11–22.

Bakhtin, M. (1981). *The dialogic imagination: four essays*. Austin: University of Texas.

Bauman, Z. (1989). *Modernity and the holocaust*. London: Polity.

Berlin, I. (1969). Two concepts of liberty. In A. Quinton (Ed.), *Political philosophy* (pp. 141–155). London: Penguin.

Bloom, P. (2017). *Against empathy: the case for rational compassion*. Northamptonshire: Random House.

Bouchall, S., Rallison, L., & Moules, N. (2015). Holding on and letting go: families' experiences of anticipatory mourning in terminal cancer. *OMEGA – Journal of Death and Dying, 72*(1), 42–68.

Bratton, M., & Chetwynd, S. (2004). One into two will not go: conceptualising conjoined twins. *Journal of Medical Ethics, 30*(3), 279–285.

Brickhill, P. (1954). *Reach for the sky: the story of Douglas Bader DSO, DFC*. London: Collins.

Brown, M. (2005). *Corporate integrity*. Cambridge: Cambridge University Press.

Buber, M. (1937). *I and thou*. Edinburgh: T and T Clark.

Burkitt, I. (2008). *Social selves: theories of self and society*. London: Sage.

Burleigh, M. (2011). *Moral combat: a history of World War II*. London: Harper Press.

Calhoun, C. (1995). Standing for something. *Journal of Philosophy, 92*(5), 235–260.

Callender, J. (2010). *Free will and responsibility*. Oxford: Oxford University Press.

Cavanaugh, T. (2006). *Double-effect reasoning: doing good and avoiding evil*. Oxford: Clarendon Press.

Cohen, S. (2001). *States of denial: knowing about atrocities and suffering*. London: Polity Press.

Cottingham, J. (2010). Integrity and fragmentation. *Journal of Applied Philosophy, 27*(1), 2–14.

Cowan, J. (2005). Atrophy of the affect. In S. Robinson, & C. Katulushi (Eds.), *Values in higher education*. Cardiff: Aureus.

Curzer, H. (2014). *Aristotle and the virtues*. Oxford: Oxford University Press.

Eisenberg, E. (1984). Ambiguity as strategy in organizational communication. *Communication Monographs, 51*, 227–242.

Epley, N. (2014). *Mindwise: how we understand what others think, believe, feel, and want*. London: Alfred A. Knopf.

Finch, J., & Mason, J. (1993). *Negotiating family responsibilities*. London: Routledge.

Fowler, J. (1996). *Faithful change*. Nashville: Abingdon.

Francis, R. (2013). *Inquiry report into Mid-Staffordshire NHS Foundation Trust*. London: House of Commons.

Gill, M. (2013). *Accountants Truth*. Oxford: Oxford University Press.

Goleman, D. (2005). *Emotional intelligence: why it can matter more than IQ*. New York: Bantam Books.

Guild of Catholic Doctors. (2000). *The Guild's stand on the High Court judgement relating to the Manchester conjoined twins*. The Guild of Catholic Doctors. Online available: http://www.cmq.org.uk/Miscellaneous/press_releaseabout_siamesetwins.htm.

Halfon, M. (1989). *Integrity: a philosophical inquiry*. Philadelphia: Temple University Press.

Harle, T. (2005). Serenity, courage and wisdom: changing competencies for leadership. *Business Ethics: A European Review, 14*(4), 348–357.

Hoffmaster, B., & Hooker, C. (2018). *Re-reasoning ethics: the rationality of deliberation and judgment in ethics*. Cambridge MA: MIT Press.

In Bruges (2008). Directed by Martin McDonagh. USA: Universal Studios.

Jonas, H. (1984). *The imperative of responsibility*. Chicago: Chicago University Press.

Ladd, J. (1980). The quest for a code of professional ethics: intellectual and moral confusion. In R. Chalk, M. Frankel, & S. Chafer (Eds.), *AAAS Professional Ethics Project* (pp. 154–159). Washington, DC: American Association for the Advancement of Science.

Lee, S. (2003). *Uneasy ethics*. London: Pimlico.

Levinas, E. (1998). *Entre nous: on thinking-of-the-other*. New York: Columbia University Press.

MacIntyre, A. (2013). *After virtue: a study in moral theory*. London: Bloomsbury.

May, L. (1992). *Sharing responsibility*. Chicago: Chicago University Press.

McKenny, G. (2005). Responsibility. In G. Meilander, & W. Werpehowski (Eds.), *Theological ethics* (pp. 237–253). Oxford: Oxford University Press.

Milgram, S. (2005). *Obedience to authority*. New York: Pinter and Martin.

Miller, W. (2003). *Integrating spirituality into treatment*. Washington: American Psychological Association.

Mustakova-Possardt, E. (2004). Education for critical moral consciousness. *Journal of Moral Education, 33*, 245–270.

National Association of Social Workers. (2017). *Code of Ethics*. Washington, DC: National Association of Social Workers. Online available: https://www.socialworkers.org/About/Ethics/Code-of-Ethics/Code-of-Ethics-English.

Nursing and Midwifery Board of Ireland. (2014). *Code of professional conduct and ethics*. Dublin: Nursing and Midwifery Board of Ireland. Online available: https://www.nmbi.ie/Standards-Guidance/Code.

Nursing and Midwifery Council. (2018). *The Code: professional standards of practice and behaviour for nurses, midwives and nursing associates*. London: Nursing and Midwifery Council. Online available: https://www.nmc.org.uk/standards/code/.

Paris, J., & Elias-Jones, A. (2001). Do we murder Mary to save Jodie? An ethical analysis of the separation of the Manchester conjoined twins. *Postgraduate Medical Journal, 77*, 593–598.

Pattison, G. (1998). *Art, modernity and faith: Restoring the image*. Norwich: SCM Press.

Pattison, S. (2001). Are nursing Codes of Practice ethical? *Nursing Ethics, 8*(1), 5–18.

Rawls, J. (1971). *A theory of justice*. Oxford: Clarendon Press.

Reid, H. (2002). Taking responsibility of life and death. In H. Reid (Ed.), *The philosophical athlete* (pp. 97–117). Durham, NC: Carolina Academic Press.

Ricoeur, P. (2000). The concept of responsibility: an essay in semantic analysis in *The Just (translated by Pellauer, D.)*. Chicago: University of Chicago Press.

Robinson, S. (2005). *Ethics and employability*. York: Higher Education Academy.

Robinson, S. (2008). *Spirituality, ethics and care*. London: Jessica Kingsley.

Robinson, S. (2016). *The practice of integrity in business*. London: Palgrave.

Rosen, M. (2012). *Dignity*. Cambridge, MA: Harvard University Press.

Schweiker, W. (2010). *Responsibility and christian ethics*. Cambridge: Cambridge University Press.

Seddon, J. (2014). *Whitehall effect*. Dorset: Triarchy Press.

Smail, D. (1984). *Illusion and reality: the meaning of anxiety*. London: Dent.

Snyder, C. (2000). The past and possible futures of hope. *Journal of Social and Clinical Psychology, 19*(1), 11–28.

Solomon, R. (2007). *True to our feelings*. Oxford: Oxford University Press.

Swinton, J. (2001). *Spirituality and mental health care*. London: Jessica Kingsley.

Tangney, J. (2000). Humility: theoretical perspectives, empirical findings and directions for future research. *Journal of Social and Clinical Psychology, 19*(1), 70–82.

Taylor, C. (1985). *Interpretation and the sciences of man*. In C. Taylor (Ed.), *Philosophical papers: Vol. 2* (pp. 15–57). Cambridge: Cambridge University Press.

Taylor, C. (1989). *Sources of the self*. Cambridge: Cambridge University Press.

Vera, D., & Rodriguez-Lopez, A. (2004). Humility as a source of competitive advantage. *Organizational Dynamics*, *33*(4), 393–408.

Verducci, S. (2000). A moral method: thoughts on cultivating empathy through method acting. *Journal of Moral Education*, *29*(1), 87–99.

Williams, B. (2005). A critique of utilitarianism. In N. Warburton (Ed.), *Philosophy: basic readings* (pp. 156–169). London: Routledge.

World Health Organisation. (1981). *International code of marketing of breast-milk substitutes*. Geneva: World Health Organisation. Online available: https://www.who.int/nutrition/publications/code_english.pdf.

The Practice of Healthcare Ethics

CHAPTER 4

Ethical Dilemmas in Practice

LEARNING OUTCOMES

When you have read and worked through this chapter, you should be able to:
- Understand why nursing ethics is relevant in everyday practice
- Explain and understand what 'care' means in the context of professional and institutionalised nursing practice
- Distinguish between the justification of particular decisions and giving reasons for a general rule or ethical policy
- Demonstrate ability to discuss the 'pros' and 'cons' of different approaches to classic issues of: capacity, concisions objection, cultural competence, end-of-life treatment decisions
- Indicate some of the common ethical features of the classic 'dilemmas' and how they differ from one another

Introduction

In previous chapters, the nature of ethics, professional/nursing values, professional relationships and institutional contexts of ethical decisions were presented. In this chapter, we examine some of the prevalent ethical dilemmas in healthcare, such as capacity, concisions objection, cultural competence and end-of-life treatment decisions. Healthcare professional face ethical dilemmas daily in their practice and in their professional relationships and decision-making roles. This raises important questions of principle and policy which must be clear and transparent. Therefore, this chapter will focus on ethical dilemmas, ethical principles, professional core values and decision-making processes within nursing practice. The principles discussed in Chapter 2, namely respect for autonomy of the patient/client, justice, beneficence, non-maleficence, veracity, fidelity, accountability, informed consent and confidentiality, should guide you as you consider the scenarios presented within this chapter.

Ethical Dilemmas in Nursing Practice

Nurses' relationship with ethics has existed within nursing since its inception – Florence Nightingale was concerned with the ethical conduct of her nurses. Her writings from the 1800s recognised that a nurse must focus foremost on the patients'/clients' recovery and comfort and be a diligent observant who is confident and knows his/her role in healthcare (Skretkowicz 2010). While nurses may not be specifically responsible for decisions within a case or scenarios, they have responsibilities and can face questions regarding care delivery and decisions made. Furthermore, nurses are regularly the carers who support patients/clients or their families, and have to deal with the aftermath of decisions made. Thus, nurses need to be actively engaged in the decision-making process and not removed from the ethical decisions/dilemmas involved in care provision, and ensure they are not mere bystanders/passengers when decisions are being made. This is vital as nurses, as members of the healthcare team, may have to perform or be instructed to carry out a task or care procedure for a patient/client based on a decision with which they have had no part in deciding or with which they disagree. Consequently, ethical dilemmas often arise as nurses encounter conflicting beliefs between their own beliefs, professional beliefs, patient/client beliefs/wishes, institutional requirements and other healthcare professionals' beliefs or instruction. Behind these conflicts may be different viewpoints on patient/client care, power inequalities, opposing goals of treatment or conflicting perspectives of the patient/client and their family. Conflict is evident when there has been an inability to reach a decision on the next step/course of action, a disagreement on what is important or goals of care. Generally, ethical situations have many potential choices and conclusions that will lead to better or worse outcomes, but rarely is there one single correct course of action and therefore the focus is on finding the best course of action.

Within modern healthcare practice, nurses face daily conflicting challenges in making ethical decisions, arising from their profession practice, where they blend professional nursing judgement with community and cultural beliefs, while appreciating individual beliefs, to bring about positive healthcare change (Bar-Yam 2006). Within a nurse's day-to-day practice, many decisions seem informal or routine; however, several of these health-related decisions may have long-standing implications for individuals and their families, and these decisions are not easily made. Although experienced nurses may have developed planning and leadership skills and can confidently make daily patient/client-centred decisions, emotional stress can affect their capacity to make balanced decisions. Healthcare ethics centres on the ethical issues and challenges that arise in healthcare practice and, while health professionals may differ in regards to these issues due to the focus of their roles and responsibilities, they share many similarities.

Codes of ethics, as noted in Chapter 3, have been promoted and published by many professional groups worldwide. The first international code of ethics for nurses was approved by the International Council of Nurses (ICN) in 1953 (ICN 2012), and national codes exist across countries such as the American Nurses Association (ANA 2015), Canadian Nurse Association (CNA 2017), Nursing and Midwifery Council (NMC 2018) and the Nursing and Midwifery Board of Ireland (NMBI 2014). These codes shape how nurses act ethically within their profession and offer guidance on how to respond to obstacles precluding nurses accomplishing their professional responsibilities. Furthermore, these codes support nurses in their practice and aim to reduce emotional stress through expressing the ethical and professional standards of the profession (Zahedi et al. 2013). Ethical codes express the aims of the professions and the ethical responsibilities expected of their members. Ideally, codes guide professionals in determining an ethically suitable course of action to be taken when ethical dilemmas occur. Regulatory bodies such as in the United Kingdom and Ireland (NMC, NMBI) have a remit to reprimand any nurse who is deemed to have failed in their professional responsibilities through their Fitness to Practice Committees. However, as noted in Chapter 3, they cannot offer detailed direction for each and every situation that may arise in practice. Moreover, some professionals and patients/clients may disagree with the duties imposed in certain circumstances such as the Irish Supreme Court (2015) and the status of Artificial Nutrition and Hydration (https://www.mondaq.com/ireland/Food-Drugs-Healthcare-Life-Sciences/448094/Withdrawal-Of-Artificial-Nutrition-And-Hydration-Who-Decides).

In short, ethical practice and codes of ethics overlap, with ethical practice focusing on the tools that enable professionals to critically consider the aims, duties, and consequences of professional codes.

Although ethical dilemmas are entwined within daily practice, many patients/clients are not immediately concerned about the ethical aspects of their care/treatment or the way care/treatment decisions are made for or with them, as they are generally more concentrated on getting through their care/treatment, managing their illness or focusing on their recovery. Hence, when we talk of ethics, we are referring to our decisions regarding what is right or wrong, and how we defend those decisions to ourselves, our profession and others. In practice, ethical dilemmas are more evident in the care of patients/clients who are more vulnerable such as:

- those moving towards the end of their life,
- frailty issues for older persons,
- resuscitation decisions,
- insertion of a feeding tube (e.g. person with severe advanced dementia),
- consent issues,
- refusal of treatment,
- assisted suicide,
- high-tech interventions,
- chemotherapy decisions for a person with advanced stage cancer
- decision making in times of scarce resource (Leuter et al. 2013).

These situations are ethically challenging, as they often involve incongruity or ambiguity as to what is best for the person, and this uncertainty cannot be fixed merely by referring to medical facts and statistics, as people have diverse views about what is good or bad, beneficial or harmful, contingent on their life experience and belief systems (Campbell and McCarthy 2018). In addition, a patient's/client's own view on the quality of their life may differ from the healthcare professionals view as to what is in their best medical interests, and this may generate strain or conflict, even where there is good communication between the patient/client, family and healthcare team (Campbell and McCarthy 2018). There may also be situations where a patient/client is too incapacitated to express wishes, and this can be challenging for staff and family members who have to make a treatment decision on the patient's/client's behalf. While the law does offer some direction in this area, it cannot apply to every detailed situation, and health professionals frequently want additional guidance and support. In line with this issue, clinical ethics has gained considerable attention where health professionals from a variety of disciplinary backgrounds, including ethicists, collaborate to address and, where possible, resolve ethical dilemmas arising in practice.

This collaboration generally involves a structured process, where a specific clinical ethics committee meets regularly to consider cases referred to it by staff, patients/clients or families and, although they review or provide guidance on multifaceted decisions, their job is not to police decision making or to replace the essential role of clinical decision-makers (Campbell and McCarthy 2018). Rather, their role is to support and advise professionals and ensure the lines of communication are open to ensure that all relevant parties are involved in the decision (including patients/clients) with the focus once more on open dialogue and being heard. Some health professionals and hospital directors are cynical about the usefulness and validity of clinical ethics as an approach to solving ethical dilemmas in healthcare. They argue that clinical ethics intrudes on the authority of clinical decision-makers, interferes with patient/client care and is hindered by a lack of expert clinical knowledge of committee members. These arguments raise questions about whether a focus on addressing ethical challenges in healthcare provision can actually improve the quality of patient/client care (Campbell and McCarthy 2018). However, supporters of clinical ethics contend that developing the capacity among healthcare professionals to make ethically competent decisions can benefit patients/clients, reduce staff burnout and streamline care. Ultimately, a lot depends on how the clinical ethics committee is viewed within the organisation, as a committee cannot be operational if it does not have the backing it requires from the management of the organisation and its workforce.

What is clear is that increasing importance is being placed on the development of ethical and professional competencies among health professionals, where we have seen a mounting appreciation of the importance of ethics training in medical, nursing and allied health curriculums at both undergraduate and postgraduate levels, with ethics more evident and structured within programmes. Ethics is an essential element in the foundation of nursing practice and, over time, nurses have developed strategies to overcome ethical dilemmas, guided by the nursing code of ethics (Mallari and Tariman 2016; Badzek 2008). Nursing is embedded with a concern for the welfare of the sick, injured and vulnerable persons in society (ANA 2015) and is responsible for providing their patients/clients with high-quality care (Johnstone 2016). Therefore, nurses need ethical knowledge to conduct their role in managing situations and providing safe, legal and ethical care in today's ever-changing world (Beth 2017).

Nursing ethics is an area of investigation that focuses on the moral problems and challenges faced by nurses in the course of their work. It encompasses an investigation and analysis of the assumptions, beliefs, attitudes, values, emotions, disagreements and relationships that underpin nursing ethical decisions (see Chapter 2). As ethical issues and challenges occur in institutional environments, nursing ethics takes into consideration the quality of the ethical climate of the institution. In some ways, nursing ethics can be viewed as one area of healthcare ethics alongside others, such as medical ethics and dental ethics. Like these, nursing ethics focuses on ethical issues that arise in patient/client professional relationships, such as consent, autonomy, confidentiality and veracity. It also considers obstacles to good care that health professionals must grapple with, such as a failure to achieve respectful and ongoing communication between families and nurses, patients/clients and physicians. The power of such communication lies in mitigating the negative consequences of moral disagreements that can readily impact on good patient/client care. Nursing ethics can also be understood as separate from other fields in healthcare ethics in important ways. Nursing ethics is linked with the unique history, goals and practices of nursing. In addition, many nurse ethicists pay particular attention to the quality of the relationship the nurse has with patients/clients, and this relationship can provide a type of embodied knowing (Wright and Brajtman 2011).

Over the past 30 years, the field of healthcare ethics in general has grown in order to try to address the moral and philosophical seismic shifts that have arisen as a result of technological developments at the beginning and end of life. In today's terms, humans can create life, modify life and prolong life in ways that make science fiction stories sound timid. Professional associations guidelines, clinical ethics committees and research ethics committees and commissions have developed to respond to the moral uncertainty and challenges that go along with such rapid advancements and changes. Nursing ethics can also be seen as part of this process of development that addresses these challenges. To meet these challenges, 'ethical fitness' is required, which includes reflecting on and practising ethics daily, engaging in ethical discussions and forums and discussing barriers to ethical practice (Storch 2010). While within practice, nurses may not be directly responsible for clinical decisions, they are regularly the professional group tasked with having to support patients/clients and their relatives, and deal with the 'fallout' from such decisions, while providing care afterwards. Nurses may have strong convictions about ethics in certain situations, for example abortion, euthanasia and compulsory psychiatric treatment, and may feel frustrated that they cannot do more to influence the outcome of decisions. However, they are not mere bystanders when decisions are taken; they are members of the team and may have to perform an activity for a patient/client following a decision with which they disagree. Whilst nurses may not influence the decision directly, they should contribute their observations to the clinical assessments that are being made, and should try to effect general policy and decision-making procedures on these matters, so as to safeguard that the ethical concerns of all stakeholders are taken into account before decisions are made.

Nursing Core Principles and Codes of Conduct

Nurses interact with vulnerable individuals due to illness, disease or life circumstances (Sellman 2011), and nursing care includes psychosocial support and acknowledgment of the patient/client as a whole person with psychological, social and physical care needs (Ausserhofer et al. 2014). Nursing is a clinical practice that comprises a methodical problem-solving (the nursing process) and nursing management approach to patient/client needs and, within this approach, conflict may arise between parties regarding healthcare decisions (Kayser 2014). However, listening to and discussing our reactions with others, assists us to express our own values and possibly review our viewpoints (Olpin and Hesson 2016). There is a need to recognise the context of nursing practice and the impact of this context on nursing practice and the fact that there may also be a corporate responsibility, as in situations such as those reported in Mid Staffs (Francis 2010; 2013), for a lack of humane competent nursing care (see Chapter 1).

Codes of conduct are examples of the nursing profession collectively attempting to express its underlying values and, along with the ethical principles set out in Chapter 2 and summarised in Table 4.1, guide its practice. The institution within which the nurse works can either help or hinder the actual expression of these values in nursing practice and patient/client care.

TABLE 4.1 ■ **Nursing Ethical Principles**

Justice	Concerns fairness, i.e. care must be fairly, justly and equitably distributed among a group of patients/clients.
Beneficence	Concerns doing good and the right thing for the patient/client.
Non-maleficence	Concerns doing no harm, where harm can be intentional or unintentional.
Accountability	Concerns accepting responsibility for one's own actions. Nurses are accountable for their nursing care and other actions.
Fidelity	Concerns keeping one's promises. The nurse must be faithful and true to their professional promises and responsibilities by providing high quality, safe care in a competent manner.
Autonomy and self-determination	Concerns accepting the patient/client as a unique person who has the innate right to have their own opinions, perspectives, values and beliefs. Nurses support patients/clients to make their own decision without any judgments or coercion, and the patient/client has the right to accept or reject any or all treatments.
Veracity	Concerns being completely truthful with patients/clients; nurses must not withhold the whole truth from patients/clients, even when it may lead to patient/client anxiety.

TABLE 4.2 ■ Professional Core Values and Principles

UK Core Values (Cummings and Bennett 2012)		Ireland Core Values (Department of Health (DoH) 2016)
Care	Communication	Compassion
Compassion	Courage	Care
Competence	Commitment	Commitment
Core Principles (NMC 2018)		**Core Principles (NMBI 2014)**
Prioritise people		Respect for the dignity of the person
Practise effectively		Professional responsibility and accountability
Preserve safety		Trust and confidentiality
Promote professionalism and trust		Collaboration with others

Nurses have the responsibility to recognise and identify ethical matters that affect patients/clients and staff, and nurses can take the necessary actions when confronted with an ethical dilemma by understanding and applying the ethical guidelines provided by professional and regulatory bodies and considering their professional values. Over the years, professional and regulatory bodies have developed and revised their core values that reflect the purpose of the profession, and Table 4.2 highlights the UK and Ireland's recent updates (see Chapter 1 for a detailed analysis of the UK's six Cs).

These core values and principles are important in promoting quality of care, increasing patients/clients understanding, increasing job satisfaction and for the retention of nursing staff (Schmidt and McArthur 2018; DoH 2016). These values and principles span across all areas of practice and all activities within practice, not just the activities we can quickly identify as an ethical challenge, and general activities related to one's professional responsibilities need also to be considered. With this in mind, we invite you to consider the Pause for Thought scenarios and explore your thoughts, feelings and decision-making skills if faced with a similar situation.

4.1 PAUSE FOR THOUGHT

Practice Situations

A man diagnosed with pneumonia and dehydration has been admitted to your care from a long-term care facility, and a nurse from the long-term care facility phones you for an update on his status.
- Can you share this information?
- You are both health information custodians; can they assume they have a patient's/client's implied consent to share the personal information?
- Can you give updates, as the purpose is to assist in providing healthcare?
- Do you need to be made aware if the patient/client or substitute decision-maker has specifically requested not to share information?

A nurse posted a comment on social media: 'Can't wait for this shift to be over its been such a hectic day, my head is done in and gone demented from this dementia group'.
- Can a post reveal the identity of the patient/client even without using names?
- Can posts be visible to others – can privacy settings guarantee that other will not see your posts?
- What could be the possible outcomes of posting inappropriate content on social media?
- Anything posted on the Internet is there forever and can be retrieved even after you have deleted it.

In an era where documenting one's life on social medial is a societal and personal norm, how does this challenge professional responsibility? This requires caution from healthcare professionals with regards to the distinction between one's professional principles and social norms. We draw your attention to some healthcare cases that resulted in sanctions, such as: the Swedish nurse who was suspended from her job after posting on Facebook pictures of a brain surgery she was involved in (Salter 2008); four nursing students who were expelled for posting pictures on Facebook of themselves with a human placenta (Gibson 2011); and the Mexican anaesthesiologist who was fired for publishing on Facebook pictures that depicted a child being immobilised prior to surgery, the amputated legs of an elderly woman, and surgery patients' pictures where their faces were visible (Vivas 2012).

Care and Caring in Nursing Practice

The act of caring is at the very heart of nursing practice (McDonough 2019). Caring is focused on action and is a core value for nursing, demonstrated by a concern and empathy for others, through having and showing compassion for others (The Free Dictionary 2019). Nurses need to cultivate a holistic approach, which integrates practical competence, empathic understanding and technical knowledge to deliver humane, responsive and sensitive care. Nurses need to be aware of caring and the attitudes needed to practise this, respecting the dignity of everybody involved (Hemingway 2013; Watson 2008).

4.2 PAUSE FOR THOUGHT

Your Values

- What is the most important element in what nurses do?
- Is this element based on the concept of treating others as valued human beings?
- What attitudes do you hold as an individual and professional that enable you to value each human being?
- Consider how, in your practice, you use a head, hand and heart approach to preserve a person's dignity.

When we deliver nursing in a respectful way, with dignity and care, then everything we do reflects that, and the problems/concerns encountered by the patient/client will be addressed in a caring manner to the best of our ability. This can be moderated by the nurse's thoughts and actions reflecting on what would be acceptable to oneself, one's partners, one's family and one's friends, and considering one's ability to walk a mile in another's shoes. As it is essential to safeguard vulnerable ill people, everybody who works with them needs to have developed an attitude that enables them to empathise with, listen to and learn from other people's experiences (Hemingway 2013). Caring encompasses a sense of self-identity and spirit of the person and involves commitment to the patient/client within a holistic approach. Caring and nursing have always had a close association and most people select nursing as a profession because of their wish to care for others (Potter and Fogel 2013; Vance 2003).

Care as a central concept has led to the development of several theories of caring in nursing, one of the best known was developed by Watson (1979). Watson (1979) defines caring as a science that comprises humanitarian, human science orientation and human caring processes, phenomena and experiences. This is grounded in a relational ontology, of being-in-relation, and a world view of unity and connectedness of all. Transpersonal caring recognises unity of life and connections that move in coextensive circles of caring from the individual, to others, to the community, to the world, to the planet Earth and to the universe. Caring science inquiries encompass reflective, subjective and interpretative as well as objective-empirical inquiry and comprise ontological, philosophical, ethical and historical inquiry and studies. In addition, caring science embraces numerous epistemological approaches to inquiry including clinical and empirical, but is accepting of new areas of investigation that explore other forms of knowing, for example, aesthetic, narrative, intuitive, poetic, personal, evolving consciousness, kinaesthetic, intentionality, metaphysical, spiritual as well as moral–ethical knowing, and has significance to all health and human service professions and practice areas (Watson 2003). Caring behaviours in nursing are identified by Taber (2017) as:

- attentive listening,
- comforting,
- honesty,
- patience,
- responsibility,
- providing information so the patient can make an informed decision,
- touch,
- sensitivity,
- respect,
- calling the patient by name.

Watson's (1979) description of nursing is that of humanism that has a chief focus on the process of human care for individuals, families and communities with its origins in the philosophy of being and knowing (McCance et al. 1999). Within Watson's theory, the goal of nursing focuses on helping the patient/client gain a higher degree of harmony within the mind, body and soul, and this is realised through caring interactions (Potter and Fogel 2013; Vance 2003). The caring process also includes a transpersonal caring relationship which conveys a concern for the inner life, where the patient/client is viewed holistically and the nurse connects with and embraces the spirit or soul of the patient/client, through the course of caring and healing (Watson 2003). To support and enable nurses to achieve this process, Watson (1979) identified 10 carative factors (referred to as interventions of the theory) as:

- forming humanistic-altruistic value systems,
- instilling faith-hope,
- cultivating a sensitivity to self and others,
- developing a helping-trust relationship,
- promoting an expression of feelings,
- using problem-solving for decision making,
- promoting teaching-learning,
- promoting a supportive environment,
- assisting with gratification of human needs,
- allowing for existential-phenomenological forces.

Caring in the nursing profession can be seen to take place each time a nurse makes contact with a patient/client, where the nurse enters the world of the patient/client so as to know the patient/client as a caring person, and it is from this 'epistemology' that nursing caring unfolds (Potter and Fogel 2013; Schoenhofer 2002). Caring makes a difference to a patient's/client's sense of well-being as caring may occur without curing, but curing cannot occur without caring (Watson 2003). It is with this belief that nurses care for patients/clients in order to contribute to the well-being and recovery/cure of the patient/client, and within this process, hope and commitment are key elements (Nweze et al. 2015; see Chapter 3). This focus on hope enables the nurse to honour the patient/client and support them in a holistic manner, and aligns to Watson's (1979) second carative factor (see Chapter 3 for hope as a virtue). Hope is guided by our commitment as nurses to our patients/clients and can be clouded by our preconceived beliefs and the values that we are raised with; thus the development and socialisation as a professional is an important factor in the development of professional ethical practice.

Caring is a central concept to the delivery of care and patients/clients encountered can be from a variety of other settings, for example, a home environment (own, family, friend) or care environment (nursing home, retirement centres). In any healthcare context, patients/clients are frequently frightened of unfamiliar environments, potential loss of control and ultimately of dying, and rely on the nurse to deliver care, staying with them through the experience and focusing on their sense of well-being. In such episodes, one is caring and being cared for (Watson 1997), creating an interconnection between nurse and patient/client, and this human connection is at a deeper level than just a physical interaction (Watson 2003). In such situations, a nurse must have an acceptance of death and dying as part of the life cycle (Watson 2002), where caring can be directed towards a pain-free death with dignity and accepting of the patient's/client's belief regarding any spiritual transformation or journey after death (Hilbers et al. 2018). As such, caring centres on the person, maintaining dignity and humanity, and is a commitment to lessen another's vulnerabilities through responding to a person's needs and being concerned for human life (Watson 2002). This model of caring embraces the intersection of art, science, humanities, spirituality and new dimensions of mind-body-spirit medicine (Watson 2003). Spirituality in this sense is not specifically or exclusively religious, but rather generic, involving significant life meaning, which, as noted in Chapter 2, feeds into ethical meaning (Robinson et al. 2003). Religion, of course, can be a particular expression of spirituality. Caring is viewed as human behaviour that includes cognitive, affective, psychomotor and administrative skills within which professional caring may be expressed. In the modern era, caring is vital as patients/clients are often cared for through the medium of highly technological areas such as the intensive care unit (ICU) or have less contact with healthcare professionals. Care and caring are predominantly used to describe the intrinsic work of nurses, and nursing is valued as a nurturing profession of which caring is an essential component of its holistic practice and central to the social relationship between the nurse, the patient/client and their relatives. In all this, the nurse as person is as important as the nurse as technical practitioner. Hence, as Blasdell (2017) notes, the action of care transcends any particular professional task. Because of this, it is possible to see care as the basis of any normative theory of ethics, and we will examine this in more detail in Chapter 11.

We must recognise that caring is not unique to nursing and that care can also be overprotective, intrusive, overbearing and infantilising (Delmar 2012). In addition, nurses are employed to get certain work done as efficiently and effectively as possible. As a result, considerable limitations and practical constraints may be placed on the time available for caring relationships and attention to the needs of patients/clients.

It is also important to take account of the moral and legal concept of a duty of care (RCN 2019). The moral aspects of a nurse's duty of care are spelled out in the various professional codes of ethics, and specified in the rules and procedures professionals are expected to follow in their working organisation (Dowie 2017). The legal duty of care derives from the nature of the implicit or actual contract between the carer and the person for whom they care (RCN 2019). To fail in one's duty of care as a professional is not only to be morally blameworthy for a breach of trust, but also one may be legally actionable for breach of contract and culpable negligence (Water et al. 2017).

Ethical Decision-Making Process

Nurses have an obligation to inform staff and patients/clients of ethical issues that can and do affect their care and address these issues. In practice, healthcare professionals have to deal with cases such as providing care to patients/clients undergoing an abortion, which may raise ethical and moral concerns for some practitioners. Other aspects, such as a patient/client asking for assistance in their suicide at the end their life, or an inquiry about the diagnosis of another patient/client, often arise and healthcare professionals must inform the patient/client what they can and cannot do for ethical and legal reasons. Key within any ethics decision process are elements that emphasise and speak to advocacy, collaboration and dialogue with others; the dignity and worth of all human beings; the preservation of patient/client rights, such as dignity, autonomy and confidentiality; the maintenance of patient/client safety; the prohibition of any discrimination; accountability and the provision of competent, safe and high-quality care. To guide the decision-making process, one can follow the sequence of steps identified in Chapter 2, and, as with all other aspects of nursing care, any intervention to promote ethical practice and the outcome of such should be evaluated and measured. To promote this process, one should identify:

- Staff knowledge regarding ethics and ethical practice.
- If staff effectively apply ethical principles in their daily practice.
- If patients/clients have the knowledge of and have been informed of ethics and ethical practice.
- If appropriate professional resources were utilised to resolve the ethical issue.

Applying Ethics in One's Practice

In ethics, we generally look at practice issues which present moral problems and dilemmas so we can identify the ways and thoughts others have used to deal with these issues, and we can then draw on this knowledge for similar issues that arise in our own practice. As in everyday life, we learn from our own experience and, as a professional, we accumulate practical wisdom and professional and general guidance on how to act. However, general knowledge does not tell us specifically what we should do in a particular situation, and we have to decide for ourselves. But knowing what others have thought or done helps prevent us from having to start from the beginning. Thereby engaging in reviewing and understanding past situations assists practitioners in guiding their practice and making ethical decisions. Later in this chapter, and throughout this book, we present ethical cases and pause for thought moments in an attempt to provoke your thinking and encourage engagement in dialogue within the practice of ethical issues. In addition, we prompt you within these dialogues to engage in a discussion of the merits and weaknesses of the actions and decisions. Whereas scientific knowledge is general, and concerned with discovering universal laws, ethics is concerned with particulars. However, within caring, the rules are often abstract and general, whereas decisions are made within concrete circumstances with reference to specific cases and particular people. While moral rules are intended to apply universally, decisions involve applying general rules to specific situations, and are a responsible decision if they are a response to the actual needs and demands of a specific situation. We may take policy decisions about matters of a general nature, for ourselves, for a professional group or for an institution, but ethical decisions as decisions are not general. They always relate to a specific context or to a specific professional group at a particular time in a particular country, or to a particular hospital or institution. The skills and experience needed to make sound ethical decisions cannot be learned solely from theory or by discussing cases. The difficulty is not in deciding what rules or principles to apply, but rather how they should be applied in a particular case. Thus, the practical challenge is to make a judgement that leads to appropriate action in the actual situation for the specific patient/client. Making ethical decisions is prospective, that is, we must confront problems for which we do not have existing answers, and still have to find solutions in the future, from our learning and from our experience. You can only learn how to become skilled in these areas by practising the skills and virtues (see Chapter 3), exercising practical responsibility and developing competence in applied ethics in real life, and in relation to real life ethical problems. It is also important to be mindful that healthcare ethics is not confined solely to dilemmas or problems in clinical practice, but include a much wider range of ethical issues, for example personal and professional value judgement, management of conflict, inter-professional relationships and ethical policy in hospitals.

Health, Ethics and Value Judgement

We cannot avoid making value judgements about our health or debating matters of ethical policy in relation to healthcare, as the whole question of our health and well-being as individuals, in family life, in our work and in society is not a matter of indifference to us. Societies can differ in terms of what they regard as health or what they define as disease; however, all desire good health and seek to avoid injury, pain, illness, disability, disease and death. Poor health can affect the well-being of others within the family, and the cost of caring for the sick, the injured, people with mental health problems or those who are severely disabled, can be seen as a burden on society through providing primary care, hospital services and professional staff. Internationally, government policy has moved or is moving to care in the community as an alternative to hospital-based care. This community focus promotes normalisation and reduces the focus on long-stay institutional care, allowing us to consider the meaning of health and quality of life. In general, people want to be healthy, as life is more enjoyable when one is fit and healthy as opposed to unfit, ill or injured. Good health is something healthcare professionals value and is an ideal and a goal they strive to realise for themselves and others. In making decisions about our personal health, we have to make both practical and moral choices about our behaviour and lifestyle if we are to live healthy lives and avoid accidents, injury, disease or premature death.

Society is and has to be interested in the health and well-being of its members. Firstly, because we are part of one another (see Chapter 10); secondly, because the whole human family may suffer if we are unable to make or are prevented from making our own contribution to society and thirdly, because of the additional burden and cost of care and treatment that may result. Consequently, government public health measures are undertaken to prevent disease, promote the health of society and to reduce the cost of ill-health to individuals and the state (e.g. health education, immunisation, screening). From the outset, there is a potential conflict here between our personal liberty to do what we want in pursuing the lifestyle of our choice, and what is seen as societal good to guide, change or redirect our health behaviour or choices. These tensions relate to basic ethical questions about the relations of personal rights and social responsibility, of personal well-being and the wider good of society. From here, we ask you to consider some practical and health delivery situations that pose ethical issues based on advances in healthcare or due to our own professional or personal value judgements. One such issue is that of immunisation and the debate regarding individual choice and the risk that may be placed on others and compulsory immunisation as an access to crèche/schools.

At a practice level, healthcare professionals are front-line health educators with a professional responsibility to prevent disease and care for and treat those who are ill. However, healthcare professionals have to face contradictions between their own health behaviour (e.g. with regard to smoking, drug or alcohol abuse, diet, fitness, responsible sex) and what they are advising their patients/clients to do. The issues are not only about the public's expectations relating to the health professional as a role model, but also about their credibility as health educators or agents of social control. Health education can be presented in such a way as to encourage people to know more about healthy living, to make informed choices and to take responsibility for our own health and choice of lifestyle. Consider, for example, a patient/client who is a smoker and what advice/education you would give them as a healthcare professional. If the advice and support the patient/client requires is outside of one's practice, one may only just engage in a conversation about health behaviours, health risks and choices and provide the relevant support information and link to a smoking cessation service (see Chapter 10). Another healthcare professional may ensure a referral and appointment is made for the smoking cessation service. The question is, do our own values affect our decision-making process, and should they influence the care provided? What if the healthcare professional is a smoker themselves, does that shape their decision? Do they see it as a personal choice, or do they empathise with the person and, through that shared understanding, make a shared decision that meets the needs of the patient/client? What if a patient is attending a smoking cessation service and, while parking their car, sees the healthcare professional who manages the service, smoking in the car park, how does this influence the outcomes for the patient/client, what professional value does it demonstrate? These questions can be considered in all areas as a healthcare professional. Any healthcare advice that is given to guide a healthy lifestyle or change a behaviour is something all healthcare professionals need to role model themselves.

The ethical issues of greatest concern tend to be those that relate directly to professional responsibility in either direct patient/client care or management roles. Issues around communication with patients/clients (truth telling and confidentiality) and conflicts tend to predominate. Whereas nurses can be seen as not having power, as they do not necessarily make the decisions, in reality, nurses have significant power over patients/clients, and even influence over doctors. The way they organise staff time and community resources can directly influence both the quantity and quality of care given to patients/clients. They can influence the patient/client both directly and indirectly by the way they change or influence the patient's/client's environment. They can influence the decisions of doctors, paramedics and other carers by their reported observations about patients/clients and the appropriateness or inappropriateness of treatment, levels of pain control, compulsory detention in hospital or discharge. The nature and quality of their observations regarding the patient's/client's physical, emotional and psychological state may be critical in the patient's/client's care management. They can also influence nursing and hospital management about necessary organisational and institutional change, or campaign for more resources, and, in general, have a responsibility to maintain the quality and standards of patient/client care. In the cases reviewed in Chapters 2 and 3, nurses in particular could have had a significant contribution, partly by being there with family and friends, providing time for reflection and deliberation, partly by communicating the voice of the family and patient to other colleagues. All of these enable the practice of *phronesis* and other virtues.

The quest for miracle cures has driven science to extraordinary lengths to find new (and profitable) ways of treating diseases. Bioengineering has resulted in the production of aids to assist people with disabilities. Biochemistry, genetics and genetic screening build hope that genetic disorders will be eliminated, infertility treated, in vitro fertilisation and embryo transplant made safe and routine and organ donation and replacement reliable. Illich (1975) identified 'the medicalisation of life', which has meant that health professionals have inherited increasing power and control over matters of life and death, where health professionals tend to preside over the rites of passage at all key life events. The medicalisation of life and advancements in care/treatment options over time can create high risk and high cost for many life-saving interventions, and attempts to deal with human distress and unhappiness have created their own crop of unprecedented ethical quandaries. This is obvious in the case of the side effects of treatment and the questions that arise about the extent to which patients/clients should be informed of all the possible consequences of treatment, and of the difficulties of obtaining fully informed consent from anxious, traumatised patients/clients. This has resulted in a much greater emphasis on patient/client rights, the need for patient/client advocacy and representation of lay people on many management and policy-making bodies in local and national healthcare.

All healthcare advances can raise ethical issues; for example, screening may identify an individual likely to inherit a genetic defect or fatal disease, such as Huntington's chorea. This not only presents the healthcare worker with the dilemma of whether or not to tell the person involved, but also presents the patient/client with a difficult choice if they wish to have children. Although assisted reproduction techniques such as in vitro fertilisation (IVF) of previously harvested ova, or intracytoplasmic sperm injection, in severe cases of male infertility, may result after several attempts in a successful live birth, there is also a high failure rate for these expensive procedures. They not only involve serious additional risks to women in the harvesting of sufficient numbers of their ova for experimental purposes, but also raise serious questions about the long-term genetic and health consequences, and costs relative to benefits, of interventions to assist individuals with genetic defects to have children. The medicalisation of life has negative implications such as the overuse of antibiotics (creating pathogens that are immune to all available drugs), including the risks of hospital-acquired infections such as methicillin resistant *Staphylococcus aureus* (MRSA); vast numbers of patients/clients addicted to prescription drugs (particularly stimulants, antidepressants, and major tranquillisers); the risks of ovarian hyper-stimulation in the harvesting of ova in the treatment of infertility; the risks of multiple births and cerebral palsy in low-birth-weight babies associated with IVF and the risk of unscrupulous pharmaceutical research on vulnerable patients/clients in the attempt to be the first to market new wonder drugs.

The medicalisation of care, and, as we shall see in more detail in Chapter 9, the managerialist approach to healthcare delivery run the danger of crowding out the time for engaged, person-centred care. To achieve a balanced, ethical judgement about a specific situation, it may be just as important to understand the background of the person involved, as it may be important from a nursing perspective not only to know the patient's/client's medical, but also his/her personal and social history. Listening to the patient's/client's story is not just useful, and perhaps comforting, to the patient/client, but it is also essential if we are to acknowledge and respect the dignity of the individual in a genuinely person-centred manner. The concept of a health career has proved very important in health education, particularly in understanding patterns of both health-promoting and dysfunctional health behaviour (Bickel et al. 2016; Blake et al. 2017). What is ethically significant about health and illness for the person involved is that illness and injury usually involve loss of autonomy and greater dependence on other people. Making a good recovery usually means regaining more control over our lives, and being able to stand on our own feet again. A person's health is a dynamic process, involving movement or shift in responsibility from the patient/client to the healthcare professional, and back again. This is clearest in cases where individuals have emergency admissions for major injury, or for severe mental health problems, but even in the minor illnesses or ups and downs of life, there are considerable fluctuations in our need for help and support, and our capacity to stand on our own feet. Problems arise for patients/clients when professionals are either reluctant or too eager to take on responsibility for them when they are in a crisis or need help. Alternatively, professionals may be slow to give up the control that they acquire over people's lives, or too readily abandon them before they are able to take control of their own lives again. Generally, ethical codes in the caring professions have focused mainly on the responsibility the carer accepts for the patient/client; few have stressed the importance of the commitment the carer must make to return control to the patient/client as soon as they are capable of being independent (Vincifori and Min 2014; Thompson 2002). Conversely, nursing codes have emphasised the responsibility of the nurse to work to restore autonomy to the individual who has lost it as a result of illness, injury or mental health problems, and this emphasises a value fundamental to nursing ethics that appears to arise out of reflection on the distinctive nature of nursing care.

Abortion/Right to Life

Throughout history, women have sought assistance to terminate a pregnancy, whether or not this has been accepted by law or morality. Some societies have prohibited, tolerated or legislated for abortion. The liberal legislation has decriminalised abortion, making it a matter of clinical and moral responsibility for nurses/midwives (Guillaume and Rossier 2018). This raises an apparent incongruence between the obligation to protect, nurture and save the life of the child, and the obligation for the wider care of the woman. The deliberate termination of a pregnancy is regularly debated from either the pro-life point of view, in terms of the sanctity of life and the rights of the unborn child, or from a women's rights perspective, particularly their right to control their own fertility and make choices. The debate either to safeguard the rights of the unborn child or to defend the rights of the woman raises tensions between popular morality on the one hand, and the law and social policy on the other. These opposing moral beliefs are not necessarily in disagreement about fundamental values, or that termination of pregnancy is an absolute wrong or an absolute right, as both groups would probably regard it as neither a good nor an ideal solution. All groups have a right in a democratic society to campaign to have their views more widely accepted, and to influence social policy and the law. However, it cannot simply be assumed that the morality of a particular group can be legitimately imposed on the wider community, even in societies where they represent the majority (see the values conflicts referred to by Haidt in Chapter 11). Considerations of justice and equity, as well as respect for the rights and freedom of conscience of individuals, make it necessary that there is scope for dissent; otherwise the society is on course to become an authoritarian society, whether the position entrenched in law and social policy is an extreme libertarian one or strictly anti-abortion.

Within the abortion debate, the healthcare professional is often found in the middle, with a duty of care to both the mother and child, leaving them in an impossible position, for example, where they have to choose between the rights of one or the other. The conflicting demands of such a situation cannot be resolved either by consulting the law or their consciences, about which individual (mother or baby) is owed a greater duty of care. Other considerations of personal rights and justice have to be considered, and the tension between these conflicting values in real life is what makes these problems so difficult.

The sanctity of life argument raises both fundamental issues and impossible problems in ethics. If all life is sacred, where do you draw the line? With the newborn, the fetus, the conceptus, the ovum or individual sperm or where? When does life become human in the continuum between individual cell and person? This raises the major question, what is a person? This is essentially a moral question and a matter of value judgement, namely, a judgement about what in particular is to be valued about human persons (Smyth and Lane 2016). This is an ethical question, and different societies will define it differently or, most likely, fail to reach a full agreement given the diversity within societies. Personhood as defined within a society directly influences how the legal concept of a person is constructed to give concrete meaning as 'a bearer of rights and duties' and how we define the scope and limits of membership of the 'moral community' (Kerridge et al. 1998). Compounding the issue of abortion are the debates about IVF and the legal status of the unborn and where we draw the line in experiments with embryos, or the storage of embryos, where contradictory policies exist, acknowledging the right of the unborn child and, on the other hand, permitting termination of pregnancy, under specific conditions. Furthermore, within societies, confusion exists whether all people enjoy the same rights (children, people with mental health problems or intellectual disability). This discussion is not meant to decide on the abortion or deliberate termination of pregnancy issue, but rather to raise a fundamental series of ethical questions (see Pause for Thought 4.3).

In many countries, termination of pregnancy (abortion) is available on demand (Gutmacher Institute 2018), and the World Health Organization (WHO) recommends 'mid-level professionals' such as nurses/midwives as the key providers in the provision of abortion services (WHO 2012), and the International Confederation of Midwives (ICM 2014), identifying essential competencies for practice, include provision of safe abortion care (Scott 2017). In jurisdictions such as the UK and Ireland, legalised abortion occurs under the supervision of medical practitioners, and is currently permitted up to the completion of week 24/26 of pregnancy when certain criteria are fulfilled. The Acts in these countries provide for a conscientious objection, where no one is under any duty to participate, contrary to conscience, although an exemption does not apply where treatment is necessary to save the life or to prevent grave permanent injury to the physical or mental health of a pregnant woman (Fleming et al. 2018). Freedom of conscience is a core element of human rights that, in Europe, is protected since its first draft document of the European Convention on Human Rights (European Court of Human Rights 1950).

4.3 PAUSE FOR THOUGHT

What Are Your Considerations

- What do we mean by a person?
- What do we mean by respect for personal dignity and rights?
- What is the scope of the moral community?
- What criteria do we apply to determine membership of the moral community?
- What rights and responsibilities does membership entail?
- What is the moral status of a fetus?
- Does a fetus have independent rights?
- What are your ethical obligations or duties to the woman (or mother) and to the fetus (or unborn baby)?
- What will lead to the best outcomes (benefits versus harms), all things considered?
- What are the best policies for preserving the moral fabric of our communities and society?
- What polices guide you in your practice in this area?
  Consider the case of:
- The judgment of the UK Supreme Court (2014) https://www.supremecourt.uk/cases/docs/uksc-2013-0124-judgment.pdf,
- The publication Abortion in Northern Ireland and the European Convention on Human Rights: Reflections from the UK Supreme Court, doi: https://doi.org/10.1017/S0020589319000034 (Ní Ghráinne and McMahon 2019).

This all raises the question of personhood, which is the status of being a person. Defining personhood is a debated topic in both philosophy and law and is closely tied with legal and political concepts of citizenship, equality, and liberty (Taylor 1985). As personhood is recognised socially and legally, it can vary over time and across cultures, signifying the notion that personhood is not universal. Attributes common to definitions of personhood include human nature, agency, self-awareness, a notion of the past and future and the possession of rights and duties, among others (Taylor 1985). Being human has been equated with being a person where being-in-itself is the only criteria. Kitwood (1997) viewed personhood as sacred and unique, and that each person should be treated with deep respect. In some religious and spiritual beliefs, people have a kind of unique inner essence, which may even be believed to continue beyond human life. The belief in a kind 'non-material soul that still exists intact underneath all the neurological losses of dementia' (Post 2006, p. 231). However, such a belief does not necessarily guarantee one will be treated humanely and with respect. For Cooley (2007), to qualify as a person, it was necessary to possess rationality (ability to think and reason logically), and to be able to communicate this to other people. Another example of a capacity-based approach is that of Warren (1973), who defined six criteria for personhood, namely consciousness, reasoning, self-motivating activity, capacity to communicate, presence of self-concept and self-awareness. However, these definitions of personhood ignore the emotional and relational needs and capacities of people such as those with dementia, learning/intellectual disabilities or mental health problems.

Early Christianity differentiated between the terms 'individual' and 'person', whereby the latter was understood as referring to the individual in relationship to others (Allen and Coleman 2006). People are not simply biological entities; they interact within a social environment, and personhood is acknowledged and confirmed through interaction. The concept of personhood has also been linked to the different selves that a person may have. Sabat (2001) described three different selves: (1) the self of personal identity (expressed through using 'I'); (2) the self-comprised of the attributes a person possesses and (3) the self-consisting of the social self or persona presented to others through social roles. Kitwood argued that there were two aspects to the person, the adapted self and the experiential self, two ways of being. The former is described as 'highly and tightly socialised, particularly in relation to the performing of given roles' (Kitwood 1997, p. 15).

The latter arises out of simply being with people within a context of equality and mutual respect and attention. Personhood is maintained in a person whose human existence is linked to a physical body in a particular familial, cultural and historical context. This does not mean that there is no consciousness, as this can be expressed through bodily activity. In all this, the idea of a person is not simply descriptive, but also evaluative, making a value judgement about the dignity of the other over time (which may involve development or diminution of rationality), and thus requires commitment to the other. Hence, personhood is as much about relationships as about bearing any particular capacity. In the issue of abortion, this means that appeal to personhood cannot form a knock down argument for or against abortion. Dialogue is thus critical to determine how the particular decision should be made.

Truth-Telling and Confidentiality

Healthcare professionals' knowledge of health matters places them in a position of authority to assist people who are in need of care, but this also gives them power over them. Thereby, people will share or hold back information about themselves during their consultations with health professional's depending on whether or not they trust the healthcare professional, and their belief that the healthcare professional will use the information for the benefit of making a diagnosis and managing their problem. Although people are usually agreeable to divulging private and sensitive information regarding themselves to healthcare professionals, they are also aware that by doing so, this makes them vulnerable, and that the possession of such information gives health professionals added power over them. Legal safeguards to protect the confidentiality of patient/client information and records are essential to safeguard the vulnerability of patients/clients, and to ensure that the possession of personal information is not inappropriately disclosed to others or abused by those caring for them (British Medical Association 2018; Brazier and Cave 2016).

On the other hand, the extent of the information that should be disclosed to a patient/client about their diagnosis, medical condition, prognosis and treatment is also a matter of responsible and sensible judgement. This control of information and its discerning disclosure is part of the power healthcare professionals hold over patients/clients, and can be used as a means of securing their compliance to treatment. It is also an essential duty of healthcare professionals to determine when, how much and by whom, information should be divulged to patients/clients. Refusal to reveal pertinent information may deny people the control to make important decisions affecting their lives. If knowledge is power, then it can be said to withhold information is to keep the patient/client in a state of helplessness and of being controlled.

While in the past healthcare professionals may have been reluctant to fully inform patients/clients of their prognosis, it is now standard practice to provide patients/clients with the relevant information about their condition, unless they have specifically asked not to be given further information, or if it is considered that divulging the information would place the patient/client under psychological distress. Nonetheless, telling the patient/client the truth is not simply a matter of stating the facts; how the information is communicated needs to be considered as, for example, heartlessly communicating a fatal diagnosis would be insensitive and irresponsible, but could also constitute a form of abuse of a vulnerable person and as such would be an inappropriate expression of professional power. Dilemmas of truth-telling and confidentiality arise because of seeming or actual conflicts between the patient's/client's right to know and the carer's duty to care. The classic situation of whether and when to tell a dying patient/client that their condition is terminal illustrates the strain between two contrasting moral concerns: respect for the patient's/client's autonomy and right to know about their condition, and the feeling of the carer that he/she should protect the patient/client from news which might shock and distress them, perhaps causing them to lose hope and cause despair.

It may seem simplistic to say that what such situations require is honesty, and honesty demands that we honour, that is, show sensitive regard for the particular patient's/client's needs and their ability to embrace the information at that time, then we can learn to titrate the truth to the needs of the individual. Responsible and empathetic truth-telling requires experience, maturity and communication and counselling skills on the part of the healthcare professional. The situation may be further convoluted in practice by the intercession of relatives demanding to know or denying communication with the dying patient/client. Here, in the non-existence of permission from the patient/client (if they have the capacity to give consent), disclosing information about the patient's/client's condition quantifies a breach of their right to confidentiality. The various parties involved, including staff, may not be willing to acknowledge failure or to relinquish control. They may merely wish to guard themselves from the emotional drain of the dying patient's/client's grief (Smith and Parker 2015). Communication with the dying requires great sensitivity and depends on the patient's trust and confidence in the healthcare staff. The issues involved are not susceptible to universal prescriptions, and the quandary of nurses may be that, in practice, they are caught in the middle and prevented by doctor's orders from doing what they believe to be the best in the circumstances. What makes these problems recurring dilemmas is that they bring contrasting rights and duties into painful conflict with each other. Whether priority should be given to the patient's/client's right to know or to the professional's duty to protect the vulnerability of the patient/client, this cannot be decided by mere appeal to principle but has to be worked out in the complexity of each unique situation, in the way that seems most caring and responsible at the given time. Hence the truth in those situations emerges through dialogue.

Respect for a patient's/client's right to privacy is again complicated by the often overriding duty to care and to do what is in line with the will and preference of the patient/client. This may involve the carer sharing confidential information with another professional with the expectation that it will contribute to better care for the patient/client. Ideally, carers have a duty to gain the consent of persons who have confided in them prior to sharing their information, and when this is not possible, ethical dilemmas arise. What takes priority, the patient's/client's right to privacy or the professional's duty to provide the best possible care to the patient/client? Dilemmas of confidentiality generally do not occur as a result of careless disclosures of patients'/clients' information, but rather when the healthcare professional's responsibilities to their patients/clients comes into conflict with the requirements of team management of patient/client care or in sharing information with family/relatives. The issues are further complicated by the problems of shift work and lack of continuity in care, where carers need to have crucial information if they are to provide appropriate care.

Being in possession of sensitive confidential information about patients/clients is often both a burden and privilege for carers, but it also promotes a special relationship with those for whom we care. It can be a burden when it is difficult to set limits to the process of self-disclosure in a patient/client with a compulsive need to tell all. Here, the healthcare professional may have to set clear limits with the patient/client regarding what information is relevant and what is required, what information is strictly secret and what can be shared with the rest of the care team. Healthcare professionals sometimes may be inclined to guard protectively confidential information about patients/clients, and are reluctant to share it with other members of the team because it means compromising the special relationship they have with their patients/clients. Situations also change within the carer patient/client relationship; for example, as the patient/client enters a crisis and becomes increasingly dependent, the carer acquires greater power and control over the life of the patient/client. Part of this control consists in the management of the flow of information to the patient/client, from the patient/client and about the patient/client. Giving or withholding information can also be a powerful way of encouraging cooperation or compliance and maintaining control in the caring relationship (Nass et al. 2009). Because knowledge is power and to withhold information is to be kept in a state of dependence, the manner in which the information and confidences are shared is an indicator of whether professional attitudes are creating dependency or are being used to assist patients/clients towards autonomy and enabling them to retain some control of their lives.

The dilemmas of confidentiality and truth-telling, as well as general conflicts between protective beneficence and respect for a person's rights, arise in the most acute form where the patient/client lacks capacity. This is particularly the case where the patient/client is psychotic and rendered practically and legally incompetent by virtue of a severe mental health problem. Treatment of people who are suffering from a severe mental health problem/illness has developed over the years and terminology has become more person-centred to avoid stigmatising effects. However, on occasions, due to a severe mental health disorder or mental incapacity, an individual may be taken into hospital against their will, and even subjected to compulsory treatment. Deciding whether an individual should be compulsorily detained in hospital may be relatively straight forward in cases of severe dementia or severe mental illness, but the vast majority of mental health problems are not so clear-cut, and the general legal requirement that the individual must be a danger to themselves or others leaves us in a difficult position, as this is particularly difficult to assess in practice. Furthermore, individuals admitted in a severely disturbed state may recover without treatment, or may have periods of reasonable normality and periods where they are clearly incompetent. Whether the system is sensitive enough to respond to these fluctuating changes in the moral status of detained patients/clients and to respect their right to information or to be consulted about their treatment, may be questioned. In addition, the introduction of community treatment orders (CTOs), which have a legal status and require a person suffering from a serious mental illness to adhere to a plan of treatment and supervision while living in the community (Corring et al. 2017), raise questions regarding choice, autonomy and rights versus control, protection and overall good.

There are several atypical features of mental illness which create moral difficulties or dilemmas, where ambiguities in the diagnosis, treatment and rehabilitation of people with mental illness (including senile dementia and severe intellectual/learning disabilities) exists. These ambiguities are to be found in all of the following:

- the moral/legal status of the patient/client,
- the scope of definitions and diagnosis of mental illness,
- the variety of activities which count as treatment in psychiatry and rehabilitation,
- the definition of which patients/clients are the carer's responsibility.

The ambiguous moral/legal status of someone suffering from a mental illness is evident in the fact that health professionals have unique legal powers to detain and treat patients/clients who are regarded as incompetent because they are mentally ill. The principal moral paradox of psychiatry is that people may have to be deprived of their liberty and treated against their will in the hope that this will make it possible for them to regain their autonomy and resume control of their lives again. To authenticate the use of these extraordinary legal powers of professionals, most legal systems need proof that the person is either a danger to themselves or to others. Assessment of these risks is essential to warrant detention of a patient/client for treatment, and this action is justified morally on the basis of a duty of protective beneficence towards the patient/client (in protecting their health and safety, and ultimately their rights as well) and justice to the wider society (in maintaining lawful order, preventing others from harm, and defending the common good). Ensuring appropriate safeguards for patients'/clients' rights becomes a difficult ethical issue in these circumstances. Within practice, we need to ensure sufficient protections for patients'/clients' rights and apply safeguards as appropriate. This is important given the focus on community services and, while this is appropriate, there needs to be resources to support community-based services that are adequate to support individuals rather than people being recycled back into institutions, such as prisons and the criminal justice system.

In mental health, there is a further irony related to the interpretation of consent to treatment for voluntary patients, for the extent to which their participation is voluntary can be debated, and the consent they are required to give amounts to almost writing a blank cheque. What counts as treatment in psychiatry possibly covers a wider range and is perhaps more inclusive than in any other area of medicine, ranging from protective/involuntary admission, one-to-one psychotherapy to group therapy of various kinds. Also included are a range of other therapies such as electroconvulsive therapy (ECT), behaviour therapy, art therapy and music therapy. It is not always clear as to what the patient/client is consenting to or what will be included in the scope and limits of treatment in the case of any specific patient/client. There is a risk that health professionals will assume the right to simply decide what therapies are in the best interests of the patient/client without consulting the patient/client or relatives to ascertain their will and preferences. In addition, the rights of individuals who have mental health problems may be compromised within the care process such as:

- The right to be adequately informed and to give voluntary consent to treatment.
- The right to privacy and confidentiality (which may be compromised in group therapy and team management).
- The right to refuse treatment and/or to discharge themselves from hospital (where even voluntary patients may fear imposition of a compulsory order if they do not comply).
- The right to vote in general elections, to emigrate or in some cases, even to go on holiday abroad.

GIVING ADEQUATE INFORMATION TO ALLOW FOR VOLUNTARY CONSENT OR REFUSE TREATMENT

An older lady, Mary (80-year-old), has been hospitalised with anaemia, ascites and lower leg oedema. She lives alone and attends a daycare centre for older people. Mary's haemoglobin level is only 4 g/dL, and the anaemia may be caused by stomach bleeding. Examination is necessary, but when this was indicated to Mary, she refused the treatment and said she was too old and the thoughts of a camera going into her stomach terrified her, and she wanted to go home.

In this situation, would you consider this Mary's choice and respect Mary' decision? Given that Mary is anaemic (haemoglobin only 4 g/dL), could this be affecting her competence to make a decision about the situation?

The nurse should give Mary more time to think about it, give her all the relevant information and present all options and possible consequences. This may enable Mary to make an informed choice and choose an option she feels comfortable with. It is important that Mary is given time to discuss the procedure and her fears (why does she feel she is too old, does she feel she deserves treatment, does she feel she will be a burden, and why is she afraid of the camera, does she know what the procedure is and what will happen) and, if she still refuses, can she choose an alternative such as offering a blood transfusion or treatment by another route. This may lead Mary to feel better and be in a better position to make an informed decision about the option the doctor proposed. If after all this Mary still refuses, then this refusal should be accepted with the clear message that should she change her mind, she can return, and ensure that she is given a referral so she receives the help she needs to address the anaemia and enable her to feel better herself.

PRIVACY AND CONFIDENTIALITY

Jack has been attending your clinic, and he has just been told that he is HIV positive and been advised to contact his sexual partners to inform them of his status. In discussion with Jack about starting his course of treatment and informing his sexual partners, he declares he has been in a relationship with Susan for the past 2 years, and they are expecting a baby in 2 months' time.

However, prior to that relationship, Jack had a series of sexual partners. On a subsequent visit to the clinic, it becomes clear that Jack has not told Susan of his HIV status. Being aware of the imminent arrival of their baby, you reiterate to Jack that steps need to be taken to assess whether Susan is HIV positive and whether the baby is at risk so that necessary treatment may be started. Jack adamantly refuses to tell Susan, and says that if she is told without his consent, then he will stop his course of treatment.

What should you do? Can/should you inform Susan, or Jack's GP?

The principle of respect for autonomy requires that personal information should not be disclosed without consent. However, in some cases, the autonomy of another person may also be an issue (in this case Susan and previous sexual partners, as well as the baby when born). Not disclosing information may limit their ability to make decisions as to treatment and lifestyle. Although maintaining confidence of personal information may be the starting point, a balance of the benefits and harms of disclosure/non-disclosure leads to consideration of the consequences of a course of action.

In this scenario, the harms of non-disclosure relate to the risk that Susan may be HIV positive. The consequence of not providing information to enable her to be tested is that she is harmed by not knowing her HIV status and not receiving a course of treatment. If Susan is HIV positive and is not aware of the risk, the consequences are that she will not take steps to minimise the risk of infection to the baby, for example obtaining treatment during pregnancy, baby born by caesarean section, knowing not to breastfeed, prophylactic treatment. If Susan did later find out that there was a risk to her and that she was not informed, she may lose trust in the doctor or the healthcare system. There are also risks to Jack's former sexual partners who could be contacted and informed. The harms of disclosure could include that if others are informed without Jack's consent, then as a consequence of that Jack may lose trust in the healthcare system and healthcare professionals. Jack has also indicated that he will end his course of treatment, thus risking relapse and severe health problems including death. It is necessary to balance the potential harms of non-disclosure with the harms that might result from disclosure without consent in breach of the duty of confidentiality. The harm to Jack in disclosing without his consent is outweighed by the harmful consequences of not disclosing. However, health professionals working in this area may consider that more weight should be given to the loss of trust that might result from breaching confidences. Compelling ethical reasons exist for protecting the privacy of persons with HIV infection, and this justification for privacy resides in the principle of respect for autonomy. To respect the privacy of persons with HIV/AIDS is to respect their wishes not to have intimate information about themselves made available to others. Privacy also enhances the development of trust, a defining characteristic of the healthcare professional patient/client relationship involving freely sharing and giving of private information. Failure to respect the confidentiality of patients/clients can drive them away from testing, counselling and treatment, and discourages patients/clients from confiding in healthcare professionals.

Euthanasia/Right to Die

Euthanasia is a term used rather loosely and can cover situations where a carer, of their own initiative, assists a patient/client to a good death (withhold treatment – passive euthanasia) and the intentional killing of the patient/client by administering a drug or treatment to cause death (active euthanasia). However, the term euthanasia is also used where a patient/client requests assistance to put an end to their suffering (assisted suicide), or has requested in advance (advanced directive or living will) that they do not wish their life to be artificially prolonged if their condition is terminal. This kind of voluntary euthanasia involves the patient/client insisting on respect for their personal wishes and assuming the right to die, or at least demanding to be consulted about the scope and limits of what we indirectly call terminal care/end-of-life care.

Murder or intentional killing of a person with or without their instructions is illegal. Consequently, the legal definition of euthanasia as 'the intentional termination of a patient's/client's life, by act or omission, in the course of medical care' (Cohen and Chambaere 2019) makes the practice morally and legally challenging, irrespective of the overwhelming desire of the patient/client or carer to end the persons suffering and have a pain free death. This presents many ethical clashes between the compulsion to put an end to the hopeless suffering of a patient/client; the ethical duty of protective care the carer is obliged to provide to the patient/client; doing good (beneficence) and avoiding doing harm (non-maleficence) and respecting patient's/client's autonomy and right to choose. Healthcare professionals can feel pressurised by patients/clients who demand respect for their right to die, and the central question is whether we have a right to die, which raises the philosophical question regarding the difference between liberties and rights. Moral and legal rights are justified claims that entitle people to demand that others act or abstain from acting in certain ways, and rights impose either positive or negative duties on others.

In general, law and public morality acknowledges that no one has a right to demand the assistance of another person to terminate their life. In practice, healthcare professionals may feel motivated to stop treatment or life support, or may actively intervene to terminate the life of someone in extreme suffering by the administration of drugs or by other means. However, such action would be illegal, whatever the circumstances, and would be morally sanctioned because carers are expected to sustain life not to end it. Nevertheless, some countries support euthanasia (assisted suicide) and have created a legal right to die, by allowing people the liberty to seek assistance to terminate their lives, under specified conditions. For example, legalisation on euthanasia in the Netherlands is liberal and intended to formally decriminalise acts of euthanasia under certain defined conditions (Emanuel 2017). However, no law permitting voluntary euthanasia can impose a duty on the healthcare professional to perform euthanasia against their will or conscience, and neither can legislation remove the painful tension, for the healthcare professional, between their duty to care and respect for the dignity of the patient/client in a particular situation.

Countries other than Britain have made attempts to legalise euthanasia (Pereira 2011). However, arguments have arisen regarding the ability to build in adequate protections to prevent the misuse of euthanasia by possibly deceitful healthcare professionals or relatives, or both in collusion with one another, to take advantage of someone in a situation of extremity, and the view that introducing such legislation may lead 'down the slippery slope' to 'non-voluntary euthanasia' or intentional killing of the terminally ill (Beckford 2010; Lewis 2007). Such concerns have weight, given the evidence that in the early years of its introduction in the Netherlands, over a period of 15 years, there were 2300 officially notified euthanasia deaths, 4000 cases of physician-assisted suicide and 1000 cases where euthanasia was performed without evidence of a specific request from the patient/client, and in total, 10,500 cases where withdrawal of treatment or increased use of drugs had shortened life (Keown 1995).

Recently, in 2016, medical assistance in dying was legalised in Canada by an amendment to the Criminal Code that removed its prohibition (Pesut et al. 2020). This legalisation allows for healthcare professionals to be both assessors and providers of medical assistance in dying. Two actions to medically assisting the dying are permissible: (1) administering a substance to a person at their request that causes their death (euthanasia) or (2) prescribing or providing a substance to a person at their request so that they may self-administer the substance and, in so doing, cause their own death (assisted suicide) (Supreme Court of Canada 2016). To date, seven countries around the world offer a type of euthanasia: Canada, the Netherlands, Belgium, Columbia, some US states, Switzerland and Luxembourg (Dalhousie University 2019). However, morally complex, ambiguous and emotionally loaded experience and tension continue to exist between respecting an individual's autonomous decision to request euthanasia and upholding one's professional duty to prevent harm (Pesut et al. 2020). Other ethical issues raised included arguments related to ethical concepts, such as the sanctity of life, quality of life, suffering, pain management and slippery slope scenarios. It should be noted that slippery slope arguments are fallacious, in the sense that they are speculative, thus requiring later evidence. Where practised, assisted dying demands clear guidelines, including:

- The patient must have made an explicit and voluntary request for euthanasia.
- The patient must be suffering unbearably and euthanasia should, in such cases, be a last resort.
- The physician must have consulted with another medical practitioner regarding the case.
- The doctor must submit an official report that he/she had complied with the law.

In supporting the life of terminally ill patients/clients, a number of rights have been identified across member states of the European Union (Council of Europe 1999), such as the right to adequate and competent palliative care, the right to self-determination of the dying, rooted in their human dignity and the right to be protected from involuntary euthanasia, or intentional killing by any person. In addition, member states should ensure legal protection for the following rights of the terminally ill:

- The right of access to appropriate and skilled palliative and terminal care.
- The right to truthful, comprehensive, yet compassionately delivered, health information.
- Reaffirmation of the right (enshrined in Article 2 of the European Convention for the Protection of Human Rights and Fundamental Freedoms), namely, 'everyone's right to life shall be protected by law and no one shall be deprived of his life intentionally'.

One of the most commonly expressed fears of the terminally ill is the fear of losing control of their bodily functions, their lives and personal affairs and of the process of dying itself (Andorno and Baffone 2014). Dying itself therefore might be defined in terms of a progressive loss of control (Rodríguez-Prat et al. 2016). Being alive means having some degree of control over one's life and decisions: bodily functions are maintained in a balance, albeit precarious, of homeostasis, and one has some control over one's finances, property and relationships. Part of the pain of death and dying is that it is something that happens to us, it is beyond our control, bodily systems disintegrate or self-destruct, our bodies corrupt and dissolve, we lose control over our futures and fortunes (Cohen-Mansfield et al. 2017). There is even a paradox in death by suicide, as by attempting to remain in control, to assert one's autonomy by taking one's own life, we put an end to our autonomy (Sartre 1969).

We all wish to retain control over our lives for as long as possible. However, an irony arises in the ethics of terminal/hospice care, where staff seek to; respect the autonomy of dying patient/clients, discuss the implications of their impending death, support them through the pre-emptive grief and distress, consult them and respect their wishes regarding how, when and where they wish to die. In this light, good terminal/hospice care, which was supposed to be an alternative to voluntary euthanasia, actually comes closest to it. What should be done and how it should be done, and by whom, can all be agonising questions. The situation may demand that something is done (even non-action is a form of action) and, in reality, no universal prescriptions are possible in such situations, nor would they be appropriate (Hold 2017).

4.4 PAUSE FOR THOUGHT

Your Thoughts

- What does good terminal/hospice care look like?
- Does good terminal/hospice care involve assisting patients/clients to a good death?
- What would this assistance look like and what ethical issues does it create?
- What action and non-actions raise ethical issues for you in your practice?
  Consider the European Convention on Human Rights (2019) Factsheet https://www.echr.coe.int/Documents/FS_Euthanasia_ENG.pdf.

Conclusion

This chapter has examined ethical dilemmas in practice and considered professional core ethical principles and values in ethical decision making. The decision-making framework in Chapter 2 highlighted that to be more effective it involves all stakeholders. This highlights that ethics is not only about responding to difficult dilemmas one faces as an individual but also about professional practice that involves dialogue which supports ethical values and thinking. These values are rooted in professional principles and values and, at times, respecting an individual's rights has to be considered against the wider societal context such as in the case of Jack, the HIV patient/client. We will consider these issues more in the next chapter on responsibility and rights.

References

Allen, F. B., & Coleman, P. G. (2006). Spiritual perspectives on the person with dementia: identity and personhood. In J. C. Hughes, S. J. Louw, & S. R. Sabat (Eds.), *Dementia: mind, meaning, and the person* (pp. 205–221). Oxford: Oxford University Press.

American Nurses Association. (2015). *Code of ethics with interpretative statements*. Silver Spring, MD: American Nurses Association. Online available: https://www.vcuhealth.org/for-health-professionals/nursing/about-nursing-at-vcu/ana-code-ethics.

Andorno, R., & Baffone, C. (2014). Human rights and the moral obligation to alleviate suffering. In R. Green, & N. Palpant (Eds.), *Suffering and bioethics* (pp. 182–200). New York: Oxford University press.

Ausserhofer, D., Zander, B., Busse, R., Schubert, M., De Geest, S., Rafferty, A. M., et al. (2014). Prevalence patterns and predictors of nursing care left undone in European hospitals: results from the multicountry cross-sectional RN4CAST study. *BMJ Quality and Safety*, 2(23), 126–135.

Badzek, L. (2008). Legacy and vision: the perspective of the American Nurses Association on nursing and health care ethics. In W. J. E. Pinch, & A. M. Haddad (Eds.), *Nursing and health care ethics: a legacy and a vision* (pp. 3–6). Silver Spring, MD: American Nurses Association.

Bar-Yam, Y. (2006). Improving the effectiveness of health care and public health: a multiscale complex systems analysis. *American Journal of Public Health*, 96(3), 459–466.

Beckford, M. (2010). *Legal assisted suicide creates 'slippery slope' to doctors killing without consent, expert claims*. The Telegraph. Online available: http://www.telegraph.co.uk/news/uknews/law-and-order/7865305/Legal-assisted-suicide-creates-slippery-slope-to-doctors-killing-without-consent-expert-claims.html.

Beth, B. P. (2017). *Professional nursing concepts and challenge* (8th ed.). St Louis: Saunders Elsevier.

Bickel, W. K., Pope, D. A., Moody, L. N., Snider, S. E., Athamneh, L. N., Stein, J. S., et al. (2016). Decision-based disorders: the challenge of dysfunctional health behavior and the need for a science of behavior change. *Policy Insights From the Behavioral and Brain Sciences*, 4(1), 49–56.

Blake, V. K., Nehrkorn, A. M., & Patrick, J. H. (2017). Differential effects of health-promoting behaviors on wellbeing among adults. *International Journal of Wellbeing*, 7(2), 28–42.

Blasdell, N. D. (2017). The meaning of caring in nursing practice. *International Journal of Nursing and Clinical Practices*, 4, 238.

Brazier, M., & Cave, E. (2016). *Medicine, patients and the law* (6th ed.). Manchester: Manchester University Press.

British Medical Association. (2018). *Confidentiality and disclosure of health information toolkit*. London: British Medical Association. Online available: https://www.bma.org.uk/advice/employment/ethics/confidentiality-and-health-records/confidentiality-and-health-records-tool-kit.

Campbell, L., & McCarthy, J. (2018). *Working together to address ethical challenges in healthcare*. Cork: Irish Examiner. Online available: https://www.irishexaminer.com/breakingnews/views/analysis/working-together-to-address-ethical-challenges-in-healthcare-865409.html.

Canadian Nurses Association. (2017). *Code of Ethics for registered nurses Canadian nurses*. Ottawa, Canada: Canadian Nurses Association. Online available: https://www.cna-aiic.ca/~/media/cna/page-content/pdf-en/code-of-ethics-2017-edition-secure-interactive.

Cohen, J., & Chambaere, K. (2019). Euthanasia. In *Access science*. New York: McGraw-Hill Education. Online available: https://doi.org/10.1036/1097-8542.246850.

Cohen-Mansfield, J., Skornick-Bouchbinder, M., & Brill, S. (2017). Trajectories of end of life: a systematic review. *The Journals of Gerontology: Series B*, 73(4), 564–572.

Cooley, D. R. (2007). A Kantian moral duty for the soon-to-be demented to commit suicide. *The American Journal of Bioethics, 7*(6), 37–44.

Corring, D., O'Reilly, R., & Sommerdyk, C. (2017). A systematic review of the views and experiences of subjects of community treatment orders. *International Journal of Law and Psychiatry, 52,* 74–80.

Council of Europe. (1999). *Parliamentary Assembly of the Council of Europe: protection of the human rights and dignity of the terminally ill and the dying.* (Recommendation 1418). Online available: https://assembly.coe.int/nw/xml/XRef/Xref-DocDetails-en.asp?FileID=16722andlang=en.

Cummings, J., & Bennett, V. (2012). *Compassion in practice: nursing, midwifery and care staff: our vision and strategy gateway reference 18479.* London: Department of Health.

Dalhousie University. (2019). *Assisted dying: end-of-life law and policy in Canada. Halifax.* Nova Scotia: Health Law Institute Dalhousie University. Online available: http://eol.law.dal.ca/?page_id=236.

Delmar, C. (2012). The excesses of care: a matter of understanding the asymmetry of power. *Nursing Philosophy, 13*(4), 236–243.

Department of Health. (2016). *Position paper one, values for nurses and midwives in Ireland.* Dublin: Office of the Chief Nursing Officer, Department of Health.

Dowie, I. (2017). Legal, ethical and professional aspects of duty of care for nurses. *Nursing Standard, 32*(16–19), 47–52.

Emanuel, E. (2017). Euthanasia and physician-assisted suicide: focus on the data. *The Medical Journal of Australia, 206*(8), 339–340.

European Convention on Human Rights. (2019). *End of life and the European Convention on Human Rights – Judgments of the Court Factsheet.* Online available: https://www.echr.coe.int/Documents/FS_Euthanasia_ENG.pdf.

Fleming, V., Frith, L., Luyben, A., & Ramsayer, B. (2018). Conscientious objection to participation in abortion by midwives and nurses: a systematic review of reasons. *BMC Med Ethics, 19*(1), 31.

Francis, R. (2010). *Independent inquiry into care provided by Mid Staffordshire NHS Foundation Trust January 2005 – March 2009.* Vol 1. Chaired by Robert Francis QC. London: Stationary Office.

Francis, R. (2013). *Report of the Mid Staffordshire NHS Foundation Trust Public Inquiry.* Chaired by Robert Francis QC. London: Stationary Office.

Gibson, M. J. (2011). *Nursing students expelled for posting photo of a placenta on Facebook.* Time. Online available: http://newsfeed.time.com/2011/01/04/nursing-students-expelled-for-posting-photo-of-a-placenta-on-facebook/.

Guillaume, A., & Rossier, C. (2018). Abortion around the world: an overview of legislation, measures, trends, and consequences. *Population – English Edition, 73*(2), 217–306.

Gutmacher Institute. (2018). *Abortions: fact sheet.* Online available: https://www.guttmacher.org/fact-sheet/induced-abortion-worldwide.

Hemingway, A. (2013). What is nursing care and who owns it? *Nursing Times, 109*(6), 16–17.

Hilbers, J., Rankin-Smith, H., Horsfall, D., & Aoun, S. M. (2018). We are all in this together: building capacity for a community-centred approach to caring, dying and grieving in Australia. *European Journal for Person Centered Healthcare, 6*(4), 685–692.

Hold, J. L. (2017). A good death: narratives of experiential nursing ethics. *Nursing Ethics, 24*(1), 9–19.

Illich, I. (1975). The medicalization of life. *Journal of medical ethics, 1*(2), 73–77.

International Confederation of Midwives. (2014). *Position statement: collaboration and partnerships for healthy women and infants.* Online available: https://www.internationalmidwives.org/assets/files/statement-files/2018/04/collaboration-and-partnerships-eng.pdf.

International Council of Nurses. (2012). *The ICN Code of Ethics for nurses.* Online available: https://www.icn.ch/sites/default/files/inline-files/2012_ICN_Codeofethicsfornurses_%20eng.pdf.

Irish Supreme Court. (2015). *The status of artificial nutrition and hydration.* Online available: https://www.mondaq.com/ireland/Food-Drugs-Healthcare-Life-Sciences/448094/Withdrawal-Of-Artificial-Nutrition-And-Hydration-Who-Decides.

Johnstone, M. J. (2016). *Bioethics: a nursing perspective* (6th ed.). Chatswood, NSW: Elsevier.

Kayser, J. B. (2014). Ethics, communication and the ICU: charting a course for resolving conflict. *Critical Connections, 13*(4), 1–9.

Keown, J. (1995). *Euthanasia examined: ethical, clinical and legal aspects.* Cambridge: Cambridge University Press.

Kerridge, I., Lowe, M., & McPhee, J. (1998). *Ethics and law for the health professions.* Katoomba, NSW: Social Science Press.

Kitwood, T. (1997). *Dementia reconsidered: the person comes first.* Buckingham: Open University Press.

Leuter, C., Petrucci, C., Mattei, A., Tabassi, G., & Lancia, L. (2013). Ethical difficulties in nursing, educational needs and attitudes about using ethics resources. *Nursing Ethics, 20*(3), 348–358.

Lewis, P. (2007). The empirical slippery slope from voluntary to non-voluntary euthanasia. *The Journal of Law, Medicine and Ethics, 35*(1), 197–210.

Mallari, M. G. D., & Tariman, J. D. (2016). Ethical frameworks for decision-making in nursing practice and research: an integrative literature review. *Journal of Nursing Practice Applications and Reviews of Research, 7*(1), 50–57.

McCance, T. V., McKenna, H. P., & Boore, J. R. P. (1999). Caring: theoretical perspectives of relevance to nursing. *Journal of Advanced Nursing, 30*(6), 1388–1396.

McDonough, D. S. (2019). *Caring: the core of nursing practice.* Brookhaven, MS: Hurst Review services. Online available: https://www.hurstreview.com/blog/caring-the-core-of-nursing-practice.

Nass, S. J., Levit, L. A., & Gostin, L. O. (2009). The value and importance of health information privacy. In S. J. Nass, L. A. Levit, & L. O. Gostin (Eds.), *Beyond the HIPAA privacy rule: enhancing privacy, improving health through research.* Washington, DC: National Academies Press.

Ní Ghráinne, B., & McMahon, A. (2019). Abortion in Northern Ireland and the European Convention on Human Rights: Reflections from the UK Supreme Court. *International and Comparative Law Quarterly, 68*(2), 477–494.

Nursing and Midwifery Board of Ireland. (2014). *Code of professional practice and ethics for registered nurses and midwives.* Dublin: Nursing and Midwifery Board of Ireland. Online available: https://www.nmbi.ie/NMBI/media/NMBI/Code-of-professional-Conduct-and-EthicsAd_2.pdf?ext=.pdf.

Nursing and Midwifery Council. (2018). *The Code: Professional standards of practice and behaviour for nurses, midwives and nursing associates.* London: Nursing and Midwifery Council. Online available: https://www.nmc.org.uk/globalassets/sitedocuments/nmc-publications/nmc-code.pdf.

Nweze, O. J., Agom, A. D., Agom, J. D., & Nwankwo, A. (2015). A critical analysis of the concept of hope: the nursing perspective. *International Journal of Science and Research, 4*(3), 1027–1030.

Olpin, M., & Hesson, M. (2016). The importance of values. In M. Olin, & M. Hesson (Eds.), *Stress management for life: a research-based experiential approach* (pp. 134–149). Belmont, CA: Thomson Higher Education.

Pereira, J. (2011). Legalizing euthanasia or assisted suicide: the illusion of safeguards and controls. *Current Oncology, 18*(2), e38–e45.

Pesut, B., Greig, M., Thorne, S., Storch, J., Burgess, M., Tishelman, C., et al. (2020). Nursing and euthanasia: a narrative review of the nursing ethics literature. *Nursing Ethics, 27*(1), 152–167.

Post, S. G. (2006). Respectare: moral respect for the lives of the deeply forgetful. In J. C. Hughes, S. J. Louw, & S. R. Sabat (Eds.), *Dementia: mind, meaning and the person* (pp. 223–234). Oxford: Oxford University Press.

Potter, D. R., & Fogel, J. (2013). Nurse caring: a review of the literature. *International Journal of Advanced Nursing Studies, 2*(1), 40–45.

Robinson, S., Kendrick, K., & Brown, A. (2003). *Spirituality and the practice of healthcare.* London: Palgrave.

Rodríguez-Prat, A., Monforte-Royo, C., Porta-Sales, J., Escribano, X., & Balaguer, A. (2016). Patient perspectives of dignity, autonomy and control at the end of life: systematic review and meta-ethnography. *PLoS One, 11*(3), e0151435. doi: 10.1371/journal.pone.0151435.

Royal College of Nursing. (2019). *Duty of care.* London: Royal College of Nursing. Online available: https://www.rcn.org.uk/get-help/rcn-advice/duty-of-care.

Sabat, S. R. (2001). *The experience of Alzheimer's disease: life through a tangled veil.* Oxford and Malden, MA: Blackwell.

Salter, B. J. (2008). *Nurses posts brain surgery pictures on Facebook.* Telegraph.co.uk. Online available: http://www.telegraph.co.uk/news/uknews/2583411/Nurses-posts-brain-surgery-pictures-on-Facebook.html.

Sartre, J. P. (1969). *Being and nothingness: an essay on phenomenological ontology.* Oxfordshire: Routledge.

Schmidt, B. J., & McArthur, E. C. (2018). Professional nursing values: a concept analysis. *Nursing Forum, 53*(1), 69–75.

Schoenhofer, S. O. (2002). Choosing personhood: intentionality and the theory of Nursing as caring. *Holistic Nursing Practice, 16*(4), 36–40.

Scott, P. A. (2017). *Key concepts and issues in nursing ethics.* Cham: Springer International Publishing.

Sellman, D. (2011). *What makes a good nurse: why the virtues are important for nurses.* London: Jessica Kingsley Publishers.

Skretkowicz, V. (2010). *Notes on nursing, notes on nursing for the labouring classes.* New York: Springer Publishing Company.

Smith, M. C., & Parker, M. E. (2015). *Nursing theories and nursing practice.* Philadelphia: F. A. Davis.

Smyth, D., & Lane, P. (2016). Abortion in modern health care: Considering the issues for health-care professionals. *International Journal of Nursing Practice, 22*(2), 115–120.

Storch, J. L. (2010). Comment on: Pattison and Wainwright: Is the 2008 NMC code ethical? *Nursing Ethics, 17*(1), 19–21.

Supreme Court of Canada. (2016). *An act to amend the criminal code and to make related amendments to other acts (medical assistance in dying) 2016.* Online available: https://laws-lois.justice.gc.ca/eng/annualstatutes/2016_3/fulltext.html.

Taber, C. W. (2017). *Taber's Cyclopedic Medical Dictionary.* Philadelphia: F. A. Davis Company.

Taylor, C. (1985). *The concept of a person, philosophical papers* (Vol. 1). Cambridge: Cambridge University Press.

The Free Dictionary. (2019). *Caring.* Online available: https://www.thefreedictionary.com.

Thompson, F. E. (2002). Moving from codes of ethics to ethical relationships for midwifery practice. *Nursing Ethics, 9*(5), 522–536.

United Kingdom Supreme Court. (2014). *The case of Doogan and another versus the Greater Glasgow and Clyde Health Board in Scotland, judgment of the on 17 December 2014.* Online available: https://www.supremecourt.uk/cases/docs/uksc-2013-0124-judgment.pdf.

Vance, T. (2003). Caring and the professional practice of nursing. *RN Journal.* Online available: https://rn-journal.com/journal-of-nursing/caring-and-the-professional-practice-of-nursing.

Vincifori, E., & Min, M. M. (2014). Ethical code and professional identity: a survey on Italian midwives. *International Journal of Childbirth, 4*(1), 55–62.

Vivas, M. L. (2012). Cesa IMSS a anestesióloga por burlarse de pacientes en Facebook. Proceso (IMSS ceases to anesthesiologist for mocking patients on Facebook). Online available: http://www.proceso.com.mx/?p=304669.

Warren, M. A. (1973). On the moral and legal status of abortion. *The Monist, 57*, 43–61.

Water, T., Rasmussen, S., Neufeld, M., Gerrard, D., & Ford, K. (2017). Nursing's duty of care: from legal obligation to moral commitment. *Nursing Praxis in New Zealand, 33*(3), 7–20.

Watson, J. (1979). *Nursing: the philosophy and science of caring.* Boston, MA: Little, Brown and Company.

Watson, J. (1997). The theory of human caring: retrospective and prospective. *Nursing Science Quarterly, 10*(1), 49–52.

Watson, J. (2002). Intentionality and caring-healing. Consciousness: a practice of transpersonal nursing. *Holistic Nursing Practice, 16*(4), 12–19.

Watson, J. (2003). Love and caring. Ethics of face and hand—An invitation to return to the heart and soul of nursing and our deep humanity. *Nursing Administration Quarterly, 27*, 197–202.

Watson, J. (2008). *Nursing: the philosophy and science of caring.* Boulder: University Press of Colorado.

World Health Organization. (2012). *Safe abortion: technical and policy guidance for health systems.* Geneva: World Health Organisation. Online available: https://apps.who.int/iris/bitstream/handle/10665/70914/9789241548434_eng.pdf?sequence=1.

Wright, D., & Brajtman, S. (2011). Relational and embodied knowing: nursing ethics within the interprofessional team. *Nursing Ethics, 18*(1), 20–30.

Zahedi, F., Sanjari, M., Aala, M., Peymani, M., Aramesh, K., Parsapour, A., et al. (2013). The code of ethics for nurses. *Iranian Journal of Public Health, 42*(Suppl. 1), 1–8.

CHAPTER 5

Responsibilities and Rights in Nurse–Patient/Client Relationships

LEARNING OUTCOMES

When you have read and worked through this chapter, you should be able to:
- Understand the concepts of rights and duties as relevant in everyday practice
- Understand and distinguish between the concepts liberties, rights and duties
- Consider the rights and duties of nurses in dealing with patients/clients
- Consider the rights of people as patients/clients
- Illustrate the nature of patient's/client's rights by discussing examples of particular cases
- Consider conflicting rights and duties of patients/clients, staff and stakeholders in analysing work-related case studies
- Consider how changes in dependency level and power relations impact on patient/client rights

Introduction

Healthcare professionals and healthcare facilities need to recognise patients'/clients' rights and, on the other side of the coin, patients/clients need to recognise healthcare professionals' right to expect certain behaviour on the part of patients/clients. One's rights are fundamental to ethics and, within a practice context, balancing one's rights can often be difficult and requires dialogue and discussion among the key stakeholders. Modern healthcare recognises all patients'/clients' rights such as information, fair treatment and autonomy. When healthcare professionals and patients/clients understand and accept their rights and responsibilities, they become partners in care. To highlight rights issues, this chapter discusses cases related to truth telling, resuscitation, consent to treatment and oversedation.

Rights and Duties

In the previous chapter, we presented ethics of caring and general ethics based on principles, values and codes. We now look at ethics within the one-to-one relationship of the nurse and the patient/client, in hospital or community settings. To begin we consider the concepts of 'rights' and 'duties' and how these apply in various situations in nursing. Within a care context, healthcare professionals can have power over people, as the person can be at their most vulnerable and dependent; also, the healthcare professional has privileged and intimate access to patients'/clients', both in terms of their bodies and their private lives (Rowland and Kuper 2018). Thus, duty of care and other general duties of healthcare professionals are a focus for consideration. In addition, the focus on patients'/clients' rights in the context of such relationships has been emphasised since the United Nations (UN) Universal Declaration of Human Rights (UN 1948). These rights are reinforced through consumer rights and patient/client advocacy groups placing a demand for rights and equitable access to health and social services, resulting in the development of patients'/clients' rights and charters (Gilmour and Huntington 2017).

Likewise, we must recognise the rights of healthcare professionals who are expected to fulfil their duty but have had to become more vocal in campaigning for their own rights, for example wages and working conditions. In the healthcare context, the patient's/client's degree of independence or dependence impacts on the ethics of the situation and the weight given to the duties of the healthcare professional relative to the rights of the patient/client and vice versa (Stuart 2018). This is evident in practice where the balance of rights and duties change with the degree of dependency or independence/autonomy of the patient/client, for example the patient's/client's right to know will be differently interpreted if the patient/client is unconscious, very distressed or anxious, compared with when they are conscious and in possession of their full capabilities. In an emergency department, a healthcare professional's first duty to the patient/client is to respond instantly to the patient's/client's right to appropriate care and treatment. As rights are interpreted differently depending on situational demands, it is necessary to clarify what we mean by rights and duties, and how they are related and distinguished and how they apply in a healthcare context.

The Meaning of 'Rights' and 'Duties'

In the previous chapter, the issues of abortion and euthanasia raised the aspect of distinguishing between liberties and rights, and moral and legal rights were considered. Moral and legal rights are justified entitlements that permit us to demand that others either act, or abstain from acting, in certain ways. Thereby, rights can impose either positive or negative duties on others (West 2017). Thus, rights and duties are connected and, simply put, particular rights and duties exist where we are subject to rules or agreements with other people. A promise made by a healthcare professional to a patient/client creates an expectation for the patient/client that the healthcare professional will recognise this obligation and keep their promise, and failing to do so will undermine the patient's/client's trust in that healthcare professional, and possibly in healthcare professionals generally (Egener et al. 2017).

In distinguishing liberties and rights, if we concede that other people have certain rights, then recognition of their rights imposes certain duties or obligations on us, but the same is not true of our freedom or liberty to do something. For example, smokers often claim that they have a right to smoke, but we don't have a duty or obligation to enable them to indulge their habit as no one is obliged, if they do not want to, to provide us with smoking breaks or rooms in which to smoke. However, if someone is over the legal age, they do have the liberty to purchase and smoke cigarettes (and damage their health) without being restricted or prevented by others (unless their habit is harming others). Whereas there is a mutual and corresponding relationship between rights and obligations, there is no positive mutual relation between liberties and duties (Farquhar et al. 2018). A liberty is something we can do without, being subject to sanctions or physically prevented from doing it, provided that it does not interfere with the liberties of others. For example, in the previous chapter we saw that if a termination of pregnancy is permitted or has been decriminalised, then a woman has the liberty to terminate a pregnancy and to request others to assist her to do so, without being prosecuted or physically prevented from exercising this liberty. However, such permissive legislation does not create a right or entitlement of a woman to demand that termination services are provided as a public duty.

Patients/clients are regularly at risk of having their rights compromised or abused, because of their confined state as residents of organisations of various kinds (Runciman et al. 2017). Particularly vulnerable are the frail elderly, patients/clients with advanced dementia, intellectual disability or with severe mental health problems. Healthcare professionals are expected to respect the rights of patients/clients and to exercise a protective duty of care and responsibility towards patients/clients committed into their care (Kpanake et al. 2018). However, in practice, there are situations where healthcare professionals may sometimes feel that in the interests of a patient/client, rights may have to be compromised (Adshead and Davies 2016); for example, the rights to refuse treatment (or the right not to be treated without one's consent) and to not have private information shared with others, or divulged to anyone else without one's permission. These negative rights of patients/clients are also subject to legal safeguards, in such measure as treatment without consent is treated in the law as a form of criminal assault regardless of the good intentions of the healthcare professional; and breach of a patient's/client's confidences may be subject to claims for damages in a civil court. Nevertheless, there are borderline and difficult situations where healthcare professionals may have to decide to treat a patient/client against their will, or pass on confidential information, such as where the patient's/client's competence is in doubt, there is a grave risk to the life of the patient/client or where sharing the information with a professional colleague is essential for their proper care and treatment.

In the last chapter, we considered Jack (HIV case) and Mary (anaemia case). Now consider Peter, a 25-year-old man who was involved in an altercation resulting in a 7 cm laceration to his forehead. Peter presented to your emergency department with the laceration and slurred speech, and admits that he has been out drinking for the day. The emergency department is very busy with urgent cases, and Peter becomes impatient as a result of waiting and wishes to leave. He states that he will not wait any longer and intends to drive himself home. Whereas there may be little risk to Peter, as there may be few life-threatening complications from the laceration, we need to understand why Peter wishes to leave the emergency department. Does Peter fully understand the need for and the risks and benefits of the procedure? Also, is Peter competent to make this decision in an intoxicated state? Whilst life-threatening complications from the laceration are low, will not having the laceration repaired affect Peters quality of life? Could a laceration not sutured affect Peter in his job or gaining employment? Do you, as a healthcare professional, have any obligation to third parties (i.e. those who may be travelling at the same time as Peter, and who may be endangered from a safety standpoint)? The conflict in this case is between the patient's right to autonomy and self-determination and the healthcare professionals concern for his well-being and the safety of others. From both a legal and ethical standpoint, competent adults have the right to decide whether they will accept treatment. This right relates to the ethical principle of autonomy and informed consent.

From an ethical standpoint, Peter is a capable decision maker if:

- He can understand information relevant to the decision at hand.
- He can interact and communicate with caregivers about the decision.
- He can weigh the possible alternatives.

Given these guidelines, Peter is capable of refusing treatment, despite the feelings of staff about the necessity of suturing the wound. But what about the third parties who may be affected by Peter's decision to drive while intoxicated? Do healthcare professionals have a duty to prevent him from driving? In instances such as these, care providers must remember that their first duty is to the patient/client. A decision to violate patient/client confidentiality or to detain the patient/client against their will, automatically places the caregivers in a position that may require justification of actions. If the patient/client is clearly too intoxicated to drive, a prudent course of action would be to document that the patient/client was asked to stay, and that he was advised that if he chose to leave, his licence plate number would be passed on to the authorities (police). Are there policies and procedures, guidelines and protocols in your facility to assist/guide you in these situations?

Whilst protocols and codes that give guidance are important, the eventual judgement is down to the integrity of the practitioner. As noted in Chapter 3, integrity involves an integration of virtues, enabling deliberation (see also Chapter 11). Integrity is focused on the identity of the nurse and any other healthcare practitioner (Macaulay 2018). It is focused on judgement, ownership of that judgement rather than an obligation determined by ethical rules and on consistency with identity (West 2019). It links to *phronesis*, enabling judgement, and allowing the person to see him- or herself in relation to the situation. Phrases like 'I cannot see myself doing that' indicate an awareness of identity. The ethical identity of the nurse is personal, professional and in the wider institutions and healthcare project. Hence, the guidance of the profession and the institutions has to be taken into account (Barsky 2019). Another aspect of integrity and nursing is membership of the academic community, in teaching, learning and research (see Chapter 7). From a research standpoint, the professional academic discipline of healthcare research has had an official set of rules and responsibilities for its members regarding research professional behaviour with patients/clients, colleagues and other health professionals from as early as the 1950s (Epstein and Turner 2015). The principles they present tend to focus on principles and rights (respect, privacy, confidentiality, trust-rapport, etc.), safety and collaboration with participants to promote health and well-being (West 2019; Lachman et al. 2015). The intention of such rights is to contribute to integrity, not simply of the individual nurse but of the profession, and of the healthcare organisations and academic institutions in which he or she practices. Responsibility for that integrity, then, is shared across the healthcare project.

Institutional, Legal and Moral Rights

Broadly speaking, we may distinguish between institutional and legal rights on the one hand, and moral rights on the other. With reference to the patient's/client's rights, the term is being used in a double sense, both a legal and a moral sense. Legal rights must be enacted by competent legal authorities, such as parliament, regional or local authorities; or must be based on bills of rights, such as the United Nations (UN) Universal Declaration of Human Rights (UN 1948) or the European Convention on Human Rights (Council of Europe 1950). Alternatively, they must be based on common law or natural law, that is, the body of principle and precedent embodied in the legal tradition of the country. In fact, if we consider the way that the term 'rights' is used in political life, in the general rhetoric of politicians and in the activity of pressure groups, it is significant that both groups are seeking as a rule to clarify or extend the scope of the law, or to mobilise public opinion to change the law (Hall et al. 2018). Thus, debate about the woman's right to choose (to terminate a pregnancy on demand), the right to free healthcare, the rights of the unborn child or the right to die, are all concerned with the actual or possible reform of the law in the light of what people believe are their moral rights, or ones they claim on behalf of other people. Institutional rights are created by, and can be abolished by, decisions of people with competent authority (Hall et al. 2018).

5.1 PAUSE FOR THOUGHT

Moral and Legal Rights and Duties

- What situations in your practice impose either negative or positive duties or obligations on you?
- Have you ever had to deal with negative rights (e.g. the right to demand that a person or persons desist from doing something – refuse treatment), and how did you address that situation?
- How do you support positive rights (e.g. the right to some social, personal or institutional benefit or provision – supporting a peaceful death, pain relief, appropriate information, a caring and private environment)?
- How do you uphold moral rights (a justified claim that places a demand on you to act or desist from acting in certain ways, e.g. a moral right to be treated with dignity)?
- Does a moral right create a legal obligation on you to respect that right and what moral rights are legal?
- A legal right creates a legal obligation, and legal rights can also be moral rights, but not all moral rights are legal rights. Most legal rights tend to stem from negative rights rather than positive rights (cessation of unwanted interventions rather than the delivery of appropriate care). Consider what legal rights apply to your practice area?

Rights and Duties When Dealing With Patients/Clients

When we consider practice situations, they present many recurrent moral dilemmas, mainly in the healthcare professional–patient/client relationship, that raise essential questions about the rights of patients/clients and the extent and bounds of professional responsibility (Fenwick 2016). Quandaries such as to tell or not to tell, to treat or not to treat, to limit the patient's/client's freedom and which patient's/client's welfare or needs take priority, all raise questions related to patients'/clients' and the fundamental moral principles of justice, beneficence and respect for persons. One approach would be to attempt to derive patients'/clients' rights from their general human rights such as the Universal Declaration of Human Rights (UN 1948). These rights include certain health rights, but more specific rights of people as patients/clients have derived from these general rights. However, another approach might be to start with the contract-to-care between the healthcare professional and patient/client, to examine the implicit assumptions involved in such contracts and analyse their moral and legal implications. In general, when people have a health problem, they seek help and go to a healthcare service and register or are admitted. This constitutes one kind of contract, and the subject of the initial consultation relates to the boundaries of another kind of contract, that is the healthcare professional negotiation of the right to assess/interview the patient/client and record their details and history (medical, social, family), and the right to undertake an examination (physical) of the patient/client and perhaps conduct a series of tests. The patient's/client's agreement in this process consists of a recognition of the patient's/client's duty to collaborate, and all of this is crucial, but preliminary to the more formal contract-to-care. The contract-to-care only comes into existence once the healthcare professional offers a diagnosis and suggests possible options of treatment, and the patient/client accepts this opinion. The (informed) consent to treatment by the patient/client is an essential part of the contract, as the patient/client entrusts him- or herself into the professional carer's hands. The healthcare professional then takes responsibility for the care and treatment of the patient/client and decides what form this should take.

In your context, it is useful to think through the process by which a person negotiates the help they require from a specific carer, and what assumptions underlie the agreements made. In general, the specific rights of people as patients/clients flow from the kind of relationship into which they enter with the healthcare professional. The relationships between the rights and duties of patient/client and healthcare professional vary in each type of situation. When a patient/client is lucid, ambulant, continent and capable of approaching the health services autonomously for help, there is a kind of contract established in which the patient/client agrees to cooperate in investigations, treatment and rehabilitation, in return for fitting therapy and supportive care. Here, the person independently approaches the health services for help with a health problem, and an implicit or explicit contract-to-care is established through negotiation. In such a contract, there are rights and duties on the part of the patient/client and corresponding duties and rights on the part of the carer. The situation is rather different if the patient/client enters the care situation unconscious, or is unable to consult because of the specific nature of his condition, injury or severe mental illness. Here, the healthcare professional has to assume responsibility for the patient/client and rely on their own and their professional code for guidance. This situation is the traditional relationship between carer and patient/client which is one of crisis intervention, where the person is unconscious or incompetent and the healthcare professional is expected to exercise a protective duty of care towards the vulnerable patient/client, governed by the code of practice of the profession.

When a person approaches a healthcare professional for help, the healthcare professional has the right to refuse to help that particular person. They might legitimately refuse for several kinds of reasons, for example:

- if they are related to the patient/client or the patient/client is in a dependent relationship to them.
- if they have such a heavy caseload already that they could not provide adequate care and support to the particular person.
- if they do not believe they have the necessary competence.
- if the person is being abusive and unpleasant, and they do not wish to have that person as a client.

If healthcare professionals refuse patients/clients on such grounds, they would be exercising their ordinary moral rights, but they would also have a professional duty to refer the person on to someone else who might be willing and able to help the patient/client with their problem. Refusal would be justified on the grounds that carers have the right not to be exploited or to have heavier demands imposed on them than they could reasonably be expected to cope with. Furthermore, healthcare professionals have a duty, in justice to their patients/clients, not to take on more patients/clients than they could possibly provide adequate care for. So, too, in the case of difficult patients/clients; refusal to take them on may be in the patients'/clients' interests as well as the carers. In these examples, the rights in question would appear to be derivable mainly from considerations of justice, although respect for persons comes into play as well.

Once the carer agrees to take on the person seeking help, the carer acquires responsibility for the patient/client, that is, a responsibility to look after a patient's/client's interests and to protect their rights. This responsibility follows from the trust the patient/client shows in the healthcare professional, but the patient/client also has responsibilities towards the healthcare professional. This is shown as soon as the carer proceeds to assess/interview the patient/client in order to develop a proper care pathway/plan. The general expectations underpinning the application of these rights by carers are that they are eligible to these privileges of intimacy as they are exercising a beneficent duty to care (see Chapter 2), in the interests of the patient/client (Sim 1995). Patients/clients have a corresponding obligation to answer truthfully the questions asked about them and their problems, and a duty to cooperate in treatment, if they are to be entitled to healthcare assistance, treatment and care.

Healthcare professionals not only have a fundamental duty to protect the interests of and to care for people who have entrusted themselves into their care, but they also have an obligation to provide patients/clients with the relevant information concerning their diagnosis and proposed methods of care and treatment. This is in return for the patient/client cooperation and to enable the them to make an informed choice as to whether or not they wish to continue with care/treatment (Kpanake et al. 2018). Here, the health professional has a fundamental duty to safeguard that the consent to treatment given by the patient/client is both fully informed and voluntary. This means that the information provided to the patient/client must be in an accessible format, appropriate for that patient/client rather than that of professionals. The patient's/client's consent must not be obtained under pressure, when the patient/client is confused, or when subject to extreme stress or anxiety, as they are unlikely to be able to process the crucial information, even if they are capable of understanding it. Health professionals have a duty to provide patients/clients with all the necessary information they require to make an informed decision about their treatment options, or the drugs or procedures involved in their treatment, including the degree of risk and possible complications involved.

5.2 PAUSE FOR THOUGHT

Gaining Consent

Consider the consent process within your care situations:
- Is the consent gained in your practice truly voluntary or fully informed?
- What difficulties do you have in determining whether consent is voluntary or fully informed?
- Does being unwell physically or mentally place the patient/client under duress?
- What limitations are on patients/clients due to their illness that may impact on their ability to dissent from what the healthcare professional proposes by way of action/treatment?
- How do you decide how much information is enough?
- How fully must all the possible risks of treatment or side effects of treatment be discussed with a patient/client?

The Rights of People as Patients/Clients

In healthcare, caring, treating and promoting health in the preservation of human life is of significance, so patients'/clients' rights become more important and must be recognised and safeguarded. Patient/client rights include adherence to standard physical, psychological, social and spiritual needs, and healthcare systems in many countries have developed a patient/client bill of rights, which are vital responsibilities of all levels of management. In recent years, there have been significant efforts made worldwide to establish and maintain patient/client rights. This is directly related to improved overall value and respect of all persons, that is human rights, which are based on the concept that all people deserve respect. Today, patients must be involved participants in their own care, rather than just being passive receivers of services, and this requires enhanced awareness by both patients/clients and healthcare professionals.

The Universal Declaration of Human Rights (UN 1948) recognises the inherent dignity and equal and unalienable rights of all members of society, and it was based upon the concepts within the UN Declaration (dignity and equality) that the concept of patient/client rights advanced. Patients'/clients' rights differ across countries and jurisdictions, often depending upon dominant social and cultural norms and different models of professional relationships that exist, and these inform the rights to which patients/clients are entitled (Sygit and Wąsik 2016). Four such models that represent this relationship include the paternalistic model, interpretive model, informative model and deliberative model. Each model advocates different professional responsibilities towards the patient/client (Universal Patient Rights Association – UPRA 2019). For example, in the paternalistic model, the best interests of the patient/client are adjudicated by the healthcare professional, and this is valued above the provision of thorough information and decision-making power of the patient/client. In contrast, the informative model recognises the patient/client as a valued member of the process who is in the best position to judge what is in their own interest, and views the healthcare professional as primarily a provider of information (UPRA 2019).

Although debate exists as to how best to consider the relationship, there is international agreement that all patients/clients have an essential right to privacy, confidentiality, consent to or refuse treatment and to be informed about the relevant risk of treatments/procedures.

Some of the earliest attempts to formulate the rights of patients/clients was The Patients' Bill of Rights put forward by the American Hospital Association (1973 and revised 1992) and a Patient Charter (Department of Health – DoH 1991) in the United Kingdom, which has been subsequently replaced by the National Health Service (NHS) Constitution for England (DoH 2015, see Chapters 10 and 11 for discussions on patients and staff rights and responsibilities in the NHS UK Constitution). At a European level, the Charter of Patients' Rights (Active Citizenship Network 2002) identifies 14 patients' rights that together aim to assure a high level of human health protection and quality of services provided by national health services across Europe. The 14 patients' rights (Table 5.1) are an example of essential rights and are interrelated with duties and responsibilities that both citizens and healthcare professionals have to assume (Active Citizenship Network 2002).

Within practice, when a patient/client presents they are the owner of their own information and, through the assessment/interview stage, the healthcare professional gains access to private information about the patient/client. If investigations are warranted, the patient/client is entitled to be provided with the diagnosis, proposed treatment and sufficient information to enable the person to make an informed decision. As part of this process, the healthcare professional will discuss with the patient/client the proposed course of treatment/management of the health problem, and possible options and outcomes. In instances where a patient/client is dying or when bad news regarding a prognosis has to be delivered to the patient/client, a healthcare professional may feel that they have a duty to protect the patient from information which they feel may be too painful for the patient/client to bear or which the patient/client is not yet ready to receive. In such cases, there is a tension between the patient's/client's right to know and the professional's duty to care, and it can be further complicated by relatives who demand that the patient/client should not be told. How this tension is resolved in practice may be decided on an individual basis and in such cases, whose rights are to be given priority? However, even if a healthcare professional decides that providing the patient/client with the diagnosis is contraindicated because it may cause physical and/or psychological harm to the patient/client, this does not justify a professional deciding to breach the duty of confidentiality by informing the patient's/client's relatives of the diagnosis. Practice situations and the exercising of professional judgement involve practical wisdom (see Chapter 3), judgement and sensitivity to the values appropriate in a specific situation, and cannot be made a matter of law and regulation.

The right to privacy covers both the right to respect the dignity of the person (physical privacy) and respect their information (confidentiality) (Brännmark 2017). The right to privacy does not mean the right to have a private ward and, whilst most people coming into the hospital may expect some general loss of privacy, it often comes as a shock to people as to how little privacy they have. Whereas individual healthcare professionals may differ in their understanding of a patient's/client's needs, the routines and physical environment in overcrowded or mixed wards may not be conducive to provide sufficient safeguards for patient privacy, or scope for healthcare professionals to hold confidential discussions with patients/clients, family members or other healthcare staff. There can, in practice, be a tension here between the scope for individual agency and structural constraints, and even if healthcare staff recognise and wish to meet patients'/clients privacy rights, the physical and managerial structures within which care is delivered may inhibit this. However, usually people are willing to share their information, bare their bodies and expose their vulnerabilities when they need help and when they feel they can trust the person that is providing the care to assist them in their recovery. In such a situation, thoughtful carers will respect the patient's/client's confidences in them and only use patient/client information for the benefit of the patient/client and advocate on behalf of the patient/client to protect their rights and interests, in the light of what they know about the patient/client.

TABLE 5.1 ■ **Fourteen Patient Rights**

Right to preventive measures	Each patient/client has the right to an appropriate service in order to avoid illness.
Right of access	Each patient/client has the right of access to health services appropriate to their health needs. This access to health services should be assured for persons equally without prejudice or discrimination on the basis of financial, residence, illness or time of access.
Right to information	Every patient/client has the right to access all information concerning their health, the health services and the evidence from scientific research and technological innovation.
Right to consent	Every patient/client has the right of access to all information that would assist them to participate in the decision-making process pertaining to their health. This is a requirement for procedures, treatment and involvement in research.
Right to free choice	Every patient/client has the right to freely choose from different treatment options and providers based on adequate information having been provided.
Right to privacy and confidentiality	Every patient/client has the right to confidentiality, where their personal information, including information regarding their health status, diagnosis and treatment, is protected at all times.
Right to respect of patients' time	Every patient/client has the right to receive essential treatment in a timely manner within a scheduled period of time.
Right to the observance of quality standards	Every patient/client has the right to have access to a high-quality health service based on a benchmarked standard.
Right to safety	Every patient/client has the right to be free from harm and have access to services and treatments that meet high safety standards.
Right to innovation	Every patient/client has the right of access to advanced procedures, in accordance with international standards independent of economic factors.
Right to avoid unnecessary suffering and pain	Every patient/client has the right to escape as much pain and suffering as possible.
Right to personalised treatment	Every patient/client has the right to care and treatment personalised to their needs.
Right to complain	Every patient/client has the right to complain whenever they have suffered a harm and receive a response and feedback to their complaint.
Right to compensation	Every patient/client has the right to receive appropriate compensation within a reasonable time frame whenever they have suffered a harm resulting from a health service treatment.

From Active Citizenship Network. (2002). *European Charter of Patients' Rights*. Online available: http://www. ehltf.info/joomla/indexphp/en/ehltf/patients-rights/.

Healthcare professionals may be expected to reveal information if it is probable that a patient's/client's condition may put the lives of other people at risk. The patient's/client's personal right to privacy has to be balanced against protection of the right to life of others, and the question is: which right is to be given priority? In such circumstances, especially where the patient's/client's safety or welfare is at risk, the nurse may have to decide, on the principle of beneficence, that her duty to care takes priority over the patient's/client's right to forbid disclosure of vital facts (Nursing and Midwifery Council – NMC 2018). Healthcare professionals are given great power to help or harm people by the information people share with them, and with this power goes great responsibility on the part of all those in the healthcare profession (Keatings and Adams 2019).

Telling the Truth to Patients or Relatives

John was diagnosed with acute lymphoblastic leukaemia at the age of 10, and over the following 3.5 years he was admitted to hospital on many occasions, with increasing frequency in the past 12 months. The staff in the hospital had developed a good relationship with John and his family over the years and during hospital stays. As in many cases, initially John's parents had difficulty accepting the diagnosis and the fear associated with such a diagnosis, but with much support, re-assurance and information, they eventually were accepting of their situation as best as one can be. Three and a half years after John's first admission and subsequent diagnosis, John was admitted and identified as end-of-life. During the time since diagnosis, John's parents had been resolute that John should not be told what was wrong with him, only that he was sick and needed to get treatment every time he got unwell. This was still the case now, but the situation now was that John was receiving end-of-life care rather than curative or preventive care. This was discussed with John's parents and also the fact that if he enquired, it might help him to know the truth, but John's parents refused for him be told. Three days before John died, he asked outright if he was going to die as he felt he was getting worse rather than better, and he asked directly what it was like to die. In spite of John's parents' wishes, the nurse felt that they had to be truthful with John. The nurse talked about the death and explained that everyone would die eventually, and that it was ok to let go when it is too difficult to fight. The nurse and parents were with John when he passed, and he died peacefully and calmly. Here, the nurse felt they did the right thing in telling John, but felt they had betrayed the trust of his parents, which had developed over the previous 3.5 years.

Considering the situation faced by the nurse in this case, it is obvious that the nurse recognised that knowing the truth that John was dying imposed certain responsibilities on her, to protect John's vulnerability (a feeling she shared with John's parents), but she also recognised that John had a right to know the truth. The dilemma she faced was the conflict of loyalties to John and to John's parents, because of the trust and understanding that had grown between the nurse and John on one hand, and between the nurse and John's parents on the other. The problem was made more difficult by the nurse's uncertainty that it was right to tell John because he was technically still a minor, and the nurse's sense of guilt at going against the wishes of his parents. On the other hand, the nurse was also aware of having been specially chosen by John as the one to ask this momentous question. Was it not possible that the distraught parents, faced with loss of their son, were using the nurse in a vain attempt to reassert their rights over their son? In such a situation, which does the nurse put first: the rights of the parents or the rights of the patient/client? It is questionable whether doctors or nurses, or relatives, ever have a right to keep information from a dying patient. Whose death is it anyway? If the dying patient does not have a fundamental right to know that they are dying, who has? However, in this case, the patient was a child, 10 years old when lympho-blastic leukaemia was first diagnosed, and only 14 when he died. Both the nurse and the parents assumed that they had a duty to protect John from the knowledge of his impending death because John was a child. But did they have the right to deny John this knowledge? Initially as John was so young, the nurse felt that the parents were right to protect John from the painful truth, but as John grew older and his health status changed and he asked more searching questions, the nurse's attitude changed. However, did John have any more right to know at age 14 than at age 10? Are parents or relatives of dying patients entitled to withhold the truth from them however young or old they are?

The right to know arises from the principle of respect for persons. If people are to be treated as persons with rights, for example the right to make informed choices, the right to autonomy, that is, to be in control of their own lives, then they cannot be deprived of the knowledge or information which will empower them to make significant life choices. The popular catch is that ignorance is bliss, but many studies show that dying patients/clients are often frightened because they do not know what is going on, are too afraid to ask questions and are aware of the conspiracy of silence around them (Funk et al. 2018; Martín et al. 2016; Terry et al. 2006). Contrary to common belief, dying patients/clients are often comforted by knowing their prognosis, as the anxiety based on doubt and uncertainty ends, and there is evidence that the condition of patients/clients may improve (Bergqvist and Strang 2019; Clayton et al. 2008). The patient/client has a right to know (particularly if the patient/client asks), and good care accepts the knowing collaboration of the patient/client (Ewuoso et al. 2017). The conspiracy of silence around the dying patient deceives no one, except perhaps the conspirators themselves, as when patients/clients are not informed, most nevertheless know that they are dying (Atout et al. 2019; Bluebond-Langner 1978). Not surprisingly, patients pick up this information anyway from various sources: by likening their symptoms and treatment to that of other patients/clients, by what they learn from exchanges with other patients/clients and healthcare professionals, by observation of their own weakening condition and what they deduce from the non-verbal communication of healthcare professionals (hushed voices, trying to silently pass by the bed, telling looks, overattentive care). Patients/clients do not give up when they are informed that their condition is terminal, provided they are given appropriate emotional support, and time to come to terms with dying (Scambler 2018). The issue is that knowledge is power, and deliberately keeping information from another person is to deprive them of power, which results in a state of dependency and powerlessness. The attitude of John's parents had the effect of infantilising John, depriving John of the chance to discuss with them his grief and anxiety of facing death. The parent's shielding paternalism reflects the attitudes often assumed by healthcare professionals in being more concerned to safeguard patients/clients than to respect their rights as persons to know and choose for themselves.

Consider another case where a woman in labour develops complications, loses consciousness and starts haemorrhaging. She was rushed to theatre and an emergency caesarean section is performed. The baby is delivered by caesarean section but is stillborn. The midwife caring for the woman and her partner is aware of the stillbirth and is present when the woman starts regaining consciousness and asking to see her baby. How, when and where does the midwife tell the mother that her baby has died? Should she tell the absent father (who was not present in theatre) first before the woman regains consciousness? Should the midwife call for the doctor and get around the difficulty that way? Should the midwife avoid telling the mother till the father is present and can comfort his wife? Should she arrange for the couple to see the baby? How does she cope with her own grief, her need to appear strong in order to comfort the parents and to continue providing care to the mother?

Here, the mother has a right to know, and the grief cannot be avoided or delayed. However, the midwife cannot simply coldly deliver the facts as they are, without considering the consequences for the mother and father. Being truthful brings with it the difficult responsibility of deciding how much truth a person can take at a given time, and how full disclosure should be delivered in specific circumstances. The questions for the midwife are whether she can cope with being the one who tells, who shares the mother's grief and the mother's likely sense of her own failure and who is available to provide ongoing support afterwards. The reservation which the midwife feels about sharing the truth in this situation, particularly if there is no convenient way out of facing the challenge, probably has more to do with her fear of accepting the responsibility for telling the truth, than any uncertainty about the mother's rights. Sharing the truth can be a costly business. Once the midwife accepts the responsibility to tell the mother, she implicitly commits herself to share her grief (and that of her partner as well). If the midwife knows anything about loss and bereavement, she will also know that telling parents that a longed-for baby has died will not only cause them immediate grief but will initiate a process, which may take many months to work through. The midwife will also know that she has a duty to continue with support for as long as possible, while the parents deal with their bereavement.

Truth sharing means accepting responsibility to share the pain and grief, anger and despair, shock and depression which knowing the truth may cause. If there is not a firm understanding of the relationship between trust and caring, or if it is not possible for the midwife to provide continuing support to the individual concerned, then telling the truth may be cruel and irresponsible (Ling et al. 2019; Tang 2019; Rising 2017). Sharing painful truth requires great sensitivity and skill in judging how, when and where it is appropriate to tell. Once the midwife accepts the responsibility to tell the mother, she also has to face the difficult practical decisions, requiring tact and judgement, of whether the mother will be most helped by being allowed to hold her dead baby, or needs to be protected from an experience which may be too painful for her to bear or which she is not yet ready for.

In healthcare, being honest with other people is a measure of how much we honour them, how much we trust and respect them as a person. The virtue of honesty, or truthfulness, is being sensitive to where other people are at, in their own present experience and ability to cope. In making an assessment of a patient/client, the nurse/midwife will not only have to rely on her own common sense, but also on the opinions of her colleagues and perhaps the relatives. But the nurse/midwife can never shelve her responsibility by relying on, or being tied by, the opinions of others. Sooner or later, all nurses/midwives will have to face situations where they have to accept responsibility for sharing the painful truth with patients/clients, and this means becoming skilled at titration of the truth to the needs of the patient/clients.

A different but related problem about sharing information arises when a dying patient/client knows the truth yet refuses to let the healthcare staff inform their loved one or family. Here, in no direct sense do the relatives have a right to know since it is not their death that is at issue, but as people who are intimately involved and likely to be affected by the patient's/client's death, the nurse/midwife may feel that they ought to be told. As we do not exist in isolation from other people, least of all from our families in most cases, family members also have a right to know (though in an extended sense of right) based on both considerations of compassion and the reciprocal responsibilities which are obtained in families and close communities. Faced with such a situation, a nurse may be assisted by discussing the matter with the person forbidding the disclosure of information, to raise awareness of how the interests of others are involved, and to help them see what comfort may be gained by sharing the truth and the grief together. From the examples above, John's parents might have been persuaded to tell John themselves (with or without the support of the medical and nursing staff); the husband might be assisted to tell his wife about the stillborn baby himself, with the midwife providing support. In the situation of dying patients not wanting their loved one or family to be informed, the nurse might need to encourage and assist them to share their anxieties about dying with their loved one and family and to set their affairs in order. However, if they still refuse, the nurse may be able to gain moral support from discussion with other members of staff. This dynamic of reflection and consultation reinforces the point that care is essentially shared amongst the different stakeholders, with each making sense of the situation and how they respond to it.

In the end, the nurse may have to make her own painful decision whether or not to tell. Here, the nurse has to balance several conflicting interests and duties: her responsibility to her patient/client against her wider responsibilities to the patients/clients loved one and family. If this course is taken by the nurse, she has to recognise that it is a breach of the duty of confidentiality and may be called to account by their regulatory body, for example the Nursing and Midwifery Council (NMC 2018). There is also the possibility of disciplinary action being taken by the nurse's employer if a complaint is made either by the patient or healthcare staff (NHS 2019). In such cases, there is also the possibility of legal action being taken by the patient in relation to the breach of confidentiality. In the cases considered, it can readily be seen that dilemmas about truth-telling relate to the rights of patients/clients (e.g. the right to know and the right to privacy) and to the tensions between these rights and the duties of nurses (e.g. the duty to protect the vulnerable patient/client from knowledge too painful to bear, or the duty, in fairness to others, to share information that may affect them) (Browne 1998). Here, we see that considerations other than respect for persons and their individual rights come into play. The principles of beneficence and justice are also involved, and it is precisely this actual or apparent conflict of principles which makes these present as moral dilemmas, and which makes decisions in these areas difficult, painful and uncertain (Ewuoso et al. 2017).

Resuscitation of a Baby

A 30-year-old woman in her third pregnancy presented to the maternity hospital at 21 + 2 weeks' gestation with spontaneous rupture of membranes. She was counselled that labour and delivery would be uncertain, and that the general risks of delivery prior to 26 weeks' gestation are very high. She was advised of the risks to the child's survival and chances of discharge from hospital for infants born at 23 weeks' gestation, and the risk of disability if they did survive. The healthcare team explains that for a baby born at 23–24 weeks' gestation or in very poor health, they would resuscitate depending in part on parental wishes and status of the baby. There are, broadly speaking, two schools of thought in this case, one that emphasises the rights of the baby, and the one that emphasises the responsibility of the healthcare team. In principle, the baby has the same right to life and right to treatment as anyone has, and the law safeguards these rights for infants and other vulnerable individuals. The parents do not have a moral right to refuse the treatment that their child requires for survival, but neither can they be forced to care for the child. If, as a society, we recognise that the child has a right to treatment, then we must also recognise that society has an obligation to provide adequate care and support for the child and possibly the parents (Johnstone 2016; Melia 1994). In practice, the situation is complicated, balancing the desire for a baby, the rare but actual fact that some babies do survive without issues, the implications of survival and the unknown health issues and lasting cognitive and physical disabilities (Patel et al. 2016). Compassion for the parents, who, understandably, may feel unable to cope, and compassion for the healthcare team, who are faced with immediate decisions about care and treatment for the child, may point to letting nature take its course and allowing the child to die (Jeremy et al. 2017). In reality, the healthcare team and the parents have to try to resolve the situation in the most responsible way (Boyle et al. 2004). In this case, the risks of medical intervention are that the child would have severe disabilities and require constant care and support and the parents would almost inevitably have to carry the burden of caring for the child. These have to be weighed up against the rare but occasional case of survival with no contraindications, for example see the miracle baby: born at 21 weeks, she may be the most premature surviving infant (Pawlowski 2017, update 2018).

Therefore, decisions in such cases are not clear-cut, whilst past experience may show that there is little hope for such children, or that interventions can be successful in ensuring survival and reasonable quality of life. Medical or practice evidence will not be enough to resolve such moral dilemmas, as quality of life is subjective, and its judgement cannot be made solely on medical grounds. Deciding what is appropriate in such a case is bound to be difficult and morally ambiguous (Guillén et al. 2015). The distinction drawn by moral theologians between 'ordinary' and 'extraordinary' means is often invoked to deal with such situations. The healthcare team are obliged to give a child in such a case the ordinary means of assistance but not obliged to employ extraordinary means in an attempt to save the child's life (Jeremy et al. 2017). However, it is doubtful that this distinction solves the moral dilemma in such cases and there is a need for decisions to be based in practical wisdom, and due regard for the circumstances and needs of the patient/client, and of all other stakeholders. Leaving nature to take its course seldom means doing nothing more for the affected infant; it would normally mean continuing to give fluids, nourishment and drugs to suppress hunger and keep the infant comfortable and free from pain.

Treatment Without Consent

A 10-year-old child, whose parents are Jehovah's Witnesses and who has been involved in a road traffic accident which has resulted in severe injuries and blood loss, has arrived by ambulance to the emergency department. The child's parents are insistent that the child should not be given a blood transfusion or any blood products. Diagnostic procedures/tests are performed, and the parents were asked to wait in the waiting area while X-rays etc. were performed. During the procedures, it became obvious that the child would not survive without an immediate blood transfusion, and this was given without the parents being informed. This case raises, in its acute form, questions of whether parents have the right to choose for their children in such vital matters as those affecting the child's right to life and whether the parents' wishes can prevail over the ordinary human rights of the child. This situation illustrates some of the issues of parental rights versus the rights of the child. In the case of the Jehovah's Witness parents, the medical and nursing staff acted as a law unto themselves, whether for the best of intentions or not. In seeking to protect the rights of the child, it could be said that they failed to show due regard for the moral and legal rights of the parents. The healthcare team colluded, in this case, in deceiving the parents so as to ensure that the child was given the necessary life-saving blood transfusions. They might have applied to a judge and had the child made a ward of court, a more formal and proper procedure, not least to protect themselves from litigation. However, even if the healthcare team had obtained the proper legal authority, their actions in this case of not involving the parents leaves much to be desired. They made assumptions about Jehovah's Witnesses which might in this case have been unfounded, and they failed to consider or address the issue of what the parents might do if they discovered what had been done, without their knowledge or consent. A more sensible course would have been to present and negotiate with the parents about the available options, and failing all attempts to persuade them, only then would recourse to the courts have been justified. Where parents and professionals do not share the same beliefs or value system, the interpretation of rights and responsibilities can become a matter of great difficulty. Common examples in work with people of different ethnic and cultural backgrounds may arise in relation to dietary or dress taboos, or particular sensitivity about issues of privacy or related to sexual health or reproduction. The value of institutions such as the courts is that they remove the problem from the domain of private professional responsibility, and enable discussion to take place in a public arena, where the parties involved in the disagreement both have the right to legal representation and the responsibility to present arguments and evidence to enable the court to make a reasonable decision in the public interest. However, in a life-and-death crisis, the urgency to act may lead the team (as possibly was the case here) to act on their own judgement, but this would be unwise unless they had sought approval from higher medical authority. Given that emergencies do arise, there is an onus on healthcare professionals to keep abreast of these issues and decision-making frameworks that would assist an ethical decision be made that upholds the respect, rights and dignity of all parties.

Gillon (2000) and Robinson (2008) argue that a respectful challenge of a religious position might, first of all, reflect on the decision-making process, involving all the stakeholders. Second, the patient might be referred to the different views within the religion about this practice. Religions all involve a diversity of ethical views (see Chapter 11). In the case of the belief system held by Jehovah's Witnesses about blood transfusion, there is evidence of debate within the community that a patient can be referred to (Elder 2000; Muramoto 1998). See also Conti et al. (2018) on blood transfusion in children, the refusal of Jehovah's Witness parents, Redmann et al. (2018) on transfusion choices, Jehovah's Witnesses and postoperative haemorrhage in paediatric otolaryngology and

Russell and Wallace (2017) on Jehovah's Witnesses and the refusal of blood transfusions, focusing on a balance of interests.

Struggles Over Sedation

Joan was admitted to the unit suffering from cirrhosis of the liver and resulting oesophageal varices, and a portacaval shunt was chosen by her consultant in her treatment. Post-surgery, Joan's condition deteriorated, and she was reporting considerable pain. However, Joan's consultant was insistent that Joan remain drug-free in order to rest the liver, and the resident doctor subsequently refused to prescribe pain relief medication, and instructed that a placebo only be given. Joan was in considerable pain and experienced a distressing night. The nursing manager and the nurses discussed Joan's care, and the nursing manager advised that pain relief medication should be given in order to make Joan as comfortable as possible. This was at odds with the consultant, whose concern seemed to be with ensuring the treatment/operation would be a success. As Joan's condition continued to deteriorate, and Joan was coming close to death, the consultant conceded that Joan should be given adequate sedation. This situation illustrates some of the struggles that may arise over sedation. In the conflict between the nurses and the doctors over the level of pain control to be given to Joan, we encounter a common problem in doctor–nurse relationships in terminal care. The problem relates to the different functions of the nurse and the doctor, and their perceived roles in relation to the severely ill patient/client, the nurse being more concerned with the comfort and well-being of the patient/client, whereas the doctor focuses on the medical problems. However, conflicts also tend to arise in the pre-terminal stage, when it is as yet unclear whether a patient is dying or their life could be saved. While there is hope, curative measures are appropriate, even to the point of denying pain relief if this may jeopardise the possibility of a cure. Once the situation is recognised to be hopeless in therapeutic terms, then appropriate palliative care should be given. Deciding when it is appropriate to switch from therapeutic to palliative measures may be difficult and fraught with uncertainty for the doctor, and faced with possible charges of negligence if he misses something.

Although hospital and medical practice may have changed in some cases, with more ready recognition of the need for palliative care, this historical case still raises the same substantive issues about who decides on the levels of pain-control that are appropriate and under what conditions. The anxiety of the medical staff not to be found wanting has tended to drive them to do all that is possible, whilst the anxiety of the nursing staff at having to cope with the distress of the patient/client (and relatives) may drive them to demand that they should provide palliative care instead. The doctor's experience that patients/clients may sometimes be snatched from the jaws of death has to be balanced by the insight of experienced nurses that patients/clients have turned the corner never to return. Decisions about the type of management that is appropriate may have to be taken under pressure from 'rebellious nurses', or by doctors asserting their medical authority. However, decisions do have to be taken by someone, and usually that is a doctor, because of their ultimate legal responsibility.

A common dilemma in such circumstances relates to the use of powerful pain-controlling drugs such as diamorphine, which can have dangerous side effects such as the suppression of respiration which may hasten a patient's death or make them more susceptible to infections which may cause their death. Some nurses object to giving diamorphine to dying patients/clients even if they are in great pain, because they regard this as a form of euthanasia. Even more nurses are afraid of being the one who administers the last injection and thus appearing to be responsible for the death of the patient/client. Clearly, a nurse has a moral right to refuse to do something that violates their conscience, but they may not have a legal right to refuse to carry out a doctor's orders. The principle of double effect (see Chapter 3) has sometimes been invoked to help provide common-sense guidance for action in such circumstances. When nurses are confronted with situations demanding action which they can foresee will have two effects, one good (such as relieving a patient's/client's pain) and the other bad (putting the patient/client at risk of an earlier death), they would be justified in performing the action subject to the conditions identified by Allmark et al. (2010) as:

- The action of administering opioids to relieve suffering is, in itself, good.
- The intent of administering opioids is for the good effect of pain relief, not the bad effect/ intention of hastening death.
- The pain relief (good effect) is not achieved by shortening life (bad effect).

As already indicated, the right to treatment is a fundamental right of people as patients/clients, regardless of their age and whether or not they can speak for themselves. Problems arise in interpreting this right, because of the varying degrees of competence of patients/clients to make decisions for themselves. Not only do different patients/clients differ in the degree of competence that can be attributed to them, but depending on the severity of their illness, injury or mental disorder, their degree of competence may vary from one stage of their illness to another. Given that dying and pain continually arise within one's practice, there is an onus on healthcare professionals to engage with the evidence and be well-informed on the issues in order to uphold the respect, rights and dignity of all parties (see Henry 2016 on a review on the ethics of palliative sedation; Rodrigues et al. 2018 on palliative sedation for existential suffering; Wright et al. 2019 on moral identity and palliative sedation; and McLean 2016 on terminal sedation, involving good medicine, ethics and law).

Right to Treatment

The least problematic situation is where an independent adult, in full possession of his senses, enters into a care situation. However, given the changing population landscape such as the increasing number of older people and people with dementia, along with people with intellectual/learning disabilities and children/infants, there is a greater need to ensure their rights and entitlements are upheld to the same standards as anyone else. A person's vulnerability whether from reasons of physical or mental illness, places them in a dependent or semi-dependent position where others often take decisions about their care and treatment. Here, the vulnerable person is relying on others to protect their rights and dignity and ensure that they get adequate treatment and care. Over the years, national and international policy has supported and guided the protection of vulnerable people's rights (UN Convention on the Rights of the Child 1989; Department of Health Mental Capacity Act 2005; UN Convention on the Rights of Persons with Disabilities 2006; Government of Ireland (GoI) Assisted Decision Making (Capacity) Act 2015). In addition, special tribunals have been set up in special circumstances, for instance, to oversee the care and management of compulsory psychiatric patients/clients. Thus, the courts have a specific responsibility to protect the rights of vulnerable individuals, and these safeguards are to protect both the individual's rights and the healthcare workers from criticism and litigation or dismissal.

A difficulty often arises due to the ambiguity regarding treatment, and what we refer to as treatment and one's right to treatment. Treatment can encapsulate any kind of intervention or care episode. Therefore, it is important to be clear about what is being referred to in a particular context, as there are important ethical differences between therapeutic measures or palliative care measures (Schildmann et al. 2012). Generally, the purpose of an operation may be to cure, by repairing injury, removing diseased tissue or preventing the spread of infection. However, for some, surgery may be palliative in nature, to relieve pain or delay the spread of malignant disease. Alternatively, an operation may be medically unnecessary, but indicated for psychological or social reasons, for example, gender realignment or cosmetic surgery. Therefore, in each individual care situation, right to treatment will have different ethical significance.

As treatment often is taken to include both cure and care, it may in practice be difficult to separate one from the other. When a patient/client has a potentially fatal disease, which might be curable or at least treatable, it may be extremely difficult for the healthcare team to decide when further therapeutic measures are no longer justifiable and it is time to provide palliative care. For the caring team to be clear about when a patient/client has reached the pre-death stage is vitally important for good end-of-life care. However, if a change of management from a therapeutic regime to palliative care is indicated, the patient/client has a right to be consulted about this change. This may be particularly difficult if the patient/client or relatives are desperately demanding that everything possible should be done, or that all treatment should be stopped. Nonetheless, the importance of dialogue remains.

Conclusion

Within this chapter, the areas and cases above have focused on rights and responsibilities. Both are aspects of freedom and autonomy. Rights focus on individual freedom, and responsibilities focus on the social context of freedom and autonomy (relationships which call for responsibilities). Hence, the ethical task is to work through both rather than simply defend one or the other. As the issues were worked through in the cases, several aspects emerged:

- The ethical decision-making framework. The framework is not used statically, but rather emerges in response to the situation and the relationship with the patient. Hence, there is no simplistic starting point for the process. The important thing is enabling the process of reflection, and thus empowering the patient. This means, for instance, that the decision-making process may begin in the second of third part, and then move back to the first to ensure that the situation and principles are properly engaged.
- The final ethical judgement may have to be rapid or may take time. In John's case, the judgement and the decision tell the truth was focused on the nurse's relationship with him, and in response to the patient's demand for the truth. Other cases may have deadlines which demand more immediate judgement. In the Jehovah's Witness case, this leads to a broadening and sharing of responsibility, drawing in management and legal advice. This reinforces the point that ethical awareness and the practice of ethical skills and virtues are needed across the organisation. Hence, the need for broad procedures based in accumulated wisdom.
- The nature of the different principles emerged through the dialogue of the caring relationship. Parents and family, for instance, may have a strong sense of duty and the principle of care. Dialogue can enable them to reflect on what their view of care is and what the consequences of that are. This includes sharing with them the nurses focus on truth and enabling autonomy in caring. Any dissonance, affective or cognitive, that emerges can enable self-challenge and learning.
- The cases all demanded the practice of the virtues, not least courage. Courage is critical to raising the issues and to enable dialogue, partly because of the fear that this may involve conflict. This reinforces the point that feelings underlie any dialogue about values. The virtues of temperance and patience enable the nurse to keep her underlying feelings from taking over, or from rushing any ethical judgement. The virtue of humility enables the nurse to recognize when another colleague may need to be consulted or involved.
- Through dialogue, each of the parties can begin to take responsibility for their actions, in relation to the core purpose of care and the ethical principles.
- None of this, as the cases show, is easy, in the sense of providing simple solutions. Indeed, it may give rise to the experience of moral distress, and we will consider this in the next chapter, which addresses conflicting demands in patient groups.

References

Active Citizenship Network. (2002). *European Charter of Patients' Rights*. Online available: http://www.ehltf. info/joomla/indexphp/en/ehltf/patients-rights/.

Adshead, G., & Davies, T. (2016). Wise restraints: ethical issues in the coercion of forensic patients. In B. Völlm, & N. Nedopil (Eds.), *The use of coercive measures in forensic psychiatric care: legal, ethical and practical challenges* (pp. 69–86). Cham: Springer.

Allmark, P., Cobb, M., Liddle, B. J., & Tod, A. M. (2010). Is the doctrine of double effect irrelevant in end-of-life decision-making? *Nursing Philosophy, 11*, 170–177.

American Hospital Association. (1973). *American Hospital Association*. Chicago: American Hospital Association.

American Hospital Association. (1992). *American Hospital Association*. Chicago: American Hospital Association.

Atout, M., Hemingway, P., & Seymour, J. (2019). The practice of mutual protection in the care of children with palliative care needs: a multiple qualitative case study approach from Jordan. *Journal of Pediatric Nursing, 45*, e9–e18.

Barsky, A. E. (2019). *Ethics and values in social work: an integrated approach for a comprehensive curriculum*. Oxford: Oxford University Press.

Bergqvist, J., & Strang, P. (2019). Breast cancer patients' preferences for truth versus hope are dynamic and change during late lines of palliative chemotherapy. *Journal of Pain and Symptom Management, 57*(4), 746–752.

Bluebond-Langner, M. (1978). *The private worlds of dying children*. Princeton: Princeton University Press.

Boyle, R. J., Salter, R., & Arnander, M. W. (2004). Ethics of refusing parental requests to withhold or withdraw treatment from their premature baby. *Journal of Medical Ethics, 30*(4), 402–405.

Brännmark, J. (2017). Respect for persons in bioethics: towards a human rights-based account. *Human Rights Review, 18*(2), 171–187.

Browne, N. (1998). Truth-telling in palliative care. *European Journal of Oncology Nursing, 2*(4), 218–224.

Clayton, J. M., Hancock, K., Parker, S., Butow, P. N., Walder, S., Carrick, S., et al. (2008). Sustaining hope when communicating with terminally ill patients and their families: a systematic review. *Psycho-Oncology: Journal of the Psychological, Social and Behavioral Dimensions of Cancer, 17*(7), 641–659.

Conti, A., Capasso, E., Casella, C., Fedeli, P., Salzano, F. A., Policino, F., et al. (2018). Blood transfusion in children: the refusal of Jehovah's Witness parents. *Open Medicine, 13*(1), 101–104.

Council of Europe. (1950). *European Convention on Human Rights*. Strasbourg Cedex, France: Council of Europe.

Department of Health. (1991). *The patient's charter*. London: HMSO.

Department of Health. (2005). *Mental Capacity Act*. London: HMSO.

Department of Health. (2015). *The NHS Constitution: the NHS belongs to us all*. London: Department of Health.

Egener, B. E., Mason, D. J., McDonald, W. J., Okun, S., Gaines, M. E., Fleming, D. A., et al. (2017). The charter on professionalism for health care organizations. *Academic Medicine, 92*(8), 1091–1099.

Elder, L. (2000). Why some Jehovah's Witnesses accept blood and conscientiously reject official Watch Tower Society blood policy. *Journal of Medical Ethics, 26*, 375–380.

Epstein, B., & Turner, M. (2015). The nursing code of ethics: its value, its history. *OJIN. The Online Journal of Issues in Nursing, 20*(2), 1–10.

Ewuoso, C., Hall, S., & Dierickx, K. (2017). How do healthcare professionals manage ethical challenges regarding information in healthcare professional/patient clinical interactions? A review of concept-or argument-based articles and case analyses. *South African Journal of Bioethics and Law, 10*(2), 75–82.

Farquhar, C., Nduati, R. W., & Wasserheit, J. N. (2018). Ethical obligations in short-term global health clinical experiences: the devil is in the details. *Annals of Internal Medicine, 168*(9), 672–673.

Fenwick, T. (2016). *Professional responsibility and professionalism: a sociomaterial examination*. London: Routledge.

Funk, L. M., Peters, S., & Roger, K. S. (2018). Caring about dying persons and their families: interpretation, practice and emotional labour. *Health and Social Care in the Community, 26*(4), 519–526.

Gillon, R. (2000). Refusal of potentially life-saving blood transfusions by Jehovah's Witnesses: doctors should explain why not all JWs think it is religiously required. *Journal of Medical Ethics, 26*, 299–301.

Gilmour, J., & Huntington, A. (2017). Power and politics in the practice of nursing. In J. Daly, S. Speedy, & D. Jackson (Eds.), *Contexts of nursing: an introduction* (5th ed.). Chatswood, NSW: Elsevier.

Government of Ireland. (2015). *Assisted Decision Making (Capacity) Act 2015*. Dublin: Stationary Office.

Guillén, U., Weiss, E. M., Munson, D., Maton, P., Jefferies, A., Norman, M., et al. (2015). Guidelines for the management of extremely premature deliveries: a systematic review. *Pediatrics*, *136*(2), 343–350.

Hall, M. A., Orentlicher, D., Bobinski, M. A., Bagley, N., & Cohen, I. G. (2018). *Health care law and ethics*. New York: Wolters Kluwer Law and Business.

Henry, B. (2016). A systematic literature review on the ethics of palliative sedation: an update (2016). *Current Opinion in Supportive and Palliative Care*, *10*(3), 201–207.

Jeremy, R., Garrett, B., Carter, S., & Lantos, J. D. (2017). What we do when we resuscitate extremely preterm infants? *The American Journal of Bioethics*, *17*(8), 1–3.

Johnstone, M. J. (2016). *Bioethics: a nursing perspective* (6th ed.). Chatswood, NSW: Elsevier.

Keatings, M., & Adams, P. (2019). *Ethical and legal issues in Canadian nursing* (4th ed.). Mosby Canada: Imprint.

Kpanake, L., Tonguino, T. K., Sorum, P. C., & Mullet, E. (2018). Duty to provide care to Ebola patients: the perspectives of Guinean lay people and healthcare providers. *Journal of Medical Ethics*, *44*(9), 599–605.

Lachman, V., Swanson, E., & Winland-Brown, J. (2015). The new 'code of ethics for nurses with interpretative statements' (2015): practical clinical application, part II. *Medsurg Nursing*, *24*(5), 363–368.

Ling, D. L., Yu, H. J., & Guo, H. L. (2019). Truth-telling, decision-making, and ethics among cancer patients in nursing practice in China. *Nursing Ethics*, *26*(4), 1000–1008.

Macaulay, M. (2018). Ethics and integrity. In E. Ongaro, & S. Van Thiel (Eds.), *The Palgrave handbook of public administration and management in Europe* (pp. 279–289). London: Palgrave Macmillan.

Martín, J. M., Olano-Lizarraga, M., & Saracíbar-Razquin, M. (2016). The experience of family caregivers caring for a terminal patient at home: a research review. *International Journal of Nursing Studies*, *64*, 1–12.

McLean, S. (2016). Terminal sedation: good medicine, good ethics, good law. *QUT L. Rev*, *16*, 113.

Melia, K. M. (1994). The task of nursing ethics. *Journal of Medical Ethics*, *20*(4), 7–11.

Muramoto, O. (1998). Bioethics of the refusal of blood by Jehovah's Witnesses. *Journal of Medical Ethics*, *24*, 223–230.

National Health Service. (2019). *Managing safeguarding allegations against staff policy*. Sussex and East Surrey: Sussex and East Surrey Sustainability and Transformation Partnership (STP).

Nursing and Midwifery Council. (2018). *The code professional standards of practice and behaviour for nurses, midwives and nursing associates*. London: Nursing and Midwifery Council. Online available: https://www.nmc.org.uk/globalassets/sitedocuments/nmc-publications/nmc-code.pdf.

Patel, P. N., Banerjee, J., & Godambe, S. V. (2016). Resuscitation of extremely preterm infants-controversies and current evidence. *World Journal of Clinical Pediatrics*, *5*(2), 151–158.

Pawlowski, A. (2017; update 2018). *Miracle baby: born at 21 weeks, she may be the most premature surviving infant*. Online available: https://www.today.com/health/born-21-weeks-she-may-be-most-premature-surviving-baby-t118610.

Redmann, A. J., Schopper, M., Antommaria, A. H. M., Ragsdale, J., de Alarcón, A., Rutter, M. J., et al. (2018). To transfuse or not to transfuse? Jehovah's Witnesses and postoperative hemorrhage in pediatric otolaryngology. *International Journal of Pediatric Otorhinolaryngology*, *115*, 188–192.

Rising, M. L. (2017). Truth telling as an element of culturally competent care at end of life. *Journal of Transcultural Nursing*, *28*(1), 48–55.

Robinson, S. (2008). *Spirituality, ethics and care*. London: Jessica Kingsley.

Rodrigues, P., Crokaert, J., & Gastmans, C. (2018). Palliative sedation for existential suffering: a systematic review of argument-based ethics literature. *Journal of Pain and Symptom Management*, *55*(6), 1577–1590.

Rowland, P., & Kuper, A. (2018). Beyond vulnerability: how the dual role of patient-health care provider can inform health professions education. *Advances in Health Sciences Education*, *23*(1), 115–131.

Runciman, B., Merry, A., & Walton, M. (2017). Safety and ethics in healthcare: a guide to getting it right. CRC Press.

Russell, G. K., & Wallace, D. (2017). Jehovah's Witnesses and the refusal of blood transfusions: a balance of interests. *The Catholic Lawyer*, *33*(4), 361–381.

Scambler, G. (2018). Death, dying and bereavement. In G. Scambler (Ed.), *Sociology as applied to health and medicine*. London: Palgrave.

Schildmann, J., Sandow, V., Rauprich, O., & Vollmann, J. (2012). *Human medical research: ethical, legal and socio-cultural aspects*. New York: Springer Science and Business Media.

Sim, J. (1995). Moral rights and the ethics of nursing. *Nursing Ethics*, *2*(1), 31–40.

Stuart, K. (2018). Handbook for health care ethics committees. *The National Catholic Bioethics Quarterly*, *18*(1), 186–188.

Sygit, B., & Wąsik, D. (2016). Patients' rights and medical personnel duties in the field of hospital care. In A. Rosiek, & K. Leksowski (Eds.), *Organizational culture and ethics in modern medicine* (pp. 282–297). Hershey, PA: IGI Global.

Tang, Y. (2019). Caregiver burden and bereavement among family caregivers who lost terminally ill cancer patients. *Palliative and Supportive Care*, *17*(5), 515–522.

Terry, W., Olson, L. G., Wilss, L., & Boulton-Lewis, G. (2006). Experience of dying: concerns of dying patients and of carers. *Internal Medicine Journal*, *36*(6), 338–346.

United Nations. (1948). *Deceleration of human rights*. Online available: https://www.ohchr.org/EN/UDHR/Documents/UDHR_Translations/eng.pdf.

United Nations. (1989). *Convention of the rights of the child*. New York: United Nations.

United Nations. (2006). *Convention of persons with disabilities*. New York: United Nations.

Universal Patient Right Association. (2019). *History of Universal Patient Rights Association*. Online available: http://www.ehhd.eu/en/history/.

West, E. (2019). Ethics and integrity in nursing research. In R. Iphofen (Ed.), *Handbook of research ethics and scientific integrity* (pp. 1–19). Cham: Springer.

West, R. (2017). Rights, capabilities, and the good society. In T. Brooks (Ed.), *Justice and the capabilities approach* (pp. 189–220). London: Routledge.

Wright, D.K., Gastmans, C., Vandyk, A., de Casterlé, B.D. (2019). Moral identity and palliative sedation: a systematic review of normative nursing literature. *Nursing Ethics*, Early View: 0969733019876312.

Conflicting Demands in Patient/Client Groups

LEARNING OUTCOMES

When you have read and worked through this chapter, you should be able:

- To explore the concept of autonomy, common good and social justice
- To consider the rights of patients/clients versus the interests of third parties
- To consider the scope and limits of one's responsibility for patients/clients
- To consider a range of moral choices we face in practice, for example, preventing suicide, behaviour modification, health screening/prevention and counselling
- To consider the ethics of situations where nurses have to exercise authority to refuse admission or persuade patients/clients to cooperate, or make difficult decisions about the allocation of scarce resources
- To consider some of the difficulties experienced in ethical practice, focusing on moral distress and the duty of candour

Introduction

This chapter focuses on patient/client autonomy and how we as healthcare professionals support such autonomy, such as by advocating for the person. Constant within healthcare interactions is the strive to balance one's rights and autonomy against one's need for support, healthcare and the rights of society at large. This raises the question of common good and can be evident in our thoughts and approach to the involvement of patients/clients in education/teaching of healthcare professionals and the direct or indirect involvement of patients/clients in research studies or of their data in research projects.

Personal Autonomy Versus the Common Good

When healthcare professionals are compelled to weigh their responsibility for individual patients/clients against their responsibilities for groups of patients/clients, conflicts may arise between these different types of responsibility, exercised both as individuals and as a healthcare professional (Bostick et al. 2008). The authority vested in healthcare professionals, to serve the interests of their patients/clients and advocate on their behalf, may contrast with the actual or relative lack of power they have depending on their position in the hierarchy or their relationships with other professional staff. An individual's autonomy and right to choose have become central to much ethical debate, and this is evident in the change from parental authority and overprotectiveness to the championing of people's rights (Hansson 2018). In aspects of service provision, there has been a shift of emphasis from the authority and duties of the service provider to the rights of the patient/client and issues of patient/client choice. In addition, a focus on public and patient involvement within health and social research, policy design and service provision has brought patient/client rights to the fore. In conjunction with such initiatives, many countries utilise a National Patient Satisfaction/Experience Survey to ensure services are patient-/client-focused and meeting individual's needs. This focus has been a move away from the traditional emphasis on the principle of beneficence and a professional's duty of responsible care. Within a rights- and choice-based approach, the concept of what it means to be a patient/client and this modern view of the concept is important, where we no longer see the patient/client as a passive recipient of care or treatment or that the healthcare professionals know what is best for the patient/client (Filipe et al. 2017), and have moved to a viewpoint of respect for the rights of others, their need to act freely and to make their own moral choices (El-Alti et al. 2019).

Personal autonomy always stands in tension with the common good, for we do not spring ready-made out of nothing, either biologically or psychologically (Thompson 2017). Our maturation as individuals, with an identity of our own, is a product of the interaction of our growing capacities for self-determination with these forces of social determinism. In seeking to express ourselves and to realise our autonomy, we do not do this in isolation, but in action and reaction within our given and chosen moral communities in which we live and work (Arjoon et al. 2018). For this reason, my good can never be intelligibly discussed apart from yours or the common good of society, who are responsible for me and to whom I am responsible (English et al. 2016). When we speak of healthcare, we are concerned with services provided by society, for all its members and meant to contribute to the common good. Our modern state-funded or state-subsidised healthcare systems, and in particular modern welfare states, are designed to achieve a greater degree of equity for all, both in access to health services and also in the distribution of health resources (Coggon and Miola 2011).

In discussing the common good, it is important to draw attention to distributive social justice, a sense of power sharing in society, with fair and equitable distribution of benefits and burdens, resources and responsibilities (Arjoon et al. 2018). In cultures which emphasise the right to personal autonomy, there is a propensity to focus on the right to equality of opportunity for individuals, and to overlook the question of whether or not the situations in which individuals find themselves make it truly conceivable to claim their rights as in reality, one requires a certain level of education, financial self-sufficiency and social advantage to be able to claim and exercise the right to equality of opportunity (Sandman et al. 2016). A focus on equity is, therefore, needed, where we aim to achieve equality of outcome for groups and reduce social inequalities in health and access to healthcare so as to ensure greater equity in the sharing of healthcare services and resources across the whole of society, to achieve equal outcomes or benefits for all groups in society (Sandman et al. 2012). Health practitioners, in facing up to their ethical responsibilities in dealing with groups of patients/clients rather than simply with individuals, and the responsibilities of management and administration, public health and research, need to cope with the tensions between autonomy and the common good, between respect for the rights of individuals and the demands of social justice and equity (Thompson et al. 2006).

Setting Limits to the Control and Direction of Patients/Clients

Supporting and managing the needs of patients/clients is a complex art, ranging from providing information to the use of minimum restraint to protect and support persons presenting with behaviours that challenge. In mental health units, emergency departments or intellectual/learning disability services, healthcare professionals often encounter violent patients/clients who may require restraint by physical or chemical means. In such incidences, staff are permitted to use minimum force to protect the patient/client, other patients/clients and staff. Such restraint may be necessary to protect the patient/client from injury, self-injury, self-mutilation or suicide. Nurses are not only responsible for individual patients/clients and their needs, they must also protect the interests of other patients/clients. The rights of individual patients/clients may have to be limited where the rights and safety of other people are put at risk. In addition, the nurse has a responsibility to protect the interests of a patient/client who is incapable of understanding or has capacity issues; for example, if a patient/client is mentally ill, unconscious, under the influence of drugs, intoxicated or has severe intellectual/learning disability. The nurse has to decide on the person's capacity, which may be guided by whether the patient/client is competent, and the circumstances in which the patient/client came into care, or was referred for appropriate care. In general, nurses exercise responsibility for patients/clients within their care and are guided in their decisions by training and experience, professional codes and personal conscience, acting always in such a way as to protect and promote the well-being and interests of patients/clients (NMC 2018). However, legislation, such as the Department of Health Mental Capacity Act (2005) and the Government of Ireland [GoI] Assisted Decision Making (Capacity) Act (2015) moves towards the person's will and preference rather than best interests, as from a healthcare professionals' perspective, what they perceive as best interest may conflict with the patient's/client's will and preference. Therefore there is a need to exercise both clinical and moral responsibility towards the patient/client. These responsibilities need to be considered in terms of the patient's/client's rights, respect for their freedom and consideration of the wider health needs of the individual and the community. Healthcare delivery to patients/clients can involve various degrees of control as guidance is given, compliance is required and behavioural change is often required. Thereby healthcare provision, in some part at least, involves some level of control over people, and this needs to be delivered appropriately with respect to the individual's rights and needs.

One area where tensions have to be navigated is the healthcare professional's role in supporting a patient's/client's wishes. What if the patient's/client's wishes are at odds with hospital policy or meet resistance from a healthcare team? Clearly a healthcare professional acts within their role if they ensure all stakeholders are made aware of the patient's/client's wishes. But how far must a healthcare professional go to represent those wishes? At what point would a healthcare professional be overstepping their professional role, and why? This is the question of patient/client advocacy, which raises the question of the appropriate commitment of the healthcare professional, the obligations that stem from them and what to do when professional loyalties come into conflict internally or within the team.

Preventing Suicide, and the 'Right' to Die

A recent admission to your ward/unit is a 73-year-old man who has been previously diagnosed as having a drug and alcohol addiction. The man has attempted to end his life through taking an overdose on several occasions over the last 3 years. As a staff involved in his care, even though the man is sober and appears rational he is demanding to be allowed home. You fear that if he were discharged, he would return home and commit suicide, compulsory detention in the hospital on the grounds that he might commit suicide would violate his right to freedom and choice, as he has the capacity to make decisions. Consider the problem encountered here for you, faced with the possible discharge of a patient/client who you think may be at risk of committing suicide. Is there a moral or legal duty to prevent the patient/client from committing suicide? The moral quandary arises because of uncertainty in the given situation about the elderly man's mental state. Is the man capable of making rational decisions about his life? If it is decided not to discharge the patient/client, would this action be seen as protecting the patient/client or might it appear too protective and restricting of the patient's/client's liberty? It could be said that not to discharge the patient/client is a natural extension of the right to treatment and the contract of the staff to care for and protect the patient/client by offering therapy as appropriate. Here, the nurse has to exercise fiduciary responsibility on behalf of the patient/client and, illogically, that might involve restricting the patient's/client's movements, in his own best interests. This action might even be construed as a demand of protective beneficence, or as required to defend the patient's/client's rights where the patient/client appears unable to take responsible decisions for himself. Of course, this argument naturally presumes that suicide is never in the best interests of the patient/client.

A less generous view of the action could be that the decision not to discharge was made less to protect the patient/client and more so to protect the healthcare professionals against charges of negligence or the guilt which might result if the patient/client succeeded in committing suicide. The fact is that no matter what precautions are taken, some patients/clients do succeed in committing suicide, and that this does cause great distress to healthcare professionals responsible for their care. Nevertheless, defensive action and conservative measures, though somewhat repressive at times, are morally justifiable. Healthcare professionals are eligible to guard themselves, and their professional reputations, from allegations of culpable neglect of patients/clients in their care. The courage to take the risk of discharging a potentially suicidal patient/client may show commendable regard for the patient's/client's autonomy but can always be criticised as irresponsibility. Achieving a balance between both caring for and protecting patients/clients and respecting their freedom, between defensive medicine and attempted rehabilitation, is always difficult. It is a matter of risk often complicated by the threat of legal action. Thus, our attitudes to suicide are ambivalent, and this is reflected in the fact that there is generally no legal obligation on people as citizens to prevent someone attempting suicide, although they may feel that they are duty-bound to do so if they can, for a variety of moral reasons. However, the law takes a different view of the responsibilities of health care professionals who have charge of patients/clients, and as long as a person is in their care, the law requires the healthcare professional to protect the patient/client from harm including self-inflicted harm. In general, the right to die provokes many challenges across services, be it an elderly service, mental health service or any other, and the dilemma of to die or not to die is addressed by Guerra and Frezza (2017), and Sulzgruber et al. (2017) highlight the ethical dilemma between life-sustaining treatment and the right to die in the elderly.

Behaviour Modification

Another type of control that raises ethical problems is the use of rewards and punishments to reinforce behaviour modification in long-term psychiatric or intellectual/learning disability patients/clients. For example, money, treats or cigarettes may be given as rewards to encourage better self-care among patients/clients for washing, shaving, dressing, bed making or care of living area. Alternatively, sanctions may be applied by the removal of privileges such as access to television, opportunities for exercise or recreation. Are these interventions or controls, and how do they relate to one's basic rights and needs?

A healthcare professional may work with a patient/client with Diogenes syndrome, who accumulates rubbish, or people who smoke, drink alcohol or use drugs. In such cases, it is easy to rationalise the use of support, interventions, retraining measures or aversion therapy for the person on the grounds of hygiene, lifestyle and health and safety risks. These can also be easily justified if the person generally wants to overcome the condition, phobia or dependence, can be consulted about treatment and can give informed and voluntary consent. However, this has to be continually considered and balanced against the respect for the person's right to non-cooperation. We are our own guardians, we own a full, undivided bundle of rights, including all our constitutional rights and the right to make decisions, even bad ones (Graypel 2015). When the patient/client is competent to give consent, these cases are reasonably straightforward. However, the situation is much more complicated when the patient/client has an intellectual/learning disability, mental health challenge, dementia or is suffering the consequences of long-term institutionalisation. Here, there may be serious doubts whether consent can be either informed or voluntary in any true sense. Nevertheless, we need to remember that decision-making capacity can change, is situation-specific and time-specific and that failure to make a decision on one issue should not be generalised to other aspects of the person's life. Here, healthcare professionals struggle interpreting issues of duty to care, best interests of the patient, protection of rights and will and preference. Guiding the decision-making process are the Mental Capacity Bill (DoH 2005) and Assisted Decision Making (Capacity) Act (GoI 2015) key principles:

- There is a presumption of capacity: all adults have the right to make their own decisions and must be presumed to have capacity unless proved otherwise.
- Capacity is decision specific: no complete label of incapacity can be made; an individual's capacity must be assessed for the actual decision at the time the decision needs to be made.
- Participation in decision making: persons should be encouraged and assisted to make their own decisions, or to contribute as completely as conceivable in decision making, by providing them with the help and support they require to make and express their choice.
- Individuals hold the right to make what may seem as unconventional or ill-advised decisions.
- All decisions are in the person's best interests: for person's lacking capacity, decisions made should be in their best interests, considering what they would have wanted, for example, their will and preference. This challenges health care professionals, as their view of best interest may be informed by their healthcare knowledge rather than the person's actual will and preference.
- Decisions made on behalf of a person should be the least restrictive of the person's basic rights and freedoms.

The opinion that something is in the best interests of the patient/client is suitable if, and only if, it is underpinned by a proper respect for the dignity of the individual patient/client, by a concern to rehabilitate them, improve their quality of life or environment or at least to improve the general standards of patient/client care. Respect for the dignity of each persons will and preference challenge healthcare professionals to set limits to the degree of coercion employed, avoid overprotectiveness and challenge assumptions (Carney et al. 2019; Skowron 2019; Harding and

Taşcıoğlu 2018), such as a person with dementia needing support due to risks to personal safety, for example, fire safety. It is far too easy for healthcare professionals to rationalise their prejudices against people who have a particular condition, who adopt different lifestyles or standards of cleanliness and to impose a regimen on patients/clients for their own convenience rather than the real will or benefit of patients/clients. If this risk is recognised, then the use of behaviour modification techniques for the rehabilitation of those whose standards of self-care have deteriorated through illness or institutionalisation may sometimes be justified.

Public Health

To have good public health, you must have good clinical evidence, as you cannot make good decisions about public health unless you understand the disease/condition process that you are trying to treat or prevent. However, in some instances, you cannot reach the best ethical decision until you understand the context in which the decision has to be made, whereas in other instances, there may be an absence of information as to the outcomes of intervention and prevention programmes (Wall et al. 2005). Here, we think of what Sherlock Holmes said to Dr Watson (A Scandal in Bohemia), 'I have no data yet. It is a capital mistake to theorise before one has data. Insensibly, one begins to twist facts to suit theories rather than theories to suit facts'. Thus, when issues come into the public consciousness, but the limitations of data/knowledge are present, it 'requires someone to talk without knowing what he is talking about' (Frankfurt 2005). Public health issues such as infectious disease outbreaks, for example, the novel coronavirus (2019-nCoV), do not always have a distinct evidence base to guide specific treatments/interventions, yet they do require an immediate response based on infection control and public safety measures until a clear treatment option is identified.

An area of ongoing concern is that of childhood behavioural problems, mental illness and autism spectrum disorder. Consider the case of 14-year-old Shaun who is under your care. Shaun has pica where he eats random objects and dirt, has behavioural outbursts, bangs his head with his hand or off the ground, hits and bites himself and others and often tries to run away. Shaun has been assessed by a psychologist and has recently been diagnosed with autism. Shaun has been referred for behavioural therapy, but his family cannot afford this therapy, and there is an 18-month waiting list. This places Shaun's parents in a difficult situation, as his behaviour is deteriorating and he has become quite distressed, to the extent that his parents are considering surrendering their son to become a ward of state to get him the mental health services he requires.

While child mental health services and groups advocate for services, how do we balance resources, costs and public need? What are the implications if we do nothing? How should prevalence, mortality, disability and cost be factored into thinking about ways to balance short- and long-term risks and benefits to individuals and the public? What if there is a government response and child mental health services are developed, but this will require cuts in services for adults as no additional monies are allocated? What role should ethical principles such as stewardship, public health leadership, and moral courage play in this case? Public health will be examined further in Chapter 10.

Health Education

Health education, seeking to change people's attitudes and behaviour, raises ethical questions. Are healthcare professionals entitled to tell people that they should stop smoking, should not drink so much or that they should go on a diet? Or, more controversially, are healthcare professionals morally justified in advising people to practise contraception or to seek sterilisation? If so, how directive should this advice be? Should people just be given the facts and left to decide for themselves? Should healthcare professionals actively try to change people's attitudes and lifestyles?

Should they be campaigning for legislation to control advertising of alcohol and tobacco? Should they support campaigns, for example, against driving under the influence of drugs or alcohol? Should they be involved directly in community development in areas of high unemployment and social deprivation? All these questions raise issues for healthcare professionals and where one's responsibility lies and stops (see Chapter 11). At a practice level, one could argue that one performs within one's scope of practice, and at a moral, ethical and professional level, one could argue that we should advocate, campaign and influence policy and service delivery.

One of the main difficulties affecting healthcare professionals involved in health education, screening and immunisation is that proactive preventive health initiatives involve a change of mindset for the average health professional. Trained to react to crises of various kinds and to deal with the presenting symptoms, they are generally loath to seek out undisclosed pathology. To shift from a reactive mode of interaction with patients/clients to a proactive mode involves not only a change in attitude and practice, but some subtle changes in ethical orientation as well. Crisis intervention and treatment of the symptoms identified by the patient/client fits comfortably with a service ethic based on responsible care or protective beneficence. Actively seeking out undeclared morbidity, in screening for breast or cervical cancer in women and prostate cancer in men, for example, requires a different kind of ethical justification. Recruitment of people for screening, or suggesting to patients/clients that they should undergo screening, may cause people a great deal of anxiety. If the tests involve biopsies, these can be more painful and inconvenient than is generally indicated, and people can experience considerable fear and anxiety until the results are known. Given the doubts which have been raised about the effectiveness of some forms of screening, (e.g. for prostate cancer or breast screening), it can be seriously questioned whether it is ethically justifiable to put people through all this and the inconvenience involved, unless there are serious grounds for suspicion.

The costs of some methods of screening, relative to their actual benefits for patients/clients, can be seriously questioned on both ethical and medical grounds. The ethical justification for such public health measures is generally a utilitarian one, namely, that they contribute to improved health for the majority of the population, even if they cause distress or health complications for some individuals (e.g. untypical reactions to vaccines, or anaesthetics used for biopsies or painful screening procedures). Here, the principles of protective beneficence and justice may be invoked to justify interventions which, it is claimed, will contribute to the common good, but individual interest and individual rights may be compromised. Trained to care for individuals, nurses may hesitate to get involved.

Health education, if it is to be relevant, must be related to the patterns of morbidity and mortality in society. In the past, the infectious diseases and those associated with poverty were responsible for high infant and maternal mortality and the deaths of young people. These diseases have been largely controlled by general improvements in the standard of living (better housing and diet), public health measures (better sewerage disposal, cleaner water supplies) and by medical measures (immunisation and the development of effective drugs). Today, in the developed countries, the pattern of morbidity and mortality is quite different. Infant and maternal mortality rates have been dramatically reduced. There has been a vast increase in the proportion of the population over the age of 50 years, and most illness in this group is lifestyle related. Apart from accidental and violent deaths (a small proportion), the vast majority of deaths and morbidity in the population are associated with smoking, alcohol abuse, inappropriate diet and lack of exercise, and here, the contribution of alcohol and drug abuse to accidents, domestic violence and suicide is considerable. While poverty and social deprivation can be aggravating factors contributing to poor health status, the epidemic of chronic and disabling diseases of middle and later life is clearly lifestyle related. If the major causes of premature death are to be eliminated, then people's attitudes, values and lifestyles have to be changed (Green et al. 2019).

The key ethical questions about health education concern the question of means and methods: how are people's attitudes, values and lifestyles to be changed? What methods, inducements or sanctions is it ethically permissible to use to achieve the long-term goal of reduced morbidity and mortality in the general population? Is it legitimate to exploit our knowledge of psychology and of people's vulnerability to play on their anxieties, to use subliminal advertising to actively promote alternative lifestyles along with commercial marketing of health products? Subtler, but just as important, is the question of the style of education to be used. Is it to be authoritarian and guilt-inducing; take-it-or-leave-it scientific information-giving; focused on developing individual knowledge and life skills for more competent living or about community development and mobilising the resources in local communities to help themselves (World Health Organisation – WHO 1986)?

Obviously, the major ethical justification for health education is the same as that which was invoked in the 19th century to justify compulsory immunisation, notification of infectious diseases and compulsory public health measures. This was to appeal to both the principles of beneficence (to protect the health and safety of people) and justice or the common good (to ensure people have equal opportunities of access to healthcare and good health). Such action was felt to be justified even if it meant restricting the rights of some individuals and dissenting minorities. The problem facing most governments is that legal and fiscal measures cannot be forced on a community entirely without their consent, even in a totalitarian state. Public opinion has to be informed and persuaded, a consensus created, and that is a task of health education. If health educators are not to offend, they have to respect the rights and autonomy of individuals, and their right to decide on their own values and lifestyle, as people cannot be forced to take responsibility for their health.

If health education is to be effective, it may be crucial to use a wide diversity of health education measures. It will not be sufficient just to give people the facts and leave them to make up their own minds. Other forces come into play, influencing people's health choices, such as peer-group pressure and mass media advertising of products damaging to people's health (such as tobacco, alcohol and junk foods). It will not be sufficient to promote the value of positive health and healthy lifestyles through the education of individuals, when some people's social conditions mean that health has low priority in their scale of survival values, and where housing, food, clothing and employment are more urgently needed. It will not be sufficient to try to influence health behaviour through taxation and legal measures when there are huge vested interests, in terms of company profits, retrenchment of staff and government revenues in relation to the tobacco, alcohol and food industries. Advertising may need to be controlled, funds may have to be allocated for community development and the combating of social deprivation and poverty. State subsidies and tax incentives may need to be given to companies to diversify and phase out the production of things damaging health (Green et al. 2019).

If we accept the WHO's definition of health, as 'complete physical, mental and social wellbeing, and not merely the absence of disease or infirmity' (WHO 1948), then all health professionals have a fundamental responsibility for the prevention of disease, as well as its treatment, as prevention is better than cure. Healthcare professionals have both a moral and professional duty to be health educators and, whether they are on a unit or in the community, should be dedicated not only to treatment of disease but also to active health promotion. Healthcare professionals therefore have a responsibility to act as role models, and if they are overweight, heavy smokers or abuse alcohol, they cannot expect their advice on these matters to be taken seriously, as their credibility is called into question. This does not mean that all healthcare professionals have to be positive role models, but their example in taking responsibility for their own health is important, as it is closely observed by patients/clients.

Health professionals have a public responsibility for maintaining health services and cannot simply rest content with passive implementation of health policies decided by other people. As they see the casualties on the units and in the community every day, they have a responsibility to try to use their political influence actively to shape health policies. This can be activated through their professional associations and unions, as healthcare professionals have the power to influence public opinion and thus achieve by political, legislative and fiscal means what cannot be achieved simply by counselling individuals. This is not to say that counselling individuals is not important or effective for the individual patient/client. However, respect for the rights of individuals must be maintained, when pressure is being exerted on individuals and nations to change their lifestyle. The definitive justification for health education is that the rights of patients/clients demand it, particularly the right to know and the right to treatment, for good health empowers people to claim and assert their other rights. The difficulty in health education is in ensuring that patient/client education does not involve manipulation, control and coercion (Ewert 2019; Hem et al. 2018; Reach 2016).

Communication and 'Counselling'

Communication with patients/clients is not only central as a means of ascertaining or transmitting information, and as a means of conveying empathy, encouragement and personal interest, it is also the single greatest significant way of acquiring their cooperation in treatment. In other words, communication plays a vital role in the management and control of patients/clients (Hall and Hall 2016). Healthcare professionals' communication is often portrayed as a failure due to poor communication. However, many healthcare professionals are highly skilled at using language and the selective disclosure of information as a means of securing the cooperation of patients/clients, and as a means of controlling them. However, what is needed is that healthcare professionals listen to patients/clients, communicate with patients/clients as persons, understanding their personal needs and responding to their different levels of comprehension and right to information. It is therefore both a professional and moral duty of healthcare professionals to present and provide information to patients/clients so that they can, in fact, read and understand the information they are given, particularly when informed consent is required for treatment or participation in a clinical controlled trial. In an attempt to meet some of these difficulties, a move has occurred toward public and patient involvement (PPI) in the development of healthcare policy and representation on health committees (Filipe et al. 2017; Abelson et al. 2016). In addition, engagement with consumers has occurred, through focus groups and satisfaction surveys, to gain their feedback on the quality and satisfaction with services and the need for improvements.

First and foremost, all health care professionals need to develop their range of communication skills. In some circumstances, controlling and managerial communication may be required and appropriate, particularly in a crisis, but the other more sensitive communication skills, associated with counselling and helping patients/clients to sort out their own problems and assisting them to make their own decisions, require quite different training and the development of quite different skills. Modern healthcare professional's education addresses patient-/client-centred and non directive counselling (Rogers 1983, see Chapter 9 for broader communication ethics across the healthcare organisation).

However, competence in these forms of communication is required across all practice areas. Much communication between healthcare professionals and patients/clients is necessarily directive, and often involves giving specific advice or warnings, and it is generally legitimised in terms of one's duty of protective care. On the other hand, counselling requires more specialised training so as the helper facilitates patients/clients to communicate more successfully about their concerns, so as to enable them to first explain the nature of their problem(s), to spell out what choices they have and to assist them to find their own answers to their problem(s). This requires the healthcare professionals refraining themselves from giving advice, or trying to help by solving the patient's/client's problems for them. Rather, they use their skills of attentive listening, focusing and clarifying, challenging and presenting of options, and teaching problem-solving skills, to help patients/clients to address their own problems, and to empower them to claim more control over their own decision making.

As an intimate exchange of often very sensitive private information occurs, the first ethical requirement for the counselling relationship is one of clearly negotiated and agreed boundaries of confidentiality. Secondly, healthcare professionals are bound to exercise a protective duty of care towards patients/clients, both in terms of protecting their vulnerability and privacy, but also to recognise the limits of their own competence and to be prepared to refer the patient/client to an appropriate specialist, if and when necessary. Thirdly, the healthcare professional has a fundamental duty to respect the individuality and opinions of the patient/client, even if the patient/client disagrees with what the healthcare professional is saying. This non-judgemental attitude is essential if patients/clients are to feel free to explore their feelings and conflicts without fear of disapproval or subsequent discrimination. The fourth requirement of empathy is often cited as an ethical and functional requirement of counselling. This is not equivalent to sympathy, which can often be condescending, but an attempt to put oneself professionally in the patients'/clients' position and to understand things in their terms and within their frame of reference (see Chapters 3 and 11).

In general, communication between healthcare professionals and patients/clients can raise two kinds of ethical problems: first, when communication fails to demonstrate respect for the patient/client as a person and second, when the patient's/client's right to know is overlooked. The first kind of problem arises, for example, when hospital staff members talk over the heads of patients/clients or, more seriously, fail to respect their confidences. The power relationship between a patient/client and a healthcare professional is an uneven one, and communication can be used to talk down to or to control patients/clients rather than to relate to them as persons. Sick or injured patients/clients are often nervous and troubled because they do not comprehend what is happening to them or why it is happening. They are vulnerable and dependant, as not only do they need the assurance which healthcare professionals can give them, but they need information to be able to reclaim any degree of control over their lives. Healthcare professionals consequently have an obligation to share with the patient/client their understanding and specific information about that patient/client, and to share it in the most helpful and caring way.

Balancing the Rights of Patients With the Interests of Third Parties

In general, and for very good reasons, the focus of healthcare professionals' training is on direct patient/client care, on the one-to-one relationship between carer and patient/client in the clinical situation. Clinical practice is grounded on the more individual, or personalist, values of beneficence and respect for persons. The values on which the other functions of healthcare are based are the more universal values derivable from principles of justice. In practice, healthcare professionals usually have obligations to several patients/clients at the same time. Because each nurse 'has only one pair of hands' and 'cannot be in two places at once', they have to make decisions about which patients/clients should be given priority, while doing the best for all their patients/clients.

Health professionals regularly feel the greatest comfort in making ethical decisions of a personal kind relating to individual patients/clients and their health needs. Their expertise and clinical experience relate best to the treatment of individual patients/clients and decisions about their management. A personalist ethic, based on caring, seems most appropriate to such situations. The conflict between these different kinds of values, personalist and universal, comes out most clearly where the rights of individual patients/clients have to be balanced against the interests of third parties. Some situations that may serve to illustrate this will be addressed in the coming sections mainly:

- Decisions to refuse admission to a patient, either because of risk to other patients, or lack of a bed.

- Persuading patients to 'volunteer' as research subjects in clinical trials and/or non-therapeutic research.
- The use of patients as teaching material for the education of healthcare professionals.
- Decisions about the allocation of resources within the hospital or in the community.

REFUSING TO ADMIT A PATIENT

A charge nurse is faced with a difficult decision as the unit is currently short-staffed (staff sickness, absenteeism, non-recruitment, non-replacement) and operating below what would be regarded as safe staffing levels. On the day in question, an incident occurred where one patient/client caused injury to another patient/client and became very upset and aggressive towards the other patients/clients and staff. Staff worked to de-escalate the situation, talking and trying to rationalise with the patient/client and offering him some medication to assist him to gain control over his emotions and alleviate anxiety and stress. In addition, staff were faced with supporting the other patients/clients, who had now also become very agitated. At this time, the charge nurse was informed that the police were at reception with a patient/client who had attempted to slash her wrists and was being abusive and aggressive towards the police. The police were seeking to admit the woman under the Mental Health Act. The doctor on duty was undecided whether the unit could cope with the new admission, but felt he ought to accept the patient/client, as she was in need of immediate medical treatment. Under the circumstances, the charge nurse refuses, as she knew staff could not cope and that the care of the other patients/clients might be put at risk, and recommends the patient/client be given the necessary care and medication in the emergency department and taken to the police cells, until alternative arrangements could be made for her care.

A classic dilemma facing a charge nurse may be whether they can accept responsibility for another patient/client when there is an acute shortage of nurses or resources, or where a patient/client is very disturbed and disruptive or where there are too few staff to ensure management of a unit. The conflict here is between the charge nurse's straightforward duty to care for a patient/client who has been brought to the unit and the nurse's duty to provide adequate care for the other patients/clients on the unit. An alternative way of viewing the problem is to see it as a conflict between the right to treatment of an individual patient/client being admitted and the rights of those in the unit already receiving treatment. Either way, there is a dilemma to be faced. In this situation, the issues faced by the charge nurse concerned the relative weight to be given to the rights of the various patients/clients in her care and the conflict between her responsibility to a whole unit of acutely ill patients/clients and her duty to help a particular woman who clearly needed care and attention. At one level, the charge nurse's decision might appear sensible and possibly the only thing to do in the circumstances. The charge nurse did not perceive it as a moral dilemma in the strict sense, but rather as a moral problem which was solved by giving priority to the demands of justice to her staff and the patients/clients on the unit. However, it is important to tease out what ethical issues are involved and to develop models for sensible decision making in such circumstances (see Chapter 2). Some of the most critical decisions faced by healthcare staff occur in situations where there are numerous people in need of urgent attention and concurrently limited staff and resources to deal with the emergency. Part of the problem may relate to competence or psychological issues, such as the inexperience of the doctor, or the sense of helplessness of the charge nurse faced with staff shortages and an unsympathetic health authority and the arrival of another patient/client, being 'the last straw'.

The ethical questions raised by this case are of various kinds. There are the questions which relate to the rights of the various patients/clients involved, the apparent conflict between the rights of one acutely disturbed patient/client and the rights of others. Clearly, here no one patient's/client's rights are paramount. As indicated in Chapter 4, our rights are not absolute or unlimited. Provision of treatment or a bed for one patient/client, for example, may mean that another patient/client is deprived or that there are fewer resources to go around for others. Sensible decisions have to be made in the best interests of all. In some cases, this demand of distributive justice may mean that a patient/client cannot be given treatment at a particular time because all available resources are committed. Alternatively, in some situations of extreme emergency, where the life of a patient/client is at risk, less ill patients may have to suffer a degree of reduced care for the sake of saving the life of another. In one case, the demands of justice for the common good prevail, and in another the case, the rights of a particular person to treatment prevails. Both cases could be said to arise from competing demands of justice for individuals or a fair outcome for the group. In theory, we may derive most personal rights from the principle of respect for persons, but we may not be able to resolve conflicts of rights between different parties without other considerations based on justice and beneficence.

Finally, there is a whole series of ethical questions to be raised about the marginalisation of mental health and the inadequate resources provided, compared with the acute medical and surgical services, despite the large proportion of patients/clients requiring treatment for mental health problems. In spite of official recommendations to the contrary, the low priority accorded to mental health services generally raises questions about the rationality of health service planning and of justice in healthcare. The kind of crisis which makes a charge nurse refuse to admit a patient/client demands more of the healthcare professional than merely a gesture of non-cooperation. The wider political responsibilities of healthcare professionals are painfully illustrated in such situations, and organised protests to the hospital or health authority, industrial action or leaks to the press may be more effective and successful in drawing attention to the inadequacy of the service for these particularly vulnerable patients/clients who are unable to defend their own rights to have proper care and treatment.

PERSUADING PATIENTS TO 'VOLUNTEER' AS RESEARCH SUBJECTS

James is a 9-year-old boy with cystic fibrosis and is under the care of a consultant paediatrician. James has had regular hospital appointments and recently has been selected for the opportunity to be part of a new drug trial that could change the treatment of cystic fibrosis and prolong the life of suffers of the condition. As James is only 9, this opportunity is presented to James' parents by the consultant. The consultant presents that James is very lucky as he has the particular strain of bacteria that this drug treats, and that if James responds to the new drug, it will extend his life expectancy.

Given the opportunity and information that this new drug may extend James' life, the parents naturally decide to be part of the trial. The question is as to how informed this choice really is, and what are the parents agreeing to – is it being part of the drug trial or the opportunity to provide the chance of a longer life for their child? How the information is presented and the language used can influence the decisions made. The question arises as to how this information should be presented and how long should the parents have to decide to partake. But also, given that consent is not a one-off process, so too should the information provision process be more than a one-off event. Two months into the trial and after weekly visits to the consultant, with many tests and procedures performed, the consultant presents a form to the parents to sign saying this form is only so James can have the treatment and so that they can check James' data to see if the drug is working. The parents are asked to sign and, after signing, are given a copy to take home to read. How does this adhere to the ethical principles of conducting research? What vulnerabilities should be considered from the parents' perspective based on the fact that they have signed and, on the other hand, what if they had decided not to sign? What questions could it raise for the parents in terms of access to treatment, desire to support their child and future care?

Although we recognise that healthcare practice can only advance through appropriately robust scientific research, the controls required in scientific research should be both methodological and ethical. Research that is not conducted according to rigorous scientific methods is valueless, and research that is not conducted with proper respect for the rights of patients/clients may be unethical and result in inhumane treatment of research subjects. The World Medical Association's (WMA) Declaration of Helsinki (WMA 2013), on the ethical and scientific requirements for sound research involving human subjects, is of general value in discussing issues related to research in which a healthcare professional may be involved, whether as responsible investigator or in an auxiliary role. In order to be scientific, research must be based on sound scientific knowledge and proper scientific methods. This means that the research must satisfy several conditions, namely:

- Initial investigations (e.g. by data collection or literature survey) must establish what has already been done in the field, to avoid unnecessary repetition and waste of public resources.
- New research instruments must be properly pre-tested to establish their reliability and validity, or alternatively, well-tried methods should be used.
- The project must be based on sound research design, approved by one's professional peers and independent assessors and undertaken by properly qualified research staff.
- The findings of the research must be disseminated, to inform future practice, for example, by publication in a peer-reviewed journal.

These requirements are not only scientific but ethical, and researchers have a responsibility not to engage in research that is valueless (to do with healthcare purpose) and a waste of time and resources (to do with justice). This is not only because most research is funded from public money and involves the use of public resources, but also to protect research subjects from unnecessary investigations of no benefit to them or to anyone else. However, the question arises especially around the second point above, where, in new research or many trials, pre-tested or established reliability and validity or well-tried methods, may not be evident but may be the focus of the research. Thus critical consideration needs to be given to the ethical basis and implications of the research, namely, whether the proposed research satisfies the research ethical principles of beneficence/non-maleficence, justice and respect for persons (see Chapter 7).

Clinical research may be therapeutic or non-therapeutic. Therapeutic research is directly linked to the patient's/client's complaint, and the patient/client stands to benefit directly from the treatments or procedures used. Non-therapeutic research is where patients/clients participate in general investigations, for example, research aimed at improving patient/client care, techniques of management or general knowledge of the physiology or pathology of particular complaints, where the investigations are of a general nature and have neither any specific therapeutic purpose, nor are of any direct benefit to the research participant. In practice, the distinction may not be so clear-cut, for patients/clients may stand to benefit in the long-run from even the most academic studies, as they may from laboratory studies of the composition of the blood or the biochemistry of the brain. Furthermore, in randomised controlled trials using placebos, some patients/clients may receive potentially therapeutic drugs or treatment and others no effective treatment at all, and yet no progress can be made without such trials. The claimed effectiveness of drugs cannot be proved by mere accumulation of evidence without testing the evidence in rigorously controlled experiments, to exclude other possible explanations of why the health of some patients/clients appears to improve with their use (Deaton and Cartwright 2018).

However, in broad principle, the distinction between therapeutic and non-therapeutic research is a useful one even if only to emphasise that the ethical safeguards in the latter type have to be more stringent (Schildmann et al. 2012). In general, the greater risks taken in clinical research are justified on two grounds; firstly, that there may be direct benefit for the patient/client and, secondly, that the research may contribute to the benefit of humanity even if it does not directly benefit the patient/client. The right of the patients/clients to treatment includes the implicit assumption that they will cooperate in the trial of various procedures, yet have the right to withdraw if they believe they are suffering harm, or that the responsible researcher will withdraw them from the study if they are at risk of harm.

It has been argued that the right of a patient/client to benefit from research carries with it a corresponding duty to assist in research that may be of benefit to other patients/clients too. On the other hand, the patient's/client's right to care and treatment cannot rest solely on this premise. Our entitlement to treatment cannot depend on our capacity to barter for it by payment in time served as a research participant. Our entitlement to adequate care and treatment must rest on some more fundamental rights related to our right to life and membership of a moral community that cares not only for the strong, but also for the weak and vulnerable too. The duty to assist medical research by participation in clinical trials, if it is a moral duty, is so in an extended sense of the word duty, and may or may not be recognised as such by the patient/client. It is not a duty that can be forced up on anybody (Seiler 2018; Schaefer et al. 2009). Patients/clients have a right to be properly informed and to give their consent without coercion or moral blackmail. Patients/clients also have a right to be informed of the risks and possible benefits, and to withdraw from any trial or research project without prejudice to their treatment. Both requirements arise because a patient's/client's participation cannot be said to be ethical unless it is voluntary, that is free and appropriately informed.

The healthcare professional in charge of patients/clients in research trials has a special responsibility to protect the interests of the individual patients/clients, to act as their advocate advising them about the conditions of participation and their right to withdraw from the trial. Because patients/clients in the hospital are to some degree captive, it is important to ensure that they feel happy about participation in a trial, particularly if it is not one from which they stand to benefit directly, or where there is a significant degree of risk or inconvenience involved. Research ethics committees are increasingly requiring of investigators that independent assessment is made of the quality of consent given by patients/clients, and the degree of discomfort or inconvenience caused, by a competent professional not involved in the research project. However, healthcare professionals involved in the research may also have to persuade patients/clients to cooperate, and here the personal values of clinical practice and the more universal ones justifying research may come into conflict. These may be particularly acute in justifying clinical research involving children, prisoners or those who have severe mental health problems or intellectual/learning disabilities. In such cases, legal and institutional safeguards (such as proxy consent) are particularly important, to protect the wider interests of those not competent to give informed and voluntary consent whether they stand to benefit or will merely be contributing to the welfare of others (Nijhawan et al. 2013).

The issue of whether it is ethical to use children as subjects of clinical research has been hotly debated over the years. On the one hand, it has been argued that children cannot be said to give consent that is either informed or voluntary in any proper sense. Children's lack of knowledge and understanding of the implications of medical procedures, and even of the legal significance of consent, may be said to invalidate any attempt to justify their use as research participants on moral grounds. Children's dependency on adults for protection and advice makes them peculiarly vulnerable to moral pressures, and it is doubtful whether their consent could really be voluntary. The researcher has a fundamental duty to protect the rights of children, to avoid them being put at risk and to prevent their exploitation. They, therefore, fall back on the proxy consent of the parents or a relative. This can be an attempt to safeguard the interests of vulnerable individuals, but the question can be raised too whether the insistence on proxy consent is not more to protect the doctor or institution from legal action than to protect the child, and how vulnerable is the parent in the situation? However, consent is a process not a one-off event, and utilising proxy consent does not excuse the healthcare professional from including and informing the child as to their involvement and the process involved. Considering the case of James above, what actions would you consider appropriate if you were involved in such a trial, what or how would you advocate, what issues are raised about the use of James' data and what issues are raised when additional treatment is offered as part of a trial rather than standard treatment/care? We will look in more detail at research ethics in Chapter 7.

USE OF PATIENTS AS TEACHING MATERIAL

Should patients/clients be used as teaching material in the training of healthcare professionals? Should patients/clients with rare or exotic disorders or unusual complications be expected to put up with the additional inconvenience, embarrassment and even discomfort of being examined by students? In a teaching centre, where the population does not have the opportunity of being treated in non-teaching hospitals, should patients/clients be given the choice of consent or refusal to act as demonstration material for clinical tutorials without suffering prejudice in treatment? And what about the right to privacy of psychiatric patients and the dying as learning opportunities?

Healthcare training without the opportunity to work on real patients would be like learning to swim on dry land. Here, the justification for compromising the right to privacy of individual patients/clients is that the patient/client stands to benefit by having highly trained staff to care for their needs. Alternatively, it can be argued that the common good of all patients/clients is served by having properly trained staff. The requirements for the provision of sound clinical training staff tend to give greater importance to considerations of the common good than to the specific needs or interests of individual patients/clients. Justice demands that patients/clients with unusual and 'exotic' disorders should not be unduly exposed to students, with or without their consent. Even unconscious patients deserve to have their privacy respected and dignity protected. Lack of respect tends to breed insensitivity, callousness and lack of consideration in trainees. Some patients/clients, or patient/client populations, may be at risk of being over-investigated, over-scrutinised because they are interesting teaching material. Some reasonable and just limits have to be set to the demands made on such patients/clients.

It may be questioned whether it can be morally justified to place additional strain on nervous and worried patients/clients (e.g. disturbed psychiatric patients) by exposure to a group of healthcare students, even with the patient's/client's consent. One may need to decide against using particular patients/clients, however interesting, because of their vulnerability. On the other hand, it needs to be stressed that the expectations of people with regard to their privacy vary according to their situation. People tend to expect the greatest degree of privacy and strictest confidentiality to be observed when they are visited in their own homes or see health professionals in a private consultation. However, when people enter public institutions, they recognise the implicit restrictions on their rights, for in order to benefit from institutional care, they may be obliged to surrender some degree of their privacy. In an institutional setting, the health professionals may be more anxious about privacy and confidentiality than patients/clients are. Nevertheless, professionals cannot ignore the need of individuals for privacy, and they have a primary moral duty to protect the rights of the patients/clients entrusted to their care. To address these issues, there is a greater emphasis on the inclusion of patients/clients in curriculum design and delivery, which has been incorporated in healthcare professionals' education and training (Rowland et al. 2019; Hayes et al. 2018; Molley et al. 2018; Suikkala et al. 2018; Williams and Dalwood 2018), with positive outcome from both the patients/clients and students' perspectives.

Allocation of Resources

Although the ethical problems related to the allocation of human and material resources in healthcare are discussed more fully in Chapter 10, there are some issues which arise here in the context of having to balance the rights of individuals against the interests of third parties. Let us consider a few examples. Should older patients be discharged from the hospital to make way for more acute cases if there is any doubt that they will be able to cope on their own, even with domiciliary services and support? Should nursing staff be allocated according to need or according to the number of patients/clients? Should more effort be put into providing care to those who have the potential for cure, rather than individuals who have enduring conditions?

In practice, decisions have to be taken, and these may be both painful and subsequently found to be mistaken or based on inadequate knowledge. All decisions, where the rights of one patient/client have to be balanced against those of other patients/clients or third parties, may involve agonising choices. In formal terms, it may be a choice between the demands of personal care for the individual patient/client and justice for a larger group of patients/clients or society. In practical terms, it may be a matter of responding to external pressures and the internal guilt and anxiety generated by an unresolvable tension between conflicting duties. The extreme case may be a medical emergency such as a road traffic accident or train disaster in which many people are injured or dying and there are limited medical supplies and limited staff to provide care and treatment. A policy of triage may be adopted dividing the victims into three groups: those who must be left to die because they are beyond help, those who can wait for treatment later, and those who must be attended to first because they need treatment urgently and stand to benefit from it most. The question is how we reconcile the conflicting demands of the principles of beneficence, justice and respect for persons in such situations? Faced with several patients/clients with renal failure and needing urgent dialysis, with only one dialysis machine available, who is to be given priority? Generally, the decision will be the doctor's, but if there are no obvious clinical criteria which would decide the issue in favour of one patient/client rather than another, other criteria might have to be considered, and nurses might get drawn into discussion of the available options. Would the decision be made most fairly by drawing lots (Silverman and Chalmers 2001) or by adhering to a first-come, first-served basis? Would attempts to assess the usefulness, value or importance of individuals be reasonable or invidious? Attempts to involve patients/clients in group decisions about the allocation of a dialysis machine would seem to be very unfair. In such circumstances, a decision by team consensus or by outside assessors might be justified if there were objective grounds on which the choice might be made. However, the judgements would tend in practice to be based either on the assessment of probabilities, on the basis of the personal experience or on the past professional experience and subjective judgement. In the case of an intractable moral dilemma, where there are no practical strategies to avoid the problem of choice, the responsible healthcare professionals would have to be prepared to make a decision and to live with the guilt and anxiety which that responsibility entails.

In making decisions impacting the lives and well-being of individuals in their care, healthcare professionals act as protectors and advocates of the rights of all their patients/clients. They have to make decisions based on their knowledge, expertise and available resources for the common good. They will have to exercise courageous initiative and be willing to take risks as they try to affect the best concession between the demands of justice, beneficence and respect for the rights of individual patients/clients. Although a person may be fit today, they may be ill or in desperate need of treatment tomorrow. Thus, we are all potential patients/clients, so we should have an interest in protecting patient's/client's rights. The right to know, the right to privacy and the right to treatment are all better understood by healthcare professionals who have experienced the lack of power and vulnerability of being a patient/client. Healthcare professionals who take their duties seriously will also be more willing to act as advocates defending the rights and dignity of patients/clients. They will also be aware that, as public officers, they have a responsibility to uphold the common good and to promote the health of the whole community. These competing duties may indeed give rise to painful and difficult choices.

Uneasy Ethics

In recent years, there have been two areas (moral distress and the duty of candour) discussed within nursing and healthcare ethics, which have highlighted the fact that the practice of ethics is not easy.

NURSING AND MORAL DISTRESS

The term 'moral distress' originated in the 1980s, and refers to the largely psychological distress felt by a nurse who 'knows the right thing to do, but institutional constraints make it nearly impossible to pursue the right course of action' (Jameton 1984 p. 6). Such distress appears to correlate with similar experiences and affects such as compassion fatigue and burnout (Rushton et al. 2015; Maiden et al. 2011). This definition assumes that there is a right thing to do, and an external constraint prevents that judgement and action from being carried out. The case of Mid Staffs would seem to be a good example of where, because of the organisational objective and re-lated constraints, the nurses 'were not free to be moral' (Yarling and McElmurry 1986 p. 63). This is a meta-narrative, which pits nurses against the organisation. Critics, especially Paley (2004), view this bluntly as the moralising of 'whinging'. Paley suggests that the very basis of the research is problematic, simply giving space for complaint, without a critical engagement with those in-volved in the event. The underlying argument is precisely that there is no organisation which does not constrain, in some way, the moral judgement of its members, or at least be interpreted in such a way. It is the person's subjective interpretation, which Paley's research into the phenomenon reports, as not sufficient.

Johnstone and Hutchinson (2015) argue that the concept of moral distress be abandoned for several reasons:

- It perpetuates the myth that there is a simple moral judgement in any nursing situation, failing to acknowledge the possibility that there might not even be a 'morally correct' course of action (Weinberg 2009).
- It fails to understand that the process of ethical decision-making demands taking responsi-bility for working through a process of dialogue and reflection which enables all parties to contribute to the discovery of the meaning of principles in the particular situation.
- The assumption of the rightness of nurses' moral judgements (Johnstone and Hutchinson 2015) can lead to failure to nurture the skills required for ethical dialogue and to integrate this into ethical decision making.

Fourie (2015) argues that there is a legitimate understanding of moral distress, and this re-quires broadening Jameton's definition, to distress caused by any moral event. It is then possible to refer to two categories in this (Fourie 2015), 'moral-constraint distress' and 'moral-conflict distress'. Morley (2018 p. 2) expands the concept to three key ideas:

- the experience of a moral event,
- the experience of 'psychological distress', and
- a direct causal relation between these two.

However, this is so broad that the term 'moral distress' begins to lose any precise meaning. Paley's argument suggests that the underlying dynamic is to establish a 'condition' of moral dis-tress, which can then be systematically addressed. This suggests a false premise to the argument about this experience.

However, as we have argued:

- Ethical practice is not easy. Integrity (see Chapter 3) demands not simply holding fast to principles but struggling with contradictions and competing views of the good (Tigard 2018; Pianalto 2012).
- All professions operate in complex situations where competing views of the good exacerbate experiences of moral distress. It is part of professional responsibility to deal with this.
- The key problem is less about preventing the nurse's expression of what is right, and more about preventing any dialogue about the good.

This last point is echoed in Marshall and Epstein's (2016) argument that moral distress is linked to what they term 'moral hazard'. The term is derived from economics and refers to the lack of incentive to guard against risk where one is protected from its consequences, for example, by insurance. In the case of healthcare, they argue, there is no incentive to take ethical responsibility because the organisation controls ethical meaning, with the implication that professionals must live with that. Hence, empirical research suggests higher levels of 'moral distress' are often correlated with poorer perceived ethical culture (Hamric et al. 2012; Silén et al. 2011).

This asks major questions of organisational culture which fails to recognise different narratives, demanding the need:

- To develop moral resilience in nursing and all healthcare professions. This focuses directly on formation of the virtues.
- To empower healthcare professions, focused on the development of a work culture which stresses a shared moral community where critical engagement and dialogue about principles and responsibility are the norm (Traynor 2017; Rushton and Carse 2016). We will address this in more detail in Chapter 9.

DUTY OF CANDOUR

Candour is 'the quality of being honest and telling the truth, especially about a difficult or embarrassing subject' (Cambridge Dictionary). It is both a principle (honesty) and a virtue (the quality or capacity to be open and honest). The meaning of the term candour carries with it a context of difficulty, that is, something has gone wrong, and with it comes a sense of surprise, that is, that one should be open in that situation. In other words, candour is not easy. The starting point is that being open about something difficult makes one vulnerable. The Francis Report (2013) offers this definition of candour: 'the volunteering of all relevant information to persons who have or may have been harmed by the provision of services, whether or not the information has been requested and whether or not a complaint or a report about that provision has been made'. Following Francis, there was a push to extend the duty of candour to a statutory duty. Hence, the duty of candour begins to emerge in three perspectives, as discussed in the following sections.

Professional Duty

A 'duty of candour' has been a part of the medical profession for some time, supported in the 1950s by the Medical Defence Union. The General Medical Council's *Good Medical Practice* (GMC 2013) advises that doctors 'must be open and honest with patients if things go wrong'. By 2015, the GMC and NMC had issued joint guidance on the duty of candour (see https://www.gmc-uk.org/-/media/documents/openness-and-honesty-when-things-go-wrong--the-professional-duty-of-cand____pdf-61540594.pdf?la=en). This explicitly acknowledges that both medical and nursing professions are focused on the same ethical duty and sets out what to do if a patient/client suffers harm or distress.

Contractual Duty

This recognises that the different professions operate in an organisation which is the means of delivering healthcare. The organisation requires the duty to be fulfilled, partly to ensure accountability, and partly to ensure that users of the organisation can trust both the professionals involved and the internal procedures of the organisation. Hence, providers of services must comply with a contractual duty of candour. This is required by the standard NHS contract, and applies to incidents that result in moderate or severe harm or death.

Statutory Duty

This was introduced for NHS bodies in England (Trusts, Foundation Trusts and Special Health Authorities) in November 2014, in addition to the contractual duty of candour. In April 2015, it was extended to all other Care Quality Commission (CQC)-registered care providers (such as GP practices and independent practitioners in England). A statutory duty of candour has been discussed in many different contexts, not least in the Hillsborough disaster (Barlow 2017). In healthcare, it was a recommendation of the Francis Report (2013). The Mid Staffs case showed how a professional duty was not sufficient, and statutory duty shows a concern for safety standards (non-maleficence) as well as honesty. These are the standards below which care must not fall and which the CQC will investigate during an inspection to make sure they are being met in all registered healthcare organisations. Care organisations have a general duty to be open and transparent in relation to care. This involves several things:

- The duty, like the contractual one, applies to organisations rather than individuals, but staff should cooperate to make sure the organisational obligation is met.
- Patients/clients should be told of a 'notifiable safety incident' as soon as is practical.
- A notifiable safety incident has two statutory definitions, depending on whether the healthcare organisation is an NHS body or not.
- The organisation has to explain to the patient/client what is known at the time, what further enquiries will be made, offer an apology and keep a written record of the notification to the patient. Failure to do so could be a criminal offence.
- The patient/client should be given reasonable support. This could be practical (e.g. an interpreter) or emotional (e.g. counselling).
- The patient/client must get written notes of the initial discussion and of the notification, including details of further enquiries, their results and an apology. The organisation needs to keep copies of all correspondence.

Apologising

At the heart of the duty of candour is the apology. Candour is an admission that something has gone wrong, and the apology is the recognition of the consequences of this and the acceptance of responsibility. Apologies can be difficult in a professional context, not least because this might suggest legal liability.

It is important then to see the apology as part of the ongoing relationship with the patient. Respecting the patient/client involves first ensuring that the person understands the context of any mishap. For instance, if a suture needle breaks in use and becomes embedded in the wound, the patient/client can become anxious about the event. The professional would then need to explain that sutures can break in this situation, and that there was no serious problem. Given the patient's anxiety, however, it is important both to explain this and to form what is a generalised apology. This becomes part of an ongoing dialogue with the patient/client involving four stages:

- Tell the patient/client (or where appropriate their representative or family) when something goes wrong that causes, or has the potential to cause, harm or distress.
- Apologise to the patient/client or their representative. The Act is clear that an apology is not an admission of legal liability.
- Offer an appropriate remedy or support to put matters right, if that is possible.
- Explain fully the short- and long-term effects of what has happened.

All of this is part of an empathic respectful response to the patient/client. Patients/clients sometimes prefer to hear an apology from the person involved and sometimes from a member of the leadership (acknowledging the concern of the organisation as a whole). Whilst concern about legislation is understandable, the Medical Defence Union (https://mdujournal.themdu.com/issue-archive/issue-2/the-effective-apology) suggests that the opposite is often true. In a culture of openness where the patient/client or family is taken seriously, and the event is owned by those involved, timely apologies tend to lead to better resolutions. The whole process addresses several different ethical principles including:

- Respect for the patient/client and family.
- Establishing mutuality in the relationship. At the heart of the patient-/client–carer relationship is information asymmetry which has to addressed. Hence, the simple act of sharing

the truth (however messy or ambiguous) empowers patient/client or family, and helps them to make a more balanced judgement.

- Justice.
- Working to develop positive responsibility and a concern for learning.

Nonetheless, the duty remains difficult to practice in the hardest cases. Glasper (2018) argues that high profile legal cases, such as child Jack, might endanger the practice. They pit retributive justice against restorative justice.

6.1 PAUSE FOR THOUGHT

The Case of Child Jack

Consider this case
    https://www.tandfonline.com/doi/pdf/10.1080/24694193.2018.1467159
    Do you agree with Glasper, that high profile cases such as this can discourage the practice of the duty of candour?
    Consider the outcome in the case terms for Dr Bawa-Garba and Nurse Amaro. The doctor was eventually restored to the medical profession; the nurse, at the time of writing, has not been restored to the nursing profession.
    What are the justifications for the two very different judgements by the professional bodies, such as restorative justice and justice as retribution?
    Would restorative justice across both professions better serve the practice of the duty of candour?

From Glasper, E. A. (2018). Promoting honesty and truthfulness when things go wrong during care delivery for sick children. *Comprehensive Child and Adolescent Nursing, 41*(2), 83–88.

The duty of candour applies across healthcare professions, and in Chapter 9 we examine it in leadership and management.

Conclusion

Within this chapter, we identified issues around patient/client autonomy and how healthcare professionals have to move from best interest to will and preference when working with and advocating for the patient/client. Cases within this chapter challenge one to consider practice issues such as preventing suicide, health education, behaviour modification, refusal to admit and counselling patients/clients. In addition, at a wider level, we are challenged to consider general issues in public health, allocation of resources and the interests of third parties. Also, at a practice level, the issues of patients/clients volunteering for research and being part of the education and training of healthcare professionals raises questions of how we practice and engage with patients/clients. The issues of research will be further developed in the next chapter.

References

Abelson, J., Wagner, F., DeJean, D., Boesveld, S., Gauvin, F. P., Bean, S., et al. (2016). Public and patient involvement in health technology assessment: a framework for action. *International Journal of Technology Assessment in Health Care, 32*(4), 256–264.

Arjoon, S., Turriago-Hoyos, A., & Thoene, U. (2018). Virtuousness and the common good as a conceptual framework for harmonizing the goals of the individual, organizations, and the economy. *Journal of Business Ethics, 147*(1), 143–163.

Barlow, E. (2017). Hillsborough disaster: police should be forced to tell truth when tackling public tragedies, bishop's report says. The Independent 1 November 2017. Online available: https://www.independent.co.uk/news/uk/home-news/hillsborough-police-duty-of-candour-burning-injustice-cultural-change-families-tragedy-bishop-james-a8031161.html.

Bostick, N. A., Levine, M. A., & Sade, R. M. (2008). Ethical obligations of physicians participating in public health quarantine and isolation measures. *Public Health Reports, 123*(1), 3–8.

Carney, T., Then, S. N., Bigby, C., Wiesel, I., Douglas, J., & Smith, E. (2019). Realising 'will, preferences and rights': reconciling differences on best practice support for decision-making. *Griffith Law Review*, 1–23. Online available: https://doi.org/10.1080/10383441.2019.1690741.

Coggon, J., & Miola, J. (2011). Autonomy, liberty, and medical decision-making. *The Cambridge Law Journal, 70*(3), 523–547.

Deaton, A., & Cartwright, N. (2018). Understanding and misunderstanding randomized controlled trials. *Social Science and Medicine, 210*, 2–21.

Department of Health. (2005). *Mental Capacity Act*. London: HMSO.

El-Alti, L., Sandman, L., & Munthe, C. (2019). Person centered care and personalized medicine: irreconcilable opposites or potential companions. *Health Care Analysis, 27*(1), 45–59.

English, V., Mussell, R., Sheather, J., & Sommerville, A. (2016). Autonomy and its limits: What place for the public good. In S. A. M. McLean (Ed.), *First do no harm: law, ethics and healthcare* (pp. 133–146). London: Routledge.

Ewert, B. (2019). From entitled citizens to nudged consumers: re-examining the hallmarks of health citizenship in the light of the behavioral turn. *Public Policy and Administration, 34*(3), 382–402.

Filipe, A., Renedo, A., & Marston, C. (2017). The co-production of what: knowledge, values, and social relations in health care. *PLoS Biology, 15*(5), e2001403.

Fourie, C. (2015). Moral distress and moral conflict in clinical ethics. *Bioethics, 29*(2), 91–97.

Francis, R. (2013). *Report of the Mid Staffordshire NHS Foundation Trust Public Inquiry*. Chaired by Robert Francis QC. London: Stationary Office.

Frankfurt, H. (2005). *On bullshit*. Princeton, NJ: Princeton University Press.

Glasper, E. A. (2018). Promoting honesty and truthfulness when things go wrong during care delivery for sick children. *Comprehensive Child and Adolescent Nursing, 41*(2), 83–88.

General Medical Council. (2013). *Good medical practice*. Manchester: General Medical Council.

Government of Ireland. (2015). *Assisted Decision Making (Capacity) Act 2015*. Dublin: Stationary Office.

Graypel, E. A. (2015). The patient refuses to cooperate. What can you do? What should you do? *Current Psychiatry, 14*(3), e3–e4.

Green, J., Cross, R., Woodall, J., & Tones, K. (2019). *Health promotion: planning and strategies* (4th ed.). London: Sage.

Guerra, A. L., & Frezza, E. E. (2017). To die or not to die: this is the dilemma. *Journal of Epidemiology and Public Health Reviews, 2*(1.) https://sciforschenonline.org/journals/epidemiology-public-health/article-data/JEPHR-2-138/JEPHR-2-138.pdf.

Hall, M. F., & Hall, S. E. (2016). *Managing the psychological impact of medical trauma: a guide for mental health and health care professionals*. New York: Springer Publishing Company.

Hamric, A., Borchers, C., & Epstein, E. (2012). Development and testing of an instrument to measure moral distress in healthcare professionals. *AJOB Primary Research, 3*(2), 1–9.

Hansson, S. O. (2018). The ethics of making patients responsible. *Cambridge Quarterly of Healthcare Ethics, 27*(1), 87–92.

Harding, R., & Taşcıoğlu, E. (2018). Supported decision-making from theory to practice: implementing the right to enjoy legal capacity. *Societies, 8*(2), 25.

Hayes, V., Bing-You, R., Pitts, D., & Manning, L. (2018). The benefits of honoring patients as teachers: a qualitative study. *PRiMER, 2*, 4.

Hem, M. H., Gjerberg, E., Husum, T. L., & Pedersen, R. (2018). Ethical challenges when using coercion in mental healthcare: a systematic literature review. *Nursing Ethics, 25*(1), 92–110.

Jameton, A. (1984). *Nursing practice: the ethical issues*. Englewood Cliffs, NJ: Prentice Hall.

Johnstone, M. J., & Hutchinson, A. (2015). Moral distress: time to abandon a flawed nursing construct. *Nursing Ethics, 22*(1), 5–14.

Maiden, J., Georges, J. M., & Connelly, C. D. (2011). Moral distress, compassion fatigue, and perceptions about medication errors in certified critical care nurses. *Dimensions of Critical Care Nursing, 30*(6), 339–345.

Marshall, M. F., & Epstein, E. G. (2016). Moral hazard and moral distress: a marriage made in purgatory. *American Journal of Bioethics, 16*(7), 46–48.

Molley, S., Derochie, A., Teicher, J., Bhatt, V., Nauth, S., Cockburn, L., et al. (2018). Patient experience in health professions curriculum development. *Journal of Patient Experience, 5*(4), 303–309.

Morley, G. (2018). What is "moral distress" in nursing: how, can and should we respond to it. *Journal of Clinical Nursing*, *27*(19–20), 3443–3445.

Nijhawan, L. P., Janodia, M. D., Muddukrishna, B. S., Bhat, K. M., Bairy, K. L., Udupa, N., et al. (2013). Informed consent: issues and challenges. *Journal of Advanced Pharmaceutical Technology and Research*, *4*(3), 134.

Nursing and Midwifery Council. (2018). *The code professional standards of practice and behaviour for nurses, midwives and nursing associates*. London: Nursing and Midwifery Council. Online available: https://www.nmc.org.uk/globalassets/sitedocuments/nmc-publications/nmc-code.pdf.

Paley, J. (2004). Commentary: the discourse of moral suffering. *Journal of Advanced Nursing*, *47*(4), 364–365.

Pianalto, M. (2012). Integrity and struggle. *Philosophia*, *40*(2), 319–336.

Reach, G. (2016). Patient education, nudge, and manipulation: defining the ethical conditions of the person-centered model of care. *Patient Preference and Adherence*, *10*, 459.

Rogers, C. (1983). *Freedom to learn*. Columbus: Merrill.

Rowland, P., Anderson, M., Kumagai, A. K., McMillan, S., Sandhu, V. K., & Langlois, S. (2019). Patient involvement in health professionals' education: a meta-narrative review. *Advances in Health Sciences Education*, *24*, 595–617.

Rushton, C., & Carse, A. (2016). Towards a new narrative of moral distress: realizing the potential of resilience. *Journal of Clinical Ethics*, *27*(3), 214–218.

Rushton, C. H., Batcheller, J., Schroeder, K., & Donohue, P. (2015). Burnout and resilience among nurses practicing in high-intensity settings. *American Journal of Critical Care*, *24*(5), 412–420.

Sandman, L., Granger, B. B., Ekman, I., & Munthe, C. (2012). Adherence, shared decision-making and patient autonomy. *Medicine, Health Care and Philosophy*, *15*(2), 115–127.

Sandman, L., Gustavsson, E., & Munthe, C. (2016). Individual responsibility as ground for priority setting in shared decision-making. *Journal of Medical Ethics*, *42*(10), 653–658.

Schaefer, G. O., Emanuel, E. J., & Wertheimer, A. (2009). The obligation to participate in biomedical research. *JAMA*, *302*(1), 67–72.

Schildmann, J., Sandow, V., Rauprich, O., & Vollmann, J. (2012). *Human medical research: ethical, legal and socio-cultural aspects*. New York: Springer Science and Business Media.

Seiler, C. (2018). Can there be a moral obligation to participate in biomedical research. *European Journal of Clinical Investigation*, *48*(4), e12896.

Silén, M., Svantesson, M., Kjellström, S., Sidenvall, B., & Christensson, L. (2011). Moral distress and ethical climate in a Swedish nursing context: perceptions and instrument usability. *Journal of Clinical Nursing*, *20*(23–24), 3483–3493.

Silverman, W., & Chalmers, I. (2001). Casting and drawing lots: a time honoured way of dealing with uncertainty and ensuring fairness. *BMJ*, *323*(7327), 1467–1468.

Skowron, P. (2019). Giving substance to 'the best interpretation of will and preferences'. *International Journal of Law and Psychiatry*, *62*, 125–134.

Suikkala, A., Koskinen, S., & Leino-Kilpi, H. (2018). Patients' involvement in nursing students' clinical education: a scoping review. *International Journal of Nursing Studies*, *84*, 40–51.

Sulzgruber, P., Sterz, F., Poppe, M., Schober, A., Lobmeyr, E., Datler, P., et al. (2017). Age-specific prognostication after out-of-hospital cardiac arrest–the ethical dilemma between 'life-sustaining treatment' and 'the right to die' in the elderly. *European Heart Journal: Acute Cardiovascular Care*, *6*(2), 112–120.

Thompson, I. E., Melia, K.M., Boyd, K.M., and Horsburgh, D. (2006). Nursing ethics. Fifth edition. Edinburgh. Churchill Livingstone, Elsevier.

Thompson, M. J. (2017). Autonomy and common good: interpreting Rousseau's general will. *International Journal of Philosophical Studies*, *25*(2), 266–285.

Tigard, D. W. (2018). Rethinking moral distress: conceptual demands for a troubling phenomenon affecting health care professionals. *Medicine, Health Care and Philosophy*, *21*(4), 479–488.

Traynor, M. (2017). *Critical resilience for nurses: an evidence-based guide to survival and change in the modern NHS*. Oxon, UK: Routledge.

Wall, L. L., Arrowsmith, S. D., Briggs, N. D., Browning, A., & Lassey, A. T. (2005). The obstetrical vesico-vaginal fistula in the developing world. *Obstetrical and Gynecological Survey*, *60*(7), S3.

Weinberg, M. (2009). Moral distress: a missing but relevant concept for ethics in social work. *Canadian Social Work Review*, *26*(2), 139–151.

Williams, C., & Dalwood, N. (2018). Patients as 'patients' and 'educators': harnessing the power and potential of the patient's voice. *Medical Education*, *52*, 462–464.

World Health Organization. (1948). *Preamble to the Constitution of the World Health Organization as adopted by the International Health Conference*. Geneva: World Health Organization.

World Health Organization. (1986). *Ottawa Charter for Health Promotion*. Ottawa, ON: World Health Organization.

World Medical Association. (2013). *The Helsinki declaration: ethical principles for medical research involving human subjects*. Fortaleza, Brazil: 64th World Medical Association General Assembly.

Yarling, R., & McElmurry, B. (1986). The moral foundation of nursing. *Advances in Nursing Science*, *8*, 63–73.

Ethics in Healthcare Research and Teaching

LEARNING OUTCOMES

When you have read and worked through this chapter, you should be able:
- To outline a brief history of research ethics
- To examine the key underlying principles of research ethics
- To consider key protocols and governance for ethical research
- To consider research with vulnerable participants, focusing on dementia and intellectual/learning disabilities
- To examine the ethical framework of teaching

Introduction

Research in healthcare, involving people directly or indirectly, is critical for developing healthcare practice, and thus improving health for the population as a whole. As such, it is an important part of developing professional practice in all of the different aspects of healthcare provision, from effective governance to medicine or surgical techniques, and an effective means of caring. Healthcare professions work within the context of Higher Education, which focuses on research and teaching. Research and teaching are often seen as separate areas, but are, in fact, the same, simply different aspects of learning in different contexts. The concern for ethics in research has increased in recent decades partly because a rigorous examination of ethics is required by funding bodies (Economic and Social Research Council – ESRC 2015), leading to what MacFarlane (2009, p. 25) refers to as 'ethics creep', and partly because of a history of cases which ignored ethical considerations. Within this chapter, we will consider research ethics and issues of ethical concern, and examples of poor ethical practice.

The Willowbrook Studies

When the New York Willowbrook School, which included 'mentally disabled' children, suffered a hepatitis epidemic, the New York School of Medicine, led by Dr Saul Krugman, conducted studies involving children at the school. The studies commenced in the 1950s and continued for 15 years, where children from the ages of 3 to 10 years, who were housed at Willowbrook School, were the subjects of Krugman's study. Krugman observed that students who were infected with hepatitis and recovered, then seemed to be immune to further outbreaks of the disease. He decided to draw antibodies from the blood of infected children and use these antibodies to try to create immunity/protection from the hepatitis. Krugman deduced that injecting uninfected students (children) with the antibodies would kick-start their immune system, causing a milder case of hepatitis once they were exposed. In addition, the antibodies would guard the children against future outbreaks. Krugman's research involved 700 students split into two groups. Group 1 involved students already housed at Willowbrook, where some were given the protective antibodies and some were not. Group 2 involved students new to Willowbrook, and all were given the protective antibodies. Some students (children) in this group were deliberately infected with hepatitis and some were not. To introduce the infection into the study subjects, some children were fed faecal matter (Rothman and Rothman 1984). As some of the symptoms varied, Krugman learned that two forms of hepatitis existed (A and B). The students who had the protective antibodies, and who were deliberately infected with hepatitis, had mild symptoms when compared to students who acquired hepatitis naturally and who did not have the protective antibodies. This knowledge paved the way for the vaccinations for hepatitis A and B that are used today.

Although vaccinations for hepatitis A and B are useful for members of society across the world, the conduct of this research raises many ethical issues such as:

- Inducement was evident in the study as Willowbrook was at capacity however, if students participated in the research, they were given a place in Willowbrook in a newer part of the centre.
- Parents and their children were not truly informed about the risks of the study, and researchers did not fully disclose what the study entailed.
- Little consideration was given to the vulnerability of the participants, in their ability to understand the risks of the study and give consent, and parents were unduly induced to give their consent (the main school was closed to new admissions in 1964).
- Due to overcrowding, parents were told there were openings in the hepatitis unit for children who could participate in the study.
- Parents had little choice over whether or not to participate in the research, as parents who wanted care for their children may not have had any other options (accepted only if they participated in the study).

- Live hepatitis virus was fed to the intellectual/learning disability children in order to deliberately infect them.
- There is no compelling reason to study viral hepatitis in children before studying it in adults.
- None of the 1000 adults working at Willowbrook were enlisted for the study.
- The reason hepatitis was present at high levels was because of overcrowding and unsanitary conditions.
- Instead of dealing with the overcrowding and unsanitary conditions, the situation was taken advantage of to conduct an experiment.
- One of the ethical problems with the Willowbrook Hepatitis Study is that it did not protect the participants from harm – patients/clients, who were healthy, were subjected to the infectious disease.
- Researchers response was that the children would more than likely have become infected during their time at Willowbrook anyway.
- The virus was spread among the healthy participants, as they could not isolate the carriers of the disease, as they did not know who the carriers were.

The Willowbrook case reveals at least two important elements. First, it was focused on a strictly utilitarian approach. The 'end' of developing effective vaccines for hepatitis was more important than the immediate questions of how one should respect the subjects of the research, who, in this case, were given no choice. Nonetheless, the researchers might have been concerned about maximising the good, and there is no doubt that the research at Willowbrook made an important contribution to the contemporary treatment of hepatitis. Second, it may have involved a form of scientism, a stress on the importance of scientific enquiry, and the good it can achieve, regardless of social context. Scientism involves a total focus on research regardless of any concern for the individuals in the research.

Over the years, there have been other cases that raise ethical issues with regards to the conduct of research. Examples include the Jewish Chronic Disease Hospital, where, in 1963, live cancer cells were injected into older patients to discover how healthy bodies responded to this (Katz et al. 1972); or the National Women's Hospital Auckland Study, where, in 1966, medical staff withheld treatment to women (n = 160) with abnormal cervical smears without their consent. This was to test if cervical abnormalities would lead to cervical cancer (McIndoe et al. 1984), and the practice continued over 20 years. In other cases, there was the domination of conflicting interests, such as the mind-control research of the 1950s conducted at McGill University, Montreal. Here, psychedelic drugs were administered to 52 patients without their knowledge in brainwashing experiments for the Central Intelligence Agency (CIA) (Rauh and Turner 2016). Moreover, between 1989 and 1991, newborns (n = 700) and 6-month-old children (n = 1500) were given EZ, an experimental measles vaccine. Parents were not informed of the experiment or that the vaccine was not yet licensed (Awadu 1996). Furthermore, other cases show the predominance of ideology, which dehumanised the subjects and constitutes an abuse of power. In the Tuskegee Syphilis Study, 1932–72, researchers withheld treatment from African-American (n = 339) syphilis sufferers in order to study its long-term effects (Brandt 1978). However, the worst examples of ethical violations were in the Nazi medical experiments of World War II. One such study focused on improving treatment for hypothermia, and the study involved participants being immersed in ice-water tanks or standing naked in below-freezing temperatures for several hours (Bogod 2004; Berger 1990). It is because of such cases that ongoing developments have been made with regard to research ethics codes.

Codes of Research Ethics

Concern for research ethics reaches back to the early 19th century. The first medical ethics code to refer to research was that of Thomas Percival in 1803 (Sara et al. 2018). The code was focused on the paternalistic role of the physician, and at one point focuses on informed consent and the use of a placebo. Percival argued that there was no duty to obtain a patient's informed consent if the predictable effect of a placebo exceeded that of all other treatments. Hence, in the final stages of cancer, for instance, a placebo might exceed the effect of controlled drugs (Thomas 2001). In these cases, the rational physician, Percival argued, would choose placebo treatment. This would preclude informing a patient of the placebo, as knowledge that it was a placebo treatment might compromise the treatment. Like Willowbrook, this was informed by utilitarianism.

However, systematic attempts to establish frameworks for research ethics only began with the Nuremberg Code. The Nuremberg Trials commenced on the 9th December, 1946, when an American military tribunal began criminal proceedings against leading German physicians and administrators (n = 23) for their willing participation in war crimes and crimes against humanity. Among the charges were that German physicians performed medical experiments on thousands of hostages in concentration camp without their consent. Most of the subjects of these experimentations died or were permanently disabled as a result.

As a consequence of the trial, the Nuremberg Code (1947) was established, identifying that the voluntary consent of the human subject is unquestionably essential, making it clear that subjects of research should give their consent freely, and that the benefits should outweigh the risks of the research.

Although it did not carry the weight of law, the Nuremberg Code was the first international document advocating an ethical framework as:

- The voluntary consent of the human subject is absolutely essential. This means that the person involved should have the legal capacity to give consent; should be so situated as to be able to exercise free power of choice, without the intervention of any element of force, fraud, deceit, duress, over-reaching or other ulterior form of constraint or coercion and should have sufficient knowledge and comprehension of the elements of the subject matter involved, as to enable him/her to understand and make an enlightened decision. This latter element requires that, before the acceptance of an affirmative decision by the experimental subject, there should be made known to him the nature, duration and purpose of the experiment; the method and means by which it is to be conducted; all inconveniences and hazards reasonably to be expected and the effects upon his/her health or person, which may possibly come from his/her participation in the experiment. The duty and responsibility for ascertaining the quality of the consent rests upon each individual who initiates, directs or engages in the experiment. It is a personal duty and responsibility, which may not be delegated to another with impunity.
- The experiment should be such as to yield fruitful results for the good of society, unprocurable by other methods or means of study and not random and unnecessary in nature.
- The experiment should be so designed and based on the results of animal experimentation and a knowledge of the natural history of the disease or other problem under study, that the anticipated results will justify the performance of the experiment.
- The experiment should be so conducted as to avoid all unnecessary physical and mental suffering and injury.
- No experiment should be conducted where there is an a priori reason to believe that death or disabling injury will occur, except, perhaps, in those experiments where the experimental physicians also serve as subjects.
- The degree of risk to be taken should never exceed that determined by the humanitarian importance of the problem to be solved by the experiment.
- Proper preparations should be made and adequate facilities provided to protect the experimental subject against even remote possibilities of injury, disability or death.
- The experiment should be conducted only by scientifically qualified persons. The highest degree of skill and care should be required through all stages of the experiment of those who conduct or engage in the experiment.
- During the course of the experiment, the human subject should be at liberty to bring the experiment to an end, if he/she has reached the physical or mental state where continuation of the experiment seemed to him/her to be impossible.

- During the course of the experiment, the scientist in charge must be prepared to terminate the experiment at any stage if he/her has probable cause to believe, in the exercise of the good faith, superior skill and careful judgement required of him/her, that a continuation of the experiment is likely to result in injury, disability or death to the experimental subject.

Helsinki Code

The World Medical Association (WMA 1964) developed recommendations to guide medics conducting biomedical research involving human subjects. The Declaration of Helsinki governs international research ethics and defines rules for research combined with clinical care and non-therapeutic research. To ensure good practice, the Declaration of Helsinki is revised on a continual basis, with the last version being in 2013 (WMA 2013), and issues addressed in the declaration of Helsinki include:

- Research with humans should be based on the results from laboratory and animal experimentation.
- Research protocols should be reviewed by an independent committee prior to initiation.
- Informed consent from research participants is necessary.
- Research should be conducted by medically/scientifically qualified individuals.
- Risks should not exceed benefits.

Belmont Report

The Belmont Report (1979) attempted to summarise the basic ethical principles acknowledged by the Belmont Commission. Alongside the principles was their stress on the fact that ethics was not an individual activity but rather one involving all parties concerned. The individual healthcare researcher has to take responsibility for research which focuses on the legitimate research question(s), on how the research participants are treated and on the effective and beneficent impact of the research. To achieve this, however, requires careful deliberation, which demands a phase in the process where the wider healthcare organisation also reflects on the proposal to confirm its ethical propriety. Here, then, responsibility for the research is also shared by those in the wider project of healthcare, demanding a clear framework of governance. Hence, Richards and Schwartz (2002) summarise the Commission's demand for research to:

- Be subject to scrutiny by an independent ethics committee/board.
- Be scientifically sound.
- Be conducted by researchers who are supervised or have adequate expertise.
- Adhere to ethical principles throughout the research process.

Underlying Principles

The underlying principles for healthcare research ethics correlate with those of healthcare and medical ethics. Within the research context, we will address respect for the autonomy of the participants and all involved in the process; beneficence and non-maleficence of participating in research and justice for participants. Emerging from these principles are veracity, fidelity, confidentiality and vulnerability of participants. The responsibility in developing such a research ethics is shared by the research community and professional bodies, with guidance for nurses in particular, included by the Canadian Nurses Association (CNA 2008); Royal College of Nursing (RCN 2009); American Nurses Association (ANA 2010); Australian Nursing Federation (ANF 2012); International Council of Nurses (ICN 2012) and the Nursing and Midwifery Board of Ireland (NMBI 2015).

RESPECT FOR AUTONOMY

Respect for autonomy demands that participants should be able to make their own choices and express their concerns, free of any coercion or influence, to participate (Butts and Rich 2013). As the Belmont Report (1979) sets out, autonomy should involve four elements: information, comprehension, competency and voluntariness (see also Beauchamp and Childress 2012), whereas Gillon (1985) argues that consideration be given to three types of autonomy: autonomy of thought (choice) or thinking for oneself; autonomy of will (capacity) or freedom to do something based on one's own deliberations and autonomy of action (sovereignty: governing oneself) or freedom to act as one wishes. Participants must receive full disclosure of information outlining the nature of the study, their right to withdraw at any time without consequence and an identification of the risks/benefits to facilitate an informed choice (Polit and Beck 2013). Templates or guidance for participant information sheets and consent forms are generally provided by research ethics committees and Tables 7.1 and 7.2 below give an example from Doody and Noonan (2016) and University Hospitals, National Health Service – NHS (2018).

These templates underline the importance of details if the participant is to trust the process and researchers. The details enable the construction of a narrative, enabling the participant to identify with the process and begin to take responsibility for it. The consent form builds on this information and signing this, in effect, confirms a contract, that the participant:

- Has read the information and has been given the opportunity to consider the information, and ask questions that have been answered satisfactorily.
- Understands that participation is voluntary and involves freedom to withdraw at any time without giving any reason, without their medical care or legal rights being affected.
- Gives permission for relevant sections of medical notes and data collected during the study to be looked at by individuals from the Sponsor, from regulatory authorities, where it is relevant to the participant taking part in this research.
- Agrees (where appropriate) to provide a sample(s) as part of their involvement in this study, to audio/video recording and the use of anonymised quotes in research reports and publications or to the General Practitioner being informed of their participation in the study.
- Understands how data will be stored in and in what format.
- Understands and agrees to actions that may be focused on the specific research, for example, genetic research, magnetic resonance imaging (MRI) studies or anonymised samples being used in future research.

TABLE 7.1 ■ **Elements Participants Must Be Aware of to Give Informed Consent**

- Title of study	- How data will be stored
- Name, place of work, qualifications and contact details of researcher(s)	- Who will have access to data
- Study population	- Participation is voluntary
- Purpose of study	- Participant has the right to refuse to participate or withdraw at any time
- Study procedures and steps for data collection	- Participant can choose not to answer any question, stop or cease their involvement at any stage
- Potential risks	
- Potential benefits	
- How anonymity or confidentiality will be upheld	- Opportunity to ask the researcher questions related to the study
- How data will be collected	- How participant can obtain the results of the study
- Who will collect data	- Both parties will receive a signed and dated consent form

From Doody, O., & Noonan, M. (2016). Nursing research ethics, guidance and application in practice. *British Journal of Nursing, 25* (14), 803–807.

TABLE 7.2 ■ Participant Information Sheet and Consent Form Templates

• Study title	• What will happen to the samples I give?
• What is the purpose of the study?	• What will happen to my data?
• Why have I been invited?	• What will happen if I do not want to carry on with
• Do I have to take part?	the study?
• What will happen to me if I decide to take part?	• What will happen to the results of this study? Alter-
• What should I consider?	natively: What happens at the end of the study?
• Are there any possible disadvantages or risks	• What if we find something unexpected?
from taking part?	• What if there is a problem?
• What are the possible benefits of taking part?	• How have patients and the public been involved
• Will my General Practitioner/family doctor	in this study?
(GP) be informed of my participation?	• Who is organising and funding the study?
• Will my taking part in the study be kept	• Who has reviewed the study?
confidential?	• Participation in future research.
• Will I be reimbursed for taking part?	• Further information and contact details:

From University Hospitals, NHS. (2018). https://www.ouh.nhs.uk/researchers/planning/documents/participant-information-sheet.pdf. Accessed 20 March 2020.

Participants' opportunity to withdraw may not always be plausible, such as after analysis and publication, or if they answered an unidentifiable questionnaire. In some cases, people may have reduced levels of autonomy (e.g. babies, those with dementia, or intellectual/learning disability) and need added safeguards due to their level of ability to give informed consent in order to guard their autonomy (Polit and Beck 2013; Newell and Burnard 2011). We will discuss an example of research ethics in dementia below and discuss the use of gatekeepers as a safeguard. As we noted in Chapter 2, autonomy is not a discrete capacity but is rather a function of dialogue. Hence, for participants to appreciate fully what is being requested of them, and the effect involvement will have on them, they must also be afforded the opportunity to ask questions before/during/after the study. Informed consent may also have cultural issues and the cultural context of informed consent needs to be considered. For example, in Lee's (1998) study of women factory workers in Hong Kong and China, it was hard for her to get across to her co-workers what she was actually doing. This was partially because of the academic term 'thesis', of which they had little understanding. In dialogue with the women, a substitute explanation was developed, involving the idea that Lee was writing a novel based on her experiences as a worker 'toiling side by side with "real" workers' (1998, p. 173). This illustrates that it is not always possible for a researcher to fully explain the purposes and nature of the research, and sometimes a compromise understanding is arrived at.

BENEFICENCE

Beneficence seeks to do good or to benefit those involved in the research. This includes benefits of the research to the individual participants and society in general (Parahoo 2014; Beauchamp and Childress 2012). Beneficence requires researchers to take action to benefit and promote the welfare of participants (Butts and Rich 2013). Researchers should ponder on what benefit will occur for those being asked to participate and society in general. To ensure this, a risk-benefit analysis should be performed, considering all possible and perceived benefits. For example, a participant may overestimate the benefits of taking part in an experimental treatment in order to gain a chance to participate and receive the experimental treatment (Wertheimer 2013). While it is usual in qualitative research that participants may not directly benefit from their involvement, it is worth identifying that participants regularly experience a cathartic effect from telling and having their story heard (Rossetto 2014; Elmir et al. 2011; Davies and Gannon 2006). Beneficence of any action can be extremely personal and may differ between individuals, where what benefits one person might not benefit another.

Frequently, benefit is construed in the broadest sense and not always as a direct benefit of participating in the research; consequently, it is common and acceptable for researchers to propose a greater probable benefit to society rather than to individual participants. Where enticements are being offered for participation, they need to be considered in terms of risk–benefit analysis, as enticements may affect the participant's ability to make a truly autonomous decision to partake in the research. This applies especially to financial enticements, as offering research participants financial enticements is a common practice. It is successful in boosting recruitment, but raises ethical concerns, including undue incentive; manipulation of those with limited finances and biased enrolment. Resnik (2015) argues that researchers and oversight committees need to address the broad issues of beneficence and include articulation of the core aspects of justice and appropriate compensation, including: the amount of time participants spend on research activities; the risk, pain, discomfort and inconvenience associated with research procedures; travel costs; recruitment issues and the characteristics of the study population (e.g. income, age and mental health status). To us, these issues suggest a clear demand for the development of policy on compensation both financial and non-financial.

NON-MALEFICENCE

Researchers have a responsibility for assessing the key risks in any research situation to safeguard participants (Parahoo 2014). This includes the nature of any unnecessary physical, emotional or psychological strains placed on participants (Polit and Beck 2013). Physical harm may be easily recognised and consequently evaded or reduced; emotional, social or economic aspects may be less obvious. In Haney et al.'s (1973) prison experiments, where students were involved over several days in a role play as prisoners and guards, several participants experienced severe emotional reactions, including mental breakdown. Many of the participants in the Milgram (1963) research on obedience to authority experienced high levels of stress and anxiety as a result of being impelled to administer electric shocks. Although these studies would no longer receive ethical approval as the risks are clear, it is not always possible to anticipate all risks. For this reason, researchers should ensure that support mechanisms such as counselling or professional/workplace advice are in place in case any participant becomes distressed (during or after) as a result of the research experience, especially in relation to any potentially sensitive areas of research. In addition, the researcher should ensure that participants can cease their involvement at any time and only resume if and when they are ready (Burns and Grove 2013).

In certain areas of research, not least into views about ethical meaning and ongoing ethical practices in the workplace, there may be the possibility that misconduct or unethical practices could be disclosed. This demands that researchers are familiar with the governing body's policy guidelines in these situations to determine if there is any ethical imperative to disclose such information. The NMBI (2015) has highlighted that the researcher should have a clear reason for the disclosure and seek support from their supervisor, ethics committee and other relevant people, and that all decisions are clearly documented. This demands a careful examination of the effect of the consequences of any action upon the different stakeholders, not least the reputation of the organisation. In parallel situations, such as counselling, the stress is on the autonomy of participants, enabled through developing their own response and disclosure (Robinson 2008, see below on inclusion).

Often overlooked is the risk to the researchers themselves; for example, researchers working with participants in dangerous venues, such as a female researcher researching emergency medical work in Syria. This involves risk from the conflict and from cultural issues around single women.

Generally, researchers should adhere to their local health authority lone worker policy and maintain a visit proforma that is accessible to colleagues/supervisors monitoring their visits. In circumstances where researchers do not work within a health authority, they should check guidance from the ethics review committee/institutional review board, seek out and consult with their supervisors/colleagues and maintain a visit proforma monitoring their visits. Other potential harm to the researcher may be involved through exposure to a fieldwork setting and certain research methods, such as auto-ethnography. This may carry a greater risk of emotional or professional harm because the researcher's own self-disclosures are the basis for the analysis (Doloriert and Sambrook 2009) and might be made public. Doloriert and Sambrook (2009) argue that this is a particular concern for student researchers whose work will be examined by more experienced and more powerful senior researchers.

JUSTICE

The principle of justice demands fairness and equity throughout the research study. It demands fair recruiting mechanisms, providing equal chance to participate in research and ensuring anonymity, privacy and fair treatment (Dempsey and Dempsey 2000). Within the principle of justice, the researcher is obliged to distribute benefits and risks equally, without bias, and specific individuals, groups or communities should not bear an unfair share of the burden nor be unfairly omitted/excluded from the possible benefits of participation. Much of the issue of justice in research is answered if the researchers stay focused on the core purpose of the research, maintaining an attitude of disinterestedness and thus research integrity, leading to equality and equity (Alperovitch et al. 2009). Research participants in studies should be similar to those who may benefit from the outcome of that research, and be selected for reasons related to the phenomenon being investigated, rather than for convenience (Pratt and Loff 2011). As Doody and Noonan (2016) note, it can be challenging for researchers to ensure that all groups in society, regardless of perceived vulnerability, are able to benefit from being involved in research. Avoiding, including or making it difficult to include, any group in research based on perceived vulnerability could be described as 'unjust', as it could be argued that all participants in research are vulnerable because of the possible power relationship between them and the researchers (Karnieli-Miller et al. 2009; Riley et al. 2003).

VERACITY

Veracity requires the researcher to tell the truth about the study (Parahoo 2014). This involves clear communication about the purpose of the research and what the implications are for the participants. Participants should be cognisant of the anticipated involvement, duration (i.e. time commitment), what happens to their information and who will have access to their information. The principle of veracity is often thought of as a secondary principle. It is grounded in respect for the autonomy of the person and the principle and virtue of honesty. It is also grounded in the modes of responsibility, enabling clarity and logical thinking about core purpose and values; dialogue which enables accountability and some sense of shared responsibility for the enterprise. For a person to make a choice, they must have the appropriate information to make their decision. This should be clear, logical and truthful, and this involves avoiding academic jargon.

There have been many famous research projects in the past that would not have received research ethics approval precisely because their results were based on the deception of the participants. A good example of this was the Milgram (1963) experiment where participants thought they were taking part in an experiment about learning, when in fact it was about obedience, and they were the participants. This kind of research is sometimes referred as covert, but Spicker

(2011) argues that covert and deceptive research are quite distinct. Covert research, he argues, is when the research is not disclosed to the participant. Examples of this are:

- Research involving standing and watching what people are doing, such as checking the use of mobile phones in cars.
- Research which involves observing a public event, like a trial, a football match or a political meeting, and analysing aspects of the event.

Deception, however, occurs where the nature of a researcher's action is misrepresented to the participant. Engagement in deception usually involves the researchers claiming to do one thing, when they are actually doing another (Milgram 1963). Most objections are to deceptive rather than covert research and these objections include the dangers that:

- Deception betrays trust.
- Deception spoils the research environment, leading people to be suspicious of researchers.
- The habit of deception infects the researcher's behaviour – it becomes a way of life.
- The strain of maintaining a deception may be damaging to the researcher.
- Deception is bad for the reputation of research in general.
- Use of this method may legitimise deception more widely.

Despite these general objections, it may be that deception in research can be justified. In certain cases, it may be important to withhold information and conceal the true purpose and conditions of research in order to be able to investigate the issue. This should be undertaken only in cases where the participant's knowledge of the study will alter the results. Such research should only be used when the significance of the study, including the positive consequences, is justified and there is no other alternative procedure. The process of ethical approval is of particular importance with covert research and research involving deception. Social research ethical guidelines stress that no harm should come to the participants as a result of such research methods and advise that, ideally, researchers should seek consent after the research has ended.

7.1 PAUSE FOR THOUGHT

Considering Your Research Practice

Have you ever given a patient/client a placebo, when there is an effective treatment?
Is this ethically problematic?
Are you deceiving the patient/client?
How would you justify that?

The practice of using placebos in medical practice is problematic; prescribing placebos disguised as genuine medication raises questions about respect for the autonomy of the patient/client, and, in the long-term, negatively affecting their trust in healthcare providers. In research studies, placebos can provide evidence about the effectiveness of a treatment, but this may mean some patients/clients would be denied potentially effective treatment during a trial. Hence, some would argue that justice demands existing medical treatments be used instead of placebos, avoiding some patients not receiving medicine. The use of placebos requires ethical approval, and there is no blanket argument for their use. Ethical analysis and international ethical guidance permit the use of placebo controls in research in four situations (Millum and Grady 2013):

- Where there is no proven effective treatment for the condition under study.
- Where withholding treatment poses negligible risks to participants.
- Where there are compelling methodological reasons, *and* withholding treatment does not pose a risk of serious harm to participants.
- When there are compelling methodological reasons for using placebo, *and* the research is intended to develop interventions that can be implemented in the population from which trial participants are drawn, *and* the trial does not require participants to forgo treatment they would otherwise receive.

FIDELITY

Fidelity focuses on the essential trust between the researcher and participants (Macnee and McCabe 2008). Participants experience a slightly different sense of vulnerability from ordinary patients/clients specifically because they do not know what the outcome of their involvement may be. Hence, this creates an additional duty to safeguard them. This involves fully including participants in all aspects of the study, including an understanding of both the risks and the potential benefits and understanding the safeguard to their rights (Parahoo 2014). As part of this process, participants should know they can withdraw from the research at any time without any consequences. The strength of this trusting relationship is in its mutuality. Researchers have to develop trust in participants' conditional commitment to the enterprise and their veracity about experiences or actions, such as taking medicine according to the study protocol. Participants in such a trusting relationship are more likely to continue in the study and are not shocked or startled by the burden of participation (Coghlan and Brydon-Miller 2014). This adds to the understanding of autonomy as not simply freedom of choice but also taking responsibility for choice and actions subsequent to that. It also raises the status of the participant, something examined in Chapter 10, and the idea of the gift relationship (Titmuss 1972). Titmuss argued that patients' involvement in research was part of their contribution to the wider Welfare Society.

CONFIDENTIALITY

Part of any protection of the participant is the guarantee of confidentiality about their identity and their data. There may be circumstances where confidentiality can be broken, and information passed on without the participant's consent. These include public interest and safety, where the researcher believes that there may be a danger in non-disclosure (NMBI 2015). Determining sufficient reason for this is not straightforward and requires dialogue with research supervisors or colleagues, the ethics committee or other relevant persons, and all decisions need to be clearly documented (NMBI 2015). Confidentiality can be assisted by assigning an identification number or pseudonym to participants (Polit and Beck 2013). Small samples and/or quotes in the data might lead to participants being recognised. This requires that researchers exclude individual expressions or language nuance when transcribing, analysing data and writing up findings. Raw data should comprise the name and/or identifiers (code, pseudonyms) that can be used to connect the participant's data to their name. Although researchers have access to this information, it should not be enclosed in the final report, nor should anybody other than those stated in the consent form have access to the data (Dempsey and Dempsey 2000). In addition, storage of data is a priority and data should be stored in a locked facility, and all electronic data should be password-protected. Participants should also be aware of where their data will be stored, for how long (duration stipulated by ethics boards is often 5–10 years) and how data will be destroyed after this time.

The terms 'anonymity' and 'confidentiality' are often used interchangeably, but they are not identical; anonymity is a form of confidentiality, where participants' identities are kept secret, that is, data do not include any identifiers, codes or exclusive information that can be used to identify the participant. Participants have the right to exclude themselves, or their information, and thus express themselves selectively. This tendency varies among cultures and individuals. In research, the use of interviews can pose difficulties, as the direction of questions cannot always be predicted, and probing questions are used to obtain important information about the phenomenon under enquiry (Parahoo 2014; Richards and Schwartz 2002). Therefore, participants may reveal intimate and personal details, and researchers should reassure participants that the information they disclose is confidential.

Much of this thinking, of course, is based on the assumption that research participants 'not only deserve the protection of anonymity, but that they actively desire it' (Grinyer 2002, p. 2). The allocation of pseudonyms to guard anonymity can cause unforeseen stress, as research participants sometimes feel that keeping their real names is an important recognition of their involvement in the research project (Grinyer 2002). This highlights how problematic it can be to make judgements on behalf of others, however well-intentioned, leading to the recommendation that this issue be dealt with on a case-by-case basis, through consultation with research participants throughout the research and publication process so that individuals have the freedom to make a more informed choice and are less likely to feel that they have lost ownership of their stories (Grinyer 2002).

VULNERABILITY

The risks to participants are even greater when research involves vulnerable participants, including those with dementia or intellectual/learning disability, children or those advanced in age. This may involve particular ongoing support such as ensuring an easy-read format for consent purposes, or having a familiar person present, as well as appropriate care and counselling support. Ganguli-Mitra and Biller-Andorno (2011) argue for three forms of vulnerability and related risks, which are competence, voluntariness and fairness. Competence comes into consideration when involving groups such as children or those suffering from mental or behavioural disorders that render them incapable of giving informed consent. Critical to this is the participants 'inability to assess risk' (Ganguli-Mitra and Biller-Andorno 2011). Voluntariness relates to participants who may have full cognitive capacity but be susceptible to manipulation or inducement of some form. This focuses on participants who are in a vulnerable power relationship, such as students, prisoners, junior professionals etc., and Ganguli-Mitra and Biller-Andorno (2011) argue that this can be exacerbated by social or medical experiences or conditions such as poverty or illness. Fairness amplifies the issue of power imbalances, and it targets the assumptions behind the attitude of healthcare professionals and researchers about groups in society which have been systematically excluded not just from research, but from society, including the frail older persons and people with intellectual/learning disability.

Such insights emerge from socio-political thinking such as critical thinking (Giroux 2010), and challenge us to question the power assumptions that underlie practice and research. Ganguli-Mitra and Biller-Andorno (2011) apply this thinking to research in their argument that vulnerable groups have been excluded from research partly because they have not fitted into the research agenda and partly because of paternalism that seeks to protect these groups. In making decisions about vulnerable participants in research, mainly, the research has to be focused on benefitting the group, and the means of consent has to be carefully worked through with research ethics committees. There are situations where the experience of the researcher can lead to the empowerment of participants, that is, the development of some form of agency. A good example of this is in qualitative research, which focuses on participants developing and reflecting on their narrative, and thus upon their self-image (Romanoff 2001) and the involvement of participants as co-researchers (Mockford et al. 2016).

Regulation and Governance of Research Ethics

It was after the Nuremberg trials that the WMA began developing guidelines for biomedical research, with the Geneva Declaration (WMA 1948) and the Helsinki Declaration (WMA 1964). However, as we shall see with governance in Chapter 9, none of these developments prevented the abuse of the research process in the post-war years. As a result, in 1975, the WMA recommended the establishment of independent committees of research ethics to assess all medical research involving people (WMA 1975). The practice of research ethics committees was perhaps the most effective element in both promoting good scientific and good ethical practice. What links the two once more is the practise of responsibility. The more rigorous the setting out of the research and how it relates to the social and medical environments, the more researchers practice accountability.

This underlines that research ethics committees are not simply a means of regulation. At their best, they enable dialogue, deliberation and good judgement about research practice.

The Research Governance Framework

In the United Kingdom (UK), the Department of Health (DoH) implemented the Research Governance Framework (RGF) to strengthen public trust in research (DoH 2005b). The improvements in the managing and monitoring of research precisely enabled greater accountability to all stakeholders, underscoring the integrity of the research process. The framework is key to all who are involved in research, including funders, host organisations, those carrying out the research (leaders and team members) and the participants of research. Hence all stakeholders should be familiar with the RGF and adhere to its principles. The framework relates to the key principles of a research culture in five governance domains (RCN 2009):

- Ethics.
- Science.
- Information.
- Health, safety and employment.
- Finance and intellectual property.

The ethics domain focuses on all the principles above including the dignity, rights, safety and well-being of participants as core to all research practice. As noted above, these connect to the practice of data protection, informed consent and confidentiality. It is important to note that the other domains are not separate from ethics. On the contrary, the science domain, for example, is built around core aspects of disinterestedness and justice. The principle of disinterestedness itself involves different principles, including: honesty, responsibility (confirming that the research is the result of the researchers' actual work) and accountability (to the research community, and all other stakeholders involved). Disinterestedness raises critical points about avoiding conflict of interest. The science domain also includes the ethical imperative of generating high quality research that is not duplicated. In practice, this means that existing sources of evidence should be used and all research proposals should be subject to peer review. Special guidance is given for research involving human embryos, animals, genetically modified organisms and medicines.

The information domain highlights the principles of honesty, transparency and accountability, including the need for information on research and subsequent findings to be accessible to the public through publication. The health, safety and employment domain ties into the principles of beneficence and non-maleficence. It focuses on careful adherence to health and safety regulations, including approval if new or existing medical devices need to be approved by the Medical Devices Agency. The finance and intellectual property (IP) domain requires compliance with the law and any rules for the use of public funds. Compensation is recommended for anyone harmed as a result of studies. IP is concerned with inventions, know-how (knowledge), copyrights and database rights, designs, trademarks and materials. Copyright, for instance, requires agreement about authorship and any related funds due to the author to be credited to the author from the beginning of the research. Once again, these elements relate directly to ethics, not least justice, in the sense of fair dealing, respect for individual rights and honesty.

Conflict of Interest

Conflict of interest refers to situations in which interests other than the research focus might compromise, or appear to compromise, the professional judgement of a researcher. Most conflicts of interest focus on researchers' relationship to sponsors of research, and to a reward, financial or reputational, that the researcher may have with them. It is important to note that questions of potential conflict of interest apply not just to researchers but to all involved in the research ethics process. A local research ethics coordinator (see below) might have strong financial links to a sponsor that could cause him not to question a proposal linked to that sponsor, or strong links to a group opposed to that sponsor (such as a non-governmental organisation (NGO) or advocacy group) that would affect his judgement about the involvement of the sponsor. Cancer Research UK (CRUK 2013) lists eight forms of relationship between researchers and sponsors:

- Employment, directorship or leadership position.
- Advisory role (paid or unpaid).
- Share ownership or options.
- Any other direct or indirect financial interest (e.g. via rewards to inventors).
- Honoraria-payments for specific speeches, seminar presentations or appearances.
- Research funding.
- Expert testimony.
- Other remuneration (trips, gifts, in-kind payments, etc.).

In the modern research climate, where researchers have to work with organisations outside of the academia organisation, both to justify the impact of their research and to gain needed resources for sustaining that research, it is difficult to avoid such relationships. Hence, many argue that it is better to use non-conflictual terms such as 'competing interests' (National Research Ethics Advisors' Panel – NREAP 2012). It is estimated that more than one-third of GPs in the UK had a competing interest due to investments in pharmaceutical companies (Iacobucci 2013). Key principles in managing competing interests recommended by National Research Ethics Advisors' Panel (NREAP 2012) include:

- Transparency, declaring all competing interests.
- Sharing of responsibilities with (independent) others acting as a corrective to any bias.
- Divesting responsibility of the research to (independent) others.
- Independent trial management/monitoring.
- Access to unbiased information for participants.
- Freedom of Publication. This means that all parties should be free to publish (negative) data.

In addition, limits might set on any remuneration received by the researcher. Oxford University procedures requiring disclosure of competing interests include an annual declaration of significant financial interests. A significant financial interest is said to exist if the value of any remuneration received from the entity in the 12 months preceding the disclosure, and the value of any equity interest in the entity as of the date of disclosure, when aggregated, exceeds £5000 (Oxford University Research Support 2018). CRUK requires a declaration of any of the above relationships of the investigators, their immediate family, spouses or partners and children, and limits remuneration (of all types) to less than £5000 per year, thus also requiring an annual declaration of conflict of interest. For further guidance about declaration on interests see NREAP (2012).

Key then to managing the competing interests is clarity about the nature of the different relationships. Hence, for instance, any funding must not constitute an inducement to prescribe, supply, administer, recommend, buy or sell any medicine, medical device, equipment or service. Researchers should ensure that they find out and adhere to institutional and governmental requirements for identifying, disclosing and managing conflicts of interest, and where possible, avoid or minimise contact with competing interests. Responsibility for management is shared, then, by the researcher and the research governance structure. It might also involve the broader groups such as professional bodies and Higher Education Institutes (HEIs), which host medical and healthcare research. From a publication perspective, publishers have implemented ethics in standards across their journals. In 1997, the committee on publication ethics (COPE) was created, and it developed its guidelines on good publication practice in 1999 and its code of conduct for editors in 2004. For details on COPE see https://publicationethics.org/about/our-organisation, and for a publication house, see, for example, Elsevier https://www.elsevier.com/about/policies/publishing-ethics.

Ethical Approval

Gaining ethical approval demands applying to research ethics committees (RECs) in the local Healthcare Trust. RECs are formed of voluntary members, consisting of one-third lay members, and the remainder of the committee providing medical, educational and scientific experience and expertise. Each committee is supported by a local administrator and by the National Research Ethics Service. RECs exist to safeguard the rights, safety, dignity and well-being of research participants. RECs review research proposals and give an opinion about whether the research is ethical. They also look at issues such as participant involvement in the research. The committees are entirely independent of research sponsors (the organisations responsible for the management and conduct of the research), funders and the researchers themselves. This enables them to put participants at the centre of their review. Providing the research is not a clinical trial of a new medicinal product, a study that is to be held on one site can be considered by the local research ethics committee (LREC). This may be complicated by context. For instance, if research is based in a university, then ethical approval might have to come from there as well. Again, regulations should be checked from the local healthcare organisation and the university.

LRECs have to respond within 60 days to applications. However, the whole process can be significantly longer. For example, research in sensitive contexts, for instance involving children, may need to complete an enhanced Criminal Records Bureau check or undergo occupational health screening. The British Psychological Society (2014) provides a good example of its support for research ethics in its Code of Human Research Ethics, which sum up the responsibilities of RECs as:

- Reviewing all research involving human participants conducted by individuals employed within or by that institution.
- Ensuring that ethics review is independent, competent and timely; protecting the dignity, rights and welfare of research participants; considering the safety of the researcher(s).
- Considering the legitimate interests of other stakeholders.
- Making informed judgements of the scientific merit of proposals.
- Making informed recommendations to the researcher if the proposal is found to be wanting in some respect.

The last two responsibilities are key, and the first of these underscores the importance of judging the scientific robustness of the proposal. Research which is not well thought through, including a clear understanding of context and impact, often leads directly to ethical problems. The informed recommendations are part of the ongoing dialogue learning cycle of good research. Detailed guidance about online applications is provided by the Health Research Authority (HRA 2020) and can be located at https://www.hra.nhs.uk/approvals-amendments/what-approvals-do-i-need/research-ethics committee-review/applying-research-ethics-committee/; in addition, also see Haigh (2007). The HRA (2020) in England and Wales sums up what research involves, and thus what requires approval:

- A Clinical Trial of an Investigational Medicinal Product (CTIMP) (with the exception of phase 1 trials in healthy volunteers taking place outside the NHS).
- A Clinical Investigation or other study of a Medical Device.
- A combined trial of an Investigational Medicinal Product and an Investigational Medical Device.
- A Clinical Trial to study a novel intervention or randomised Clinical Trial to compare interventions in clinical practice.
- A basic science study involving procedures with human participants.
- A study administering questionnaires/interviews for quantitative analysis, or using mixed qualitative/quantitative methodology.
- A study involving qualitative methods only.

- A study limited to working with human tissue samples (or other human biological samples) and data (specific project only).
- A study limited to working with data (specific project only).

Human Tissue Act

Clinical research nurses can be involved in research that includes the collection and storage of human tissue, though rarely as lead investigator. This may involve focusing on obtaining consent as part of a larger team, and this demands awareness of responsibilities set out under the Human Tissue Act (Human Tissue Authority – HTA 2004). The Human Tissue Act covers any material containing human cells, except gametes and fetal material outside a woman's body. This includes hair and nails from living people. The primary principle of the Act is one of explicit and appropriate consent, and the key points of the Human Tissue Act are:

- The Human Tissue Act 2004 regulates the removal, storage and use of human tissue. This is defined as material that has come from a human body and consists of, or includes, human cells.
- The Human Tissue Act 2004 creates a new offence of DNA 'theft'. It is unlawful to have human tissue with the intention of its DNA being analysed, without the consent of the person from whom the tissue came.
- The Human Tissue Act 2004 makes it lawful to take minimum steps to preserve the organs of a deceased person for use in transplantation while steps are taken to determine the wishes of the deceased, or in the absence of their known wishes, obtaining consent from someone in a qualifying relationship.

For detailed guidance on the Human Tissue Act, see Brazier and Forvargue (2006) and given that issues related to this act will be debated, challenged and reviewed, it is good to keep abreast of the issues from practice and policy. Some areas to consider reading would be articles on organ donation (Okenyi 2016); storage, retention and use of human tissue specimens (Kapila et al. 2016); right to paternity testing of tissue samples (Wilkinson and Stirton 2018) and conflicts over the excavation, retention and display of human remains (White 2019).

Internet Ethics

Recent decades have seen the development and increased use of internet-based research methods, including: web page content analysis; online focus groups; online interviews and analysis of e-conversations. Haigh and Jones (2005) have provided an analysis of the ethical dilemmas that underpin cyberspace research, and the Association of Internet Researchers (AoIR) has developed ethical guidelines (AoIR 2019) focusing on: maintaining participants' privacy and confidentiality; gaining informed consent and questions of verifying the identity of subjects in the world of online research. The responsibility of the researcher being involved in constant dialogue and deliberation with participants, not least because cyberspace is continually evolving (AoIR 2019). As well as consulting the AoIR guidance, any researcher involved in such research should also consult the research guidance of their host HEI and the ESRC (2015) ethical framework (https://esrc.ukri.org/files/funding/guidance-for-applicants/esrc-framework-for-research-ethics-2015/). Orton-Johnson (2010) argues that the ethical responses to the internet, including that of the ESRC, have too often been broad brush and negative, lacking an appreciation of cyberspace and its potential.

The Nursing Student as Research Participant

Students are often used in lecturers' research projects, not least because they are accessible and usually amenable. However, students are a captive population. The relationship of lecturer to student is one of fiduciary trust. A fiduciary relationship is one of inequality, where the more powerful actor is entrusted with the best interests of the less powerful actor (Lemmens and Singer 1998). This sets up a relationship of dependency, which demands trust, and is central to the education of students. In the context of research, this relationship is tested by the use of students as participants, because lecturers take on double agency. This refers to fulfilling two roles simultaneously in relation to the same individuals (Edwards and Chalmers 2002), teacher–student and researcher–participant. This raises potential conflicts of interest and challenges to ethical principles in the relationship (Lemmens and Singer 1998). These ethical challenges come throughout the research process: recruitment, the informed and voluntary consent process (risks and benefits), data collection, participant withdrawal, anonymity and confidentiality.

In the recruitment and voluntary consent process, there is a danger that it might unintentionally exert pressure on students to participate (Ebbs 1996), eroding any sense of actual choice. The risk of not participating may be perceived by the student as leading to a negative attitude from the lecturer/researcher, which may affect the learning relationship, including fewer learning opportunities, lower evaluative outcomes or slower progress in general, and even possible lower marks (Ferrari and McGowan 2002). At best, participation might be focused on the desire to please lecturers, rather than a careful deliberation about capacity, resources and risk. The pressure on students to participate is tangible, whether risks and benefits are real or imagined. Transparency and dialogue in the process may mitigate some of these issues. However, the usual assurance of research expectations, such as the opportunity to withdraw at any time, is of little consequence if the initial decision is focused on a student's dependency relationships with the teacher.

Students have a right to privacy as they engage in learning (Dyregrov 2004; Orb et al. 2001; Kavanaugh and Ayres 1998), and this may be compromised within the data collection process. There is a danger that, especially in qualitative research, the focus might be on personal and intimate issues that students might choose to keep private. A power difference exists between lecturer and student, where students are asked about personal information, that could influence the learning situation for that student. In turn, this affects the quality of the research. Participant withdrawal from research has similar problems to recruitment. The sense of obligation to the researcher, based on real or imagined duties, along with the knowledge of the time and effort put in by the researcher, can make it very hard to withdraw. Hence, even when the research process is arduous, distressing or inconvenient for the student participant, they may feel that withdrawal could have a negative impact on the teaching relationship.

Confidentiality and anonymity are based on the principle of respect for the dignity and autonomy of research participants. However, whilst the identity of student participants can be kept from the public, it is very difficult to maintain anonymity of participants from the researcher. Hence, the researcher is unable to maintain the confidentiality of data from those in academic and professional power, viz. themselves. It is possible to maintain anonymity with respect to other members of the faculty and trust if research techniques are rigorously followed. The need to advance the knowledge of the disciplines or the pedagogy of the disciplines is a worthy goal. Nonetheless, there will be constant tension between the roles of the researcher and the lecturer, which has to be managed. Strategies include:

- RECs will provide an independent perspective seeking to protect and support both parties.
- A primary question for researchers is whether the research goals can be achieved by involving participants who are not in dependent relationships with the researcher.
- Convenience of participants should not be a criterion.
- The frequency of research participation invites to students should be monitored. High levels could add to any sense of stress.
- Research about the experience and nature of pedagogy demands student participants. Any negative impact can be mitigated through the use of several strategies:
  - Recruit students in that programme who the researcher is not directly responsible for (Moreno 1998).

- Make use of intermediaries such as other faculty members or research assistants for recruitment, clarifications and even data gathering, including ensuring anonymity from the lead researcher (Edwards and Chalmers 2002; Bell and Nutt 1999).
- Avoid unnecessary personal disclosure by the student, including the use of reflective journals.
- Avoiding naming institutions or locations (Morse and Richards 2002), reporting the contributions of single participants so their interviews could be reconstructed or using quotations that reveal participants' roles or responsibilities are all ways in which their anonymity can remain uncompromised.

7.2 PAUSE FOR THOUGHT

Consider Your Practice Area and Research Activities

Are there situations where similar issues to those discussed above would arise between the researcher and participant?

How would this play out if you were doing a study in your area of practice and you required the participation of (1) patients, (2) students on placement, (3) fellow staff and (4) management grades?

What if your manager was doing the study and you were invited to participate, how would you decide to be involved or not?

How honest would you be with your manager if it were about practice issues or your experience?

Double Agency

The nurse as researcher is not only a teacher but is also a member of the nursing profession and this may also lead to managing different expectations. For example, you are involved in ethnographic research (the scientific description of peoples and cultures with their customs, habits and mutual differences), which involves you observing a unit. Lunch is delivered, but one elderly patient finds it hard to reach the food. The assistant asks one of the nurses to help the man sit up properly so he can reach it. The man thanks the nurse but says he cannot properly see it. The nurse does not answer, simply pushes the food a little closer, and then leaves. It takes the man several minutes to locate the cutlery, and much of the food slips off his fork. He locates his pudding, in a plastic container but finds it hard to hold the container, spilling its contents. The staff member who brought the food returns soon after. 'Well John, you've not made much of an effort have you' she says, and takes the remains of his lunch away. John does not answer.

7.3 PAUSE FOR THOUGHT

Considering the Case of John

What would your response be here?
   Is there a conflict between your researcher role and professional role?
   Does the case above involve a question of patient/client safety?
   Would you inform the unit manager, and if so, when would you do it?
   Was there any harm being caused to the patient/client?

In such situations, it is important to refer to one's code of professional practice and, for example, the Nursing and Midwifery Council (NMC 2018) code requires that there should be no delay in responding to a situation where there is risk to patient safety. Thus, if you were the researcher observing in this case and you felt there was a risk to the patient's/client's safety, your professional responsibility would take precedence over your research. The management of different interests demands the establishment of a protocol. In this case, the research protocol should have included an indication of how the observation of poor care would be managed. This may involve immediate reporting of care that required a swift response, in this case, an older patient unable to eat his lunch, and later reporting of practices which are less problematic.

Research in the Dementia Population

At the time of writing this book, there were around 850,000 people with dementia in the UK, and this is projected to rise to 1.6 million by 2040 (Alzheimer's Society 2019). One in six people over the age of 80 have dementia, and there are over 42,000 people under 65 with dementia. The total cost of care for people with dementia in the UK is £34.7 billion. This is set to rise sharply over the next two decades, to £94.1 billion by 2040. Unpaid carers supporting someone with dementia save the UK economy £13.9 billion a year. The cost of social care for people with dementia is set to nearly treble by 2040, increasing from £15.7 billion to £45.4 billion. The Alzheimer's Society (2019) suggests that research into dementia falls broadly into four categories: cause, cure, care and prevention. As well as searching for a cure and effective treatment, research is important to develop interventions that can improve quality of life. The National Institute for Health and Clinical Excellence (NICE) and Social Care Institute for Excellence (SCIE) recommend research into four areas, one to establish the usefulness of existing treatments and the other three related to drug-free interventions (Gould and Kendall 2007).

However, research which involves patients/clients with dementia is problematic as symptoms, including loss of short-term memory problems and difficulty with concentration and understanding, all of which get worse as the disease progresses, call into question the capacity for informed consent. For the most part then, as consent strictly can only come from the participant, researchers have sought assent (giving approval on behalf of another) from relatives of patients with dementia. This is not always straightforward, as it is not always clear that next of kin actually know what the patient/client would have wanted. Moreover, it is conceivable that the participant could object to the next of kin's assent (Kitwood 1995). With this in mind, the Medical Research Council (MRC 2007) guidance comes down on the wishes of the person with dementia. What needs to be considered is that dementia does not mean a person automatically lacks the capacity to consent. However, the exact nature of informed consent begins to be questioned. Does informed consent actually need the person to be fully aware of all aspects of the research in order to give consent? The stress on transparency and honesty above assumes this. However, as Pratt (2002) suggests, whilst it is not possible to be certain of informed consent with someone who has dementia, it is probably true that there is not complete certainty of informed consent from any participant. It is unlikely that all participants have been told every detail, for example, the details of the data analysis. The Mental Capacity Act (DoH 2005a) assumes capacity if the person can:

- understand information relevant to the decision, including consequences.
- retain information.
- use or weigh the information as part of the process of making the decision.
- communicate their decision.

This provides a starting point for assuring that patients/clients have protection (NMC 2018), and Dewing (2007) argues that informed consent should be seen as a process which takes account of situational complexity and, in her research, this involved:

- Gaining permission to access the patient from staff and from next of kin or named person. This involves biographical information.
- Establishing the basis for consent. This may involve discovering how the patient consents to ongoing care or activities, including consideration of the best time to approach the patient, given possible fluctuations of cognition.

- Seeking initial consent, recording non-verbal communication and once more focusing on the patient's usual means of consent. At this stage, absence of verbal objection should not be assumed as consent.
- Ongoing monitoring of consent, involving revisiting the decision with each engagement.
- Feedback to staff and next of kin.

The process is focused on constant dialogue with gatekeepers who allow access and understandings to be brought to the situation. For example, next of kin may share anxieties of the patient/client about loss of control, and staff may be able to observe how the experience negatively or positively affects the patient/client. The principle objection with the process consent method is how much time it takes to do well. It also requires high care skills from the researcher. However, such professional skills are necessary in many qualitative research processes, not least those which focus on the narrative of the patient/client. Moreover, these are necessary for the researcher to balance the principles of beneficence, non-maleficence and respect for autonomy. Hence, when conducting a study, the researcher should remain focused on other indicators of the client's general well-being, including facial expressions, to assist in identifying their capacity to consent (Dewing 2007).

Dewing (2007) notes an ethical objection, that in the early stages the researcher will be gathering some data about the patient/client without consent to the research. A more general problem is the accidental disclosure of diagnosis. The patient may not know he has the condition, and awareness of the diagnosis in a lucid period could cause intense anxiety. The principle of non-maleficence comes up against the principle of respect for autonomy. Some would argue for the avoidance of 'unnecessary truth' (Andrew 2006), whereas others (Marzanski 2000) see it as 'justifiable benevolent deception'.

The autonomy of the patient/client with dementia is, of course, problematic. However, what is clear is that knowledge of the actual diagnosis is not critical to respecting limited autonomy. Pratt (2002) in her research spoke with the patients/clients about the symptoms of dementia and did not bring up actual diagnosis unless the patient/client asked about it. Once more, autonomy emerges as a function of dialogue. The dialogue and care can be furthered by having family members or staff members well known to participants present during data collection. Acting as third parties or validator is important for identifying signs of discomfort or stress should they transpire.

This focus on the wider responsibility for care reinforces the point that research is not something that happens apart from care. Indeed, as noted above, whilst the research has a specific wider purpose, it can have strong benefits for the patient/client. These include: helping others to better understand their reality, gaining insight into the experiential nature or quality of life, understanding the embodied experience of dementia, getting the perspectives of those under-represented in public policy and discovering positive experiences of care. The simple experience of spending more time with patients/clients has a positive effect on their sense of well-being, esteem and capacity (Clark and Keady 2002; Dewing 2002; Kapp 1998). Hellstrom et al. (2007) link this to respect for the dignity of the patient/client, with inclusion enhancing that dignity. This takes us to a wider more holistic view of dignity, which is not purely based on respect for the rational capacity of the other (Rosen 2018). The focus is less on rationality than on the recognition of and response to humanity, and this emerges in relationships of mutuality and the ensuing sense of purpose and worth (Robinson et al. 2003). In order to effectively meet the care needs of people diagnosed with dementia, we must understand what those needs are, and it is clear that this information is best obtained from people with dementia themselves. Thus, research that aims to understand the experience of living with dementia will help to improve the services provided and is therefore essential in creating a better understanding of their care needs and their experiences.

Gatekeepers

Gaining access to research participants nearly always includes going through gatekeepers or facilitators and a hierarchy of gatekeepers (Goldsmith and Skirton 2015) or tiers of management (McKeown et al. 2010). Using gatekeepers typically involves the added stage of providing the gatekeeper with information about the study and asking them to suggest or contact potential participants. This involves building rapport and trust with the gatekeeper before doing so with potential/actual participants. For gatekeepers to support, they will want to be convinced of the benefits for the people they often regard as in need of their safeguarding. It is recognised that while there is a need to include individuals who may be seen as vulnerable in research, there remains a possibly negative outcome in that of exclusion for the least able through the over-protection and gatekeeping roles taken by service providers. Gatekeepers are faced with the hard decision when trying to agree to grant access but may actually block access (Morrisey 2012), rendering the person silent (Witham et al. 2015), and this shielding power can be seen as oppressive (Tew 2011). This difficult position placed upon gatekeepers may be lessened by them having access to the ethics committee's review comments and a letter of approval to support their decision making and decrease their apprehensions.

Having to negotiate access to a client group such as people with intellectual/leaning disability reveals the importance of gatekeepers when it comes to conducting research (Peel and Wilson 2008). Here, the directors of the organisation/agency act as initial gatekeeper, granting access to their facilities to conduct the study. The second layer of gatekeepers is the staff members on whom researchers rely, to approach care recipients and inquire if they would be interested in being involved and to ensure that potential participants understand the researcher's explanation of why the researcher wishes to involve them, what the research will involve and that they could withdraw at any point during the process. Gatekeepers may also enable access and have a significant role in carefully explaining to participants how research is different from intervention, with different purposes and timelines (Mumford et al. 2008). Moreover, staff are often required to remain with clients during data collection and are often too busy and tired or too suspicious of the research to want to get involved (Oye et al. 2015). Although staff members do not have the power to deny permission because the director would already have granted authority, they have power to block access to clients (Stalker 1998). The power of gatekeepers can also be explicit in their ability to make determinations about which clients may be more appropriate to participate in the research than others (Morrisey 2012). In addition, self-advocacy organisations supporting people with intellectual/learning disability can become overwhelmed by the increasing volume of opportunities to participate in research and reject approaches from some researchers.

Inclusion in Research

To draw attention to this debate, we continue with the field of intellectual/learning disability and dementia. The drive for inclusion in research developed in parallel with academic discourse and culminated with the publication of Nothing About Us Without Us (Charlton 2000), which united academics, professionals, clinicians and individuals who valued sharing research agendas. Inclusive research integrates two methodological approaches – participative research and emancipatory research (Walmsley and Johnson 2003; Chappell 2000). Participative research assists coalitions or partnerships to develop between the researcher and the participants. Within participatory research, it is important to differentiate between the level of participation, as people with intellectual/learning disability or dementia may participate, but have no control of the research process. Emancipatory research, on the other hand, enables people with intellectual/learning disability or dementia gain control of the full research process, thus leading to empowerment, social change and the emancipation of people with disabilities or dementia (Walmsley 2004; Wilkinson 2002). The participatory model, to date, has been more commonly used, endorsing partnership working by professionals and clients, whereas the aim of the emancipatory approach is for clients to have control by being involved in all decisions throughout the process (Walmsley 2004).

In comparison, emancipatory methodologies are based on the social model (creating access and removing barriers) and can utilise either qualitative or quantitative methods in the research process, where the researchers' knowledge is available for people with disability or dementia. Emancipatory research is committed to changing the circumstances of the relationship between the researcher and the researched (Oliver 1997). This form of research represents a shift from doing research on and about populations, to conducting research with populations and involving relevant patients/clients, carers or their representative groups in the design, conduct, analysis and reporting of research (DoH 2005b). Through using such methods, researchers can be best informed as to how they will frame their research questions, test the validity and acceptability of the research methodology and assist in interpretation of the findings. In these ways, inclusive approaches augment the efficacy of research and, in today's research environment, many funding agencies require an inclusive approach (Doody 2018). In addition, the United Nations' Convention on Rights for Persons with Disabilities challenges researchers to find ways to include people with intellectual/learning disability or dementia in the development of research about them and to collect data and statistics which can inform policy and practice (UN 2006).

Including people with intellectual/learning disabilities or dementia in research about their lives is widely recognised (Carey et al. 2014; Heggestad et al. 2013), and progress is evident with the promotion of inclusive research (Bane et al. 2012; Hubbard et al. 2003). To support the inclusion of people with intellectual/learning disability or dementia in research, a diversity of approaches and forms of involvement have arisen (Fudge Schormans et al. 2019; Novek and Wilkinson 2019; Murphy et al. 2015; Bigby et al. 2014; O'Brien et al. 2014; McKeown et al. 2010). Utilisation of supports are evident across the research literature such as:

- Akkerman et al. (2014) photovoice.
- Bartlett (2012) diary keeping.
- Benbow and Kingston (2016) autobiographical narrative production.
- Cannella-Malone et al. (2013) video-recording.
- Capstick and Ludwin (2015) filmmaking.
- Darewych et al. (2015) art medium.
- Jenkins et al. (2016) writing and acting.
- Manning (2009) story-telling.
- McCleery (2015) high-technology devices and supports.
- Murphy et al. (2010) talking mats.

In addition, people with intellectual/learning disability or dementia have been involved in: acting as an adviser (Ward and Campbell 2013; Nind and Vinha 2012), data collection and analysis (O Sullivan et al. 2014; Kramer et al. 2011), provision of research education and training (Cheffey et al. 2017; Salmon et al. 2014), dissemination of research findings (Wiersma 2011; Goodley and Moore 2000), identification of research questions (Digby et al. 2016; Garbutt et al. 2009), being a member of an ethics committee (McDonald and Kidney 2012) and being involved or their involvement advocated at each step of the research process (Gove et al. 2018; Tuffrey-Wijne and Butler 2010; Kramer et al. 2011). Thus, the opportunity to take part in research is increasing for many people with dementia or intellectual/learning disability (Gove et al. 2018; Roberts et al. 2011).

What must be considered is that people with dementia or intellectual/learning disability are a heterogeneous population, and within this population, many sub-groups exist depending on the level of severity or stage of the disease. Some individuals with intellectual/learning disability or dementia will have few problems understanding the nature of a research project and the implications of their involvement. They will be able to make a decision about their participation and

TABLE 7.3 ■ Ethics in Practice Guide

- How the research is to be explained to the participants?
- How participant consent (and/or proxy consent) is to be obtained?
- How participants are to be treated during the research?
- What safeguards are in place to minimise any potential harm to participants?
- What mechanisms are in place to respond to any adverse events?
- How participants' personal information and research results pertaining to them as an individual are to be kept private and confidential?
- What mechanisms are in place to report findings to the participants and allow for peer review by the scientific community?
- What mechanisms are in place to maximise any benefit to participants (and their community) of research findings?

From Dalton, A. J., & McVilly, K. R. (2004). Ethics guidelines for international, multicenter research involving people with intellectual disabilities. *Journal of Policy and Practice in Intellectual Disabilities, 1* (2), 57–70.

provide or withhold their consent. However, people whose ability and associated needs require the highest levels of continual support and care challenge our understanding of how best to support their participation in research. This group is also least equipped to understand their own situation and be able to articulate their sense of self (Doody 2018). Nevertheless, people should not be excluded, in society or in research, and the MRC (2007) noted that people who do not have the capacity to consent should not be discriminated against by being excluded from research, as this would be stopping them from participating fully in society. Any such research would, however, require appropriate safeguards due to the vulnerability of the group. Thereby careful planning by the researcher on issues, such as access to participants, consent by participants, content and appropriateness of information (written and verbal), nature and duration of data collection, support required by participants, accessibility and transport arrangements need to be considered.

Early commentators such as Oliver (1992) and Zarb (1992) advocate for an emancipatory model, framing research as an activity decided by people rather than by professional researchers, thereby creating three aspects of research ethics – consent, inclusion and review and access – all of which work for or against the interest of some individuals. To address vulnerability and the aspect of inclusion/exclusion, ethics committees/institutional review boards should have at least one member who can represent and advocate for the interests of those participants for the study. This would enable ethics committees to move away from protectionism and acknowledge the empowering potential of inclusive research (Doody 2018). To do this, it may be helpful to distinguish between procedural ethics (what happens in research design and in research ethics committees) and ethics in practice (what happens in the interactions between researcher and participants and in the way data are interpreted, communicated and used). Ethics in practice is enhanced by procedural ethics, and the underlying values are the same. Dalton and McVilly (2004) offer a guide for ethics in practice when conducting research with people with intellectual/learning disability, and similarities can be drawn for the dementia population (Table 7.3).

The Ethical Framework of Teaching

Nurse training, like the training of most professions, takes place in Higher Education. This reflects learning as complex, with higher education as instrumental both in terms of developing the capacity and enabling the well-being of the student, and also in terms of the contribution of the person to society. In resistance here with each other are the value of fitness for work, personal interest and also service to society. Beneath such values can be seen a view of humanity as interdependent, with personal ambition operating alongside contribution to the common good. As it stands, this acts as a well-balanced basis for higher education practice, which will encourage skills development and reflection on values.

Barnett (1990, 1994) argues that higher education is, in essence, emancipatory and holistic. In effect, it liberates the student from the narrow focus of the academic disciplines, enabling reflective thinking, which can critique the assumptions of the discipline and look beyond to relations with other areas. Products of this process are 'self-understanding and self-empowerment', enabling students to 'come into themselves' (Barnett 1994). In extending their argument to higher education, Barnett focuses on the meaning of 'higher', arguing that higher education requires higher order thinking, involving the development of 'analysis, evaluation, criticism and even imagination' (Barnett 1994, p. 85). This level of thinking transcends the simple acquisition of work-centred skills, developing an awareness of the wider context and the capacity to learn about learning. Inevitably, this affects the way the whole person reflects and learns.

Underlying this are some core values of the learning relationship: autonomy, collegiality and justice. Respect for the autonomy of the learner is central to the learning relationship. Important in this is the student taking responsibility for her own learning, learning how to learn rather than uncritically accepting the view of the teacher. Autonomy in such a relationship cannot be summed up in the liberal view of simply respecting the choice of the individual, not least because the traditional student is developing emotionally and intellectually, and because the student does not know as much about the area of learning as the lecturer. It could be argued that autonomy as the capacity to reflect and make decisions, therefore, is actually developed through the learning relationship. The learning experience is therefore about enabling that development. It can be risky, given the need to take responsibility for learning. In Cowan's (2005) terms, this means an environment which will provide core values of empathy, congruence and unconditional positive regard. Learning in higher education, however, takes one beyond the simple Rogerian view to a more collegial stance (Cowan 2005). This is a relationship that has a high degree of mutuality to it, albeit asymmetrical. The more the student is taking responsibility for learning, the more they move to a research mode and thus become a co-learner with the lecturer. It is all the more important for the lecturer to enable the student to take risks, and constructively learn from any mistakes. The priority here is as much on formative assessment as summative, and moves the focus on learning away from the commodification of learning to learning as a lifelong search or journey. It also acts as a balance to the exclusive focus on individual academic success.

All this points to a community of learning, which is characterised by collegiality and, in Megone's (2005) terms, the familial. In the light of such a community, the student and staff can accept their limitations, become used to mutual challenge and become reflective partners in learning. Such learning requires a contract, of a verbal or written kind, in order to clarify expectations. The contract, however, is an instrument to facilitate learning, not the end of learning. The student is not so much a customer, with service provided by the institution, as a member of a community, with all the rights and responsibilities this brings with it. Alongside autonomy and collegiality is justice. This is important in four different ways. First, if respect for autonomy is about the development of the particular person, then justice demands an equitable response to different groups of students. Second, justice demands that the particular response of the student is developed and acknowledged. Hence, plagiarism, the direct use of other people's work is wrong. Third, justice demands that all students are subject to the same criteria of judgement and discipline, and based on these, students should be rewarded according to merit. This is expressed in the many different rules of the learning community. Fourth, justice can also be based upon need, ensuring the needs of students are met. Disability and equality and diversity offices are good examples of this in action. All of these aspects of justice are important to the learning process and relationship.

Two things are of note in this overview of the principles of learning. First, these principles are, for the most part, the same ones that underlie the profession of nursing itself. Respect for autonomy and justice and related principles feeds directly into the development of disinterested and critical thinking, and of professional development, which is more than simply training. Learning which takes in the whole person leads to the development of autonomy and the capacity of justice, which, as Chapter 3 noted, are central to professional virtues. Second, these principles demand an approach to learning which is focused on a learning community, which practices reflective practice and dialogue, the marks of collegiality. Quoting Randall Collins, Ford (2004, p. 25) suggests that at the heart of collegiality is 'intensive, disciplined face to face conversation and debate between contemporaries and across generations'. It is this form of community which enables the transmission of good practice and shared values across generations. Third, such a community enables research and teaching to be united. Ford (2004) suggests that both research and teaching be seen as essentially part of the learning process. Fourth, it sets the character of any governance in Higher Education, as sustaining a culture of collegiality and a 'long term vision in the interests of future generations' (Ford 2003; see Chapter 3 on clinical governance).

Conclusion

The issue of research ethics is of vital importance, as poor ethical conduct in research has implications for patients/clients and society. To ethically conduct research, one needs to be aware and follow one's professional research codes, principles and governance frameworks. Thereby ethics is fundamental to good research practice and the protection of society. Historically, research ethics has had a chequered past, and without due consideration, there is always the potential for research to do harm. Thus, it is important to plan for and anticipate any potential or actual risks when conducting research. Researchers must always preserve participants' anonymity and confidentiality, which are at risk in research, as sensitive data are often collected and produced in outputs. As a healthcare researcher, it can be difficult to balance one's role as researcher with the responsibilities integral in one's profession, as all research can, in theory, be harmful to participants and researchers, and research should be seen as a privilege, not a right.

References

Akkerman, A., Janssen, C. G., Kef, S., & Meininger, H. P. (2014). Perspectives of employees with intellectual disabilities on themes relevant to their job satisfaction: an explorative study using photovoice. *Journal of Applied Research in Intellectual Disabilities, 27*(6), 542–554.

Alperovitch, A., Dreifuss-Netter, F., Dickele, A. M., Gaudray, P., Le Coz, P., Rouvillois, P., et al. (2009). *Ethical issues raised by a possible influenza pandemic.* Luxemburg: National Consultative Ethics Committee for Health and Life Sciences. Online available: http://tinyurl.com/z8f4z4g.

Alzheimer's Society. (2019). *What is dementia?* London: Alzheimer's Society. Online available: https://www.alzheimers.org.uk/about-us/news-and-media/facts-media.

American Nurses Association. (2010). *Code of ethics for nurses with interpretive statements.* Silver Spring, Maryland: American Nurses Association.

Andrew, A. (2006). The ethics of using dolls and soft toys in dementia care. *Nursing and Residential Care, 8*(6), 419–421.

Association of Internet Researchers. (2019). *Internet research: ethical guidelines 3.0.* Chicago: Association of Internet Researchers. Online available: https://aoir.org/reports/ethics3.pdf.

Australian Nursing Federation. (2012). *Nursing and midwifery research.* Victoria: Australian Nursing Federation. Online available: http://tinyurl.com/z8wjrxb.

Awadu, K. O. (1996). Outrage! How babies were used as guinea pigs in a LA county vaccine experiment. *The Conscious Rasta Report, 13*(6). Online available: http://www.whale.to/vaccines/awadu.html.

Bane, G., Deely, M., Donohoe, B., Dooher, M., Flaherty, J., Iriarte, E. G., et al. (2012). Relationship of people with learning disabilities in Ireland. *British Journal of Learning Disabilities, 40*(2), 109–122.

Barnett, R. (1990). *The idea of higher education.* Milton Keynes: Open University Press.

Barnett, R. (1994). *The limits of competence: knowledge, higher education and society.* Milton Keynes: Open University Press.

Bartlett, R. (2012). Modifying the diary interview method to research the lives of people with dementia. *Qualitative Health Research*, *22*, 1717–1726.

Beauchamp, T., & Childress, J. (2012). *Principles of biomedical ethics* (3rd ed.). New York: Oxford University Press.

Bell, L., & Nutt, L. (1999). Divided loyalties, divided expectations: research ethics, professional and occupational responsibilities. In M. Mauthner, M. Birch, J. Jessop, & T. Miller (Eds.), *Ethics in qualitative research* (pp. 70–90). Thousand Oaks, CA: Sage.

Belmont Report. (1979). Ethical principles and guidelines for the protection of human subjects of research, national commission for the protection of human subjects of biomedical and behavioral research. Washington: US Department of Health, Education and Welfare Publication No. (OS) 78-0014.

Benbow, S. M., & Kingston, P. (2016). Talking about my experiences at times disturbing yet positive: Producing narratives with people living with dementia. *Dementia*, *15*(5), 1034–1052.

Berger, R. L. (1990). Nazi science: the Dachau hypothermia experiments. *New England Journal of Medicine*, *322*(20), 1435–1440.

Bigby, C., Frawley, P., & Ramcharan, P. (2014). Conceptualizing inclusive research with people with intellectual disabilities. *Journal of Applied Research in Intellectual Disabilities*, *27*(1), 3–12.

Ganguli-Mitra, A. & Biller-Andorno, N. (2011). Vulnerability in healthcare and research ethics. In Chadwick, R., Ten Have, H. & Meslin, E.M. (Eds.), *The SAGE handbook of health care ethics* (pp. 239–250). London: SAGE.

Bogod, D. (2004). The Nazi hypothermia experiments: forbidden data? *Anaesthesia*, *59*(12), 1155–1156.

Brandt, A. M. (1978). Racism and research: the case of the Tuskegee Syphilis Study. *Hastings Center Report*, *8*, 21–29. Online available: https://dash.harvard.edu/bitstream/handle/1/3372911/Brandt_Racism.pdf?sequence=1&isAllowed=y.

Brazier, M., & Fovargue, S. J. (2006). A brief guide to the Human Tissue Act 2004. *Clinical Ethics*, *1*(1), 26–32.

British Psychological Society. (2014). *Code of human research ethics*. Leicester: British Psychological Society. Online available: https://www.bps.org.uk/sites/bps.org.uk/files/Policy%20-%20Files/BPS%20Code%20of%20Human%20Research%20Ethics.pdf.

Burns, N., & Grove, S. K. (2013). *The practice of nursing research: appraisal, synthesis and generation of evidence* (7th ed.). St Louis, MI: Elsevier Saunders.

Butts, J. B., & Rich, K. L. (2013). *Nursing ethics: across the curriculum and into practice* (3rd ed.). Burlington, MA: Jones and Bartlett Learning.

Canadian Nurses Association. (2008). *Code of ethics for registered nurses*. Ottawa: Canadian Nurses Association.

Cancer Research UK. (2013). *Conflict of interest for investigators participating in Cancer Research UK sponsored clinical trials*. Online available: https://www.cancerresearchuk.org/sites/default/files/conflicts_of_interest_policy.pdf.

Cannella-Malone, H. I., Brooks, D. G., & Tullis, C. A. (2013). Using self-directed video prompting to teach students with intellectual disabilities. *Journal of Behavioural Education*, *22*(3), 169–189.

Capstick, A., & Ludwin, K. (2015). Place memory and dementia: findings from participatory film-making in long-term social care. *Health and Place*, *34*, 157–163.

Carey, E., Salmon, N., & Higgins, A. (2014). Research active programme: views of service users. *Learning Disability Practice*, *17*, 22–28.

Chappell, A. (2000). Emergence of participatory methodology in learning difficulty research: understanding the context. *British Journal of Learning Disabilities*, *28*(1), 38–43.

Charlton, J. (2000). *Nothing about us without us: disability oppression and empowerment*. Berkley, CA: University of California Press.

Cheffey, J., Hill, L., McCullough, C., & McCullough, C. (2017). Can I facilitate a project when my memory lets me down: the challenges and rewards of co-producing a "living well with dementia" course. *FPOP Bulletin*, *137*, 19–25.

Coghlan, D., & Brydon-Miller, M. (2014). *The SAGE encyclopaedia of action research*. London: SAGE.

Clark, C., & Keady, J. (2002). Getting down to brass tacks: discussion of data collection with people with dementia. In H. Wilkinson (Ed.), *The perspectives of people with dementia: research methods and motivations*. London: Jessica Kingsley.

Cowan, J. (2005). The atrophy of the affect. In S. Robinson, & C. Katulushi (Eds.), *Values in higher education* (pp. 159–177). Leeds: Leeds University Press.

Dalton, A. J., & McVilly, K. R. (2004). Ethics guidelines for international, multicenter research involving people with intellectual disabilities. *Journal of Policy and Practice in Intellectual Disabilities*, *1*(2), 57–70.

Darewych, O. H., Carlton, N. R., & Wayne, K. (2015). Digital technology use in art therapy with adults with developmental disabilities. *Journal on Developmental Disabilities*, *21*(2), 95–102.

Davies, B., & Gannon, S. (2006). The practices of collective biography. In B. Davies, & S. Gannon (Eds.), *Doing collective biography: investigating the production of subjectivity* (pp. 1–15). Berkshire: McGraw-Hill Education.

Dempsey, P. A., & Dempsey, A. D. (2000). *Using nursing research: process, critical evaluation and utilization* (5th ed.). Philadelphia: Lippincott.

Department of Health. (2005a). *Mental Capacity Act*. London: HMSO.

Department of Health. (2005b). *Research governance framework for health and social care* (2nd ed.). London: Department of Health. Online available: https://assets.publishing.service.gov.uk/government/uploads/system/uploads/attachment_data/file/139565/dh_4122427.pdf.

Dewing, J. (2002). From ritual to relationship: a person-centred approach to consent in qualitative research with older people who have a dementia. *Dementia*, *1*(2), 157–171.

Dewing, J. (2007). Participatory research: a method for process consent with persons who have dementia. *Dementia*, *6*(1), 11–25.

Digby, R., Lee, S., & Williams, A. (2016). Interviewing people with dementia in hospital: recommendations for researchers. *Journal of Clinical Nursing*, *25*(7–8), 1156–1165.

Doloriert, C., & Sambrook, S. (2009). Ethical confessions of the "I" of autoethnography: the student's dilemma. *Qualitative Research in Organizations and Management: An International Journal*, *4*(1), 27–45.

Doody, O. (2018). Ethical challenges in intellectual disability research. *Mathews Journal of Nursing*, *1*(1), 5.

Doody, O., & Noonan, M. (2016). Nursing research ethics, guidance and application in practice. *British Journal of Nursing*, *25*(14), 803–807.

Dyregrov, K. (2004). Bereaved parents' experiences of research participation. *Social Science and Medicine*, *58*, 391–400.

Ebbs, C. A. (1996). Qualitative research inquiry: issues of power and ethics. *Education*, *117*(2), 217–222.

Economic and Social Research Council. (2015). *Framework for research ethics*. Swindon: Economic and Social Research Council. Online available: https://esrc.ukri.org/files/funding/guidance-for-applicants/esrc-framework-for-research-ethics-2015/.

Edwards, M., & Chalmers, K. (2002). Double agency in clinical research. *Canadian Journal of Nursing Research*, *34*(1), 131–142.

Elmir, R., Schmied, V., Jackson, D., & Wilkes, L. (2011). Interviewing people about potentially sensitive topics. *Nurse Researcher*, *19*(1), 12–16.

Ferrari, J. R., & McGowan, S. (2002). Using exam bonus points as incentive for research participation. *Teaching of Psychology*, *29*(1), 29–32.

Ford, D. (2003). *Knowledge, meaning and the world's great challenges: reinventing Cambridge University in the twenty-first Century*. Cambridge: Cambridge University Press.

Ford, D. (2004). Responsibilities of universities. *Studies in Christian Ethics*, *17*(1), 22–37.

Fudge Schormans, A., Wilton, R., & Marquis, N. (2019). Building collaboration in the co-production of knowledge with people with intellectual disabilities about their everyday use of city space. *Area*, *51*(3), 415–422.

Garbutt, R., Tattersall, J., Dunn, J., & Boycott-Garnett, R. (2009). Accessible article: involving people with learning disabilities in research. *British Journal of Learning Disabilities*, *38*(1), 21–34.

Gillon, R. (1985). Deontological foundations for medical ethics. *British Medical Journal*, *290*(6478), 1331–1333.

Giroux, H. A. (2010). Rethinking education as the practice of freedom: Paulo Freire and the promise of critical pedagogy. *Policy Futures in Education*, *8*(6), 715–721.

Goldsmith, L., & Skirton, H. (2015). Research involving people with a learning disability: methodological challenges and ethical considerations. *Journal of Research in Nursing*, *20*, 435–446.

Goodley, D., & Moore, M. (2000). Doing disability research: activist lives and the academy. *Disability and Society*, *15*(6), 86–88.

Gould, N., & Kendall, T. (2007). Developing the NICE/SCIE guidelines for dementia care: the challenges of enhancing the evidence base for social and health care. *British Journal of Social Work*, *37*(3), 475–490.

Gove, D., Diaz-Ponce, A., Georges, J., Moniz-Cook, E., Mountain, G., Chattat, R., et al. (2018). Alzheimer Europe's position on involving people with dementia in research through PPI (patient and public involvement). *Aging and Mental Health, 22*(6), 723–729.

Grinyer, A. (2002). *The anonymity of research participants: assumptions, ethics and practicalities. Social research update, issue 36.* Surrey: Department of Sociology, University of Surrey.

Haigh, C. (2007). Getting ethics approval. In T. Long, & M. Johnson (Eds.), *Research ethics in the real world: issues and solutions for health and social care* (pp. 123–138). London: Churchill Livingstone, Elsevier.

Haigh, C., & Jones, N. A. (2005). An overview of the ethics of cyber-space research and the implication for nurse educators. *Nurse Education Today, 25*(1), 3–8.

Haney, C., Banks, W. C., & Zimbardo, P. G. (1973). A study of prisoners and guards in a simulated prison. *Naval Research Review, 30*, 4–17.

Health Research Authority. (2020). *Applying to a Research Ethics.* London: Health Research Authority. Online available: https://www.hra.nhs.uk/approvals-amendments/what-approvals-do-i-need/research-ethics-committee-review/applying-research-ethics-committee/.

Heggestad, A. K. T., Nortvedt, P., & Slettebø, Å. (2013). The importance of moral sensitivity when including persons with dementia in qualitative research. *Nursing Ethics, 20*(1), 30–40.

Hellstrom, I., Nolan, M., Nordenfelt, L., & Lundh, U. (2007). Ethical and methodological issues in interviewing persons with dementia. *Nursing Ethics, 14*(5), 608–619.

Hubbard, G., Downs, M. G., & Tester, S. (2003). Including older people with dementia in research: challenges and strategies. *Aging and Mental Health, 7*(5), 351–362.

Iacobucci, G. (2013). More than a third of GPs on commissioning groups have conflicts of interest: BMJ investigation shows. *British Medical Journal, 346*, f1569.

International Council of Nurses. (2012). *Ethical guidelines for nursing research.* Geneva, Switzerland: International Council of Nurses.

Jenkins, N., Keyes, S., & Strange, L. (2016). Creating vignettes of early onset dementia: an exercise in public sociology. *Sociology, 50*, 77–92.

Kapila, S. N., Boaz, K., & Natarajan, S. (2016). The post-analytical phase of histopathology practice: storage, retention and use of human tissue specimens. *International Journal of Applied and Basic Medical Research, 6*(1), 3.

Kapp, M. B. (1998). Persons with dementia as 'liability magnets': ethical implications. *The Journal of Clinical Ethics, 9*(1), 66–70.

Karnieli-Miller, O., Strier, R., & Pessach, L. (2009). Power relations in qualitative research. *Qualitative Health Research, 19*(2), 279–289.

Katz, J., Capron, A. M., & Swift Glass, E. (1972). The Jewish Chronic Disease Hospital Case. In J. Katz, A. M. Capron, & E. Swift Glass (Eds.), *Experimentation with human beings: the authority of the investigator, subject, professions, and state in the human experimentation process* (pp. 9–66). New York: Russell Sage Foundation.

Kavanaugh, K., & Ayres, L. (1998). Not as bad as it could have been: assessing and mitigating harm during research interviews on sensitive topics. *Research in Nursing and Health, 21*, 91–97.

Kitwood, T. (1995). Positive long-term changes in dementia: some preliminary observations. *Journal of Mental Health, 4*(2), 133–144.

Kramer, J., Kramer, J. C., García-Iriarte, E., & Hammel, J. (2011). Following through to the end: the use of inclusive strategies to analyse and interpret data in participatory action research with individuals with intellectual disabilities. *Journal of Applied Research in Intellectual Disabilities, 24*(3), 263–273.

Lee, C. K. (1998). *Gender and the South China miracle: two worlds of factory women.* California: University of California Press.

Lemmens, T., & Singer, P. A. (1998). Bioethics for clinicians: 17. Conflict of interest in research, education and patient care. *Canadian Medical Association Journal, 159*(8), 960–965. Online available: https://www.ncbi.nlm.nih.gov/pmc/articles/PMC1229743/pdf/cmaj_159_8_960.pdf.

MacFarlane, B. (2009). *Researching with integrity.* London: Routledge.

Macnee, C. L., & McCabe, S. (2008). *Understanding nursing research: using research in evidence-based practice.* Philadelphia: Lippincott Williams and Wilkins.

Manning, C. (2009). My memory's back: inclusive learning disability research using ethics, oral history and digital storytelling. *British Journal of Learning Disabilities, 38*(3), 160–167.

Marzanski, M. (2000). Would you like to know what is wrong with you: on telling the truth to patients with dementia. *Journal of Medical Ethics, 26*(2), 108–113.

McCleery, J. P. (2015). Comment on technology-based intervention research for individuals on the autism spectrum. *Journal of Autism Developmental Disorder, 45*(12), 3832–3835.

McDonald, K. E., & Kidney, C. A. (2012). What is right: ethics in intellectual disabilities research. *Journal of Policy and Practice in Intellectual Disabilities, 9*(1), 27–39.

McIndoe, W. A., McLean, M. R., Jones, R. W., & Mullins, P. R. (1984). The invasive potential of carcinoma in situ of the cervix. *Obstetric Gynecology, 64*, 418–451.

McKeown, J., Clarke, A., Ingleton, C., & Reeper, J. (2010). Actively involving people with dementia in qualitative research. *Journal of Clinical Nursing, 19*(13–14), 1935–1943.

Medical Research Council. (2007) *MRC Ethics guide 2007: Medical research involving adults who cannot consent.* London: Medical Research Council.

Megone, C. (2005). Virtue and the virtual university. In S. Robinson, & C. Katulushi (Eds.), *Values in higher education* (pp. 117–132). Leeds: Leeds University Press.

Milgram, S. (1963). Behavioral study of obedience. *Journal of Abnormal and Social Psychology, 67*, 371–378.

Millum, J., & Grady, C. (2013). The ethics of placebo-controlled trials: methodological justifications. *Contemporary Clinical Trials, 36*(2), 510–514.

Mockford, C., Murray, M., Seers, K., Oyebode, J., Grant, R., Boex, S., et al. (2016). A SHARED study-the benefits and costs of setting up a health research study involving lay co-researchers and how we overcame the challenges. *Research Involvement and Engagement, 2*(1), 8.

Moreno, J. D. (1998). Convenient and captive populations. In J. P. Kahn, A. C. Mastroianni, & J. Sugarman (Eds.), *Beyond consent: seeking justice in research* (pp. 111–130). Oxford, UK: Oxford University Press.

Morrisey, B. (2012). Ethics and research among persons with disabilities in long-term care. *Qualitative Health Research, 22*, 1284–1297.

Morse, J. M., & Richards, L. (2002). *Readme first for a user's guide to qualitative methods.* Thousand Oaks: CA: Sage.

Mumford, M. D., Connelly, S., Brown, R. P., Murphy, S. T., Hill, J. H., Antes, A. L., et al. (2008). A sense making approach to ethics training for scientists: preliminary evidence of training effectiveness. *Ethics and Behaviour, 18*(4), 315–339.

Murphy, J., Gray, C., van Achterberg, T., Wyke, S., & Cox, S. (2010). The effectiveness of the Talking Mats framework in helping people with dementia to express their views on wellbeing. *Dementia, 9*, 454–472.

Murphy, K., Jordan, F., Hunter, A., Cooney, A., & Casey, D. (2015). Articulating the strategies for maximising the inclusion of people with dementia in qualitative research studies. *Dementia, 14*(6), 800–824.

Newell, R., & Burnard, P. (2011). *Research for evidence-based practice in healthcare* (2nd ed.). Oxford: John Wiley and Sons.

Nind, M., & Vinha, H. (2012). Doing research inclusively: bridges to multiple possibilities in inclusive research. *British Journal of Learning Disabilities, 42*(2), 102–109.

Novek, S., & Wilkinson, H. (2019). Safe and inclusive research practices for qualitative research involving people with dementia: a review of key issues and strategies. *Dementia, 18*(3), 1042–1059.

National Research Ethics Advisors' Panel. (2012). *Conflict of interest/competing interests: NREAP/04/2012/02/13 v1.2.* Croydon: National Research Ethics Advisors' Panel. Online available: nreap04-guidance-national-research-ethics-advisors-panel-13-february-2012.pdf.

Nuremberg Code. (1947). *Trials of war criminals before the Nuremberg Military Tribunals under Control Council Law No. 10* (Vol. 2). Washington, DC: US Government Printing Office.

Nursing and Midwifery Board of Ireland. (2015). *Ethical conduct in research: professional guidance.* Dublin: Nursing and Midwifery Board of Ireland. Online available: https://www.nmbi.ie/NMBI/media/NMBI/ethical-conduct-in-research-professional-guidance.pdf?ext=.pdf.

Nursing and Midwifery Council. (2018). *The code professional standards of practice and behaviour for nurses, midwives and nursing associates.* London: Nursing and Midwifery Council. Online available: https://www.nmc.org.uk/globalassets/sitedocuments/nmc-publications/nmc-code.pdf.

O'Brien, P., McConkey, R., & García-Iriarte, E. (2014). Core searching with people who have intellectual disabilities: insights from a national survey. *Journal of Applied Research in Intellectual Disabilities, 27*(1), 65–75.

O'Sullivan, G., Hocking, C., & Spence, D. (2014). Action research: changing history for people living with dementia in New Zealand. *Action Research, 12*, 19–35.

Okenyi, E. (2016). A reform proposal for the Human Tissue Act (2004): making it more appropriate for organ donation in 2020. *Southampton Student Law Review*, *6*(1), 11–22.

Oliver, M. (1992). Changing the social relations of research production. *Disability and Society*, *7*, 101–114.

Oliver, M. (1997). Emancipatory research: realistic goal or impossible dream. In C. Barnes, & G. Mercer (Eds.), *Doing disability research* (pp. 15–31). Leeds: The Disability Press.

Orb, A., Eisenhauer, L., & Wynaden, D. (2001). Ethics in qualitative research. *Journal of Nursing Scholarship*, *33*(1), 93–96.

Orton-Johnson, K. (2010). Ethics in online research; evaluating the ESRC framework for research ethics categorisation of risk. *Sociological Research Online*, *15*(4), 13. Online available: https://www.socresonline.org.uk/15/4/13.html.bak.

Oxford University Research Support. (2018). *Research integrity*. Oxford: University of Oxford. Online available: http://www.admin.ox.ac.uk/researchsupport/integrity/conflict/research/.

Oye, C., Sorensen, N. O., & Glasdam, S. (2015). Qualitative research ethics on the spot. *Nursing Ethics*, *23*(4), 455–464.

Parahoo, K. (2014). *Nursing research principles, process and issues* (3rd ed.). Basingstoke: Palgrave Macmillan.

Peel, N. M., & Wilson, C. (2008). Frail older people as participants in research. *Educational Gerontology*, *34*(5), 407–417.

Percival, T. (1803). *Medical Ethics: Or a Code of Institutes and Precepts Adapted to the Professional Conduct of Physicians and Surgeons*. Manchester: J Johnson.

Polit, D. F., & Beck, C. T. (2013). *Essentials of nursing research: appraising evidence for nursing practice* (8th ed.). Philadelphia: Wolters Kluwer.

Pratt, B., & Loff, B. (2011). Justice in international clinical research. *Developing World Bioethics*, *11*(2), 75–81.

Pratt, R. (2002). Nobody's ever asked how I felt. In H. Wilkinson (Ed.), *The perspectives of people with dementia: research methods and motivations* (pp. 165–182). London: Jessica Kingsley Publishers.

Rauh, J., & Turner, J. (2016). 1957-1961, Canada: MKULTRA Experiments in Montreal. Online available: http://tinyurl.com/hovufge.

Resnik, D. B. (2015). Bioethical issues in providing financial incentives to research participants. *Medicolegal and Bioethics*, *24*(5), 35.

Richards, H. M., & Schwartz, L. J. (2002). Ethics of qualitative research: are there special issues for health services research? *Family Practice*, *19*(2), 135–139.

Riley, S., Schouten, W., & Cahill, S. (2003). Exploring the dynamics of subjectivity and power between researcher and researched. *Forum Qualitative Sozialforschung/Forum: Qualitative Social Research*, *4*(2), Art 40.

Roberts, A., Greenhill, B., Talbot, A., & Cuzak, M. (2011). Standing up for my human rights: a group's journey beyond consultation towards co-production. *British Journal of Learning Disabilities*, *40*(4), 292–301.

Robinson, S. (2008). *Spirituality, ethics and care*. London: Jessica Kingsley.

Robinson, S., Kendrick, K., & Brown, A. (2003). *Spirituality and the practice of healthcare*. London: Palgrave.

Romanoff, B. D. (2001). Research as therapy: the power of narrative to effect change. In R. A. Neimeyer (Ed.), *Meaning reconstruction and the experience of loss* (pp. 245–257). Washington: American Psychological Association. Online available: https://doi.org/10.1037/10397-013.

Rosen, M. (2018). *Dignity its history and meaning*. Cambridge, MA: Harvard University Press.

Rossetto, K. R. (2014). Qualitative research interviews assessing the therapeutic value and challenges. *Journal of Social and Personal Relationships*, *31*(4), 482–489.

Rothman, D., & Rothman, S. (1984). *The Willowbrook Wars*. New York: Harper and Row.

Royal College of Nursing. (2009). *Research ethics: RCN guidance to nurses*. London: Royal College of Nursing.

Salmon, N., Carey, E., & Hunt, A. (2014). Research skills for people with intellectual disabilities. *Learning Disability Practice*, *17*(3), 27–35.

Sara, P., Giada, G., & Rosagemma, C. (2018). Thomas Percival: discussing the foundation of medical ethics. *Acta bio-medica: Atenei Parmensis*, *89*(3), 343.

Spicker, P. (2011). Ethical covert research. *Sociology*, *45*(1), 118–133.

Stalker, K. (1998). Some ethical and methodological issues in research with people with learning difficulties. *Disability and Society*, *13*(1), 5–19.

Tew, J. (2011). *Social approaches to mental distress*. Basingstoke: Palgrave Macmillan.

Thomas, W. J. (2001). Informed consent, the placebo effect, and the revenge of Thomas Percival. *Journal of Legal Medicine*, *22*(3), 313–348.

Titmuss, R. (1972). *The gift relationship*. London: Penguin.

Tuffrey-Wijne, I., & Butler, G. (2010). Co-Researching with people with learning disabilities: an experience of involvement in qualitative data analysis. *Health Expectations, 13*(2), 174–184.

United Nations. (2006). *General assembly: convention on the rights of persons with disabilities, optional protocol to the Convention*. New York: United Nations.

University Hospitals, NHS. (2018). https://www.ouh.nhs.uk/researchers/planning/documents/participant-information-sheet.pdf.

Walmsley, J., & Johnson, K. (2003). *Inclusive research with people with intellectual disabilities: past, present and futures*. London: Jessica Kingsley Publishing.

Walmsley, J. (2004). Involving users with learning difficulties in health improvement: lessons from inclusive learning disability research. *Nursing Inquiry, 11*(1), 54–64.

Ward, R., & Campbell, S. (2013). Mixing methods to explore appearance in dementia care. *Dementia, 12*, 337–347.

Wertheimer, A. (2013). Is payment a benefit? Bioethics, *27*(2), 105–116.

White, L. (2019). Conflicts over the excavation, retention and display of human remains: an issue resolved. In S. Campbell, L. White, & S. Thomas (Eds.), *Competing values in archaeological heritage* (pp. 91–102). Cham: Springer.

Wiersma, E. C. (2011). Using photovoice with people with early-stage Alzheimer's disease: a discussion of methodology. *Dementia, 10*(2), 203–216.

Wilkinson, H. (2002). *The perspectives of people with dementia: research methods and motivations*. London: Jessica Kingsley Publishers.

Wilkinson, M. J., & Stirton, R. (2018). Right to paternity testing of tissue samples should extend beyond medical necessity. *British Medical Journal, 360*, k1257.

Witham, G., Beddow, A., & Haigh, C. (2015). Reflections on access: too vulnerable to research. *Journal of Research in Nursing, 20*, 28–37.

World Medical Association. (1948). *Declaration of Geneva*. Geneva: World Medical Association General Assembly.

World Medical Association. (1964). *The Helsinki Declaration: Ethical principles for medical research involving human subjects*. Helsinki, Finland: 18th World Medical Association General Assembly.

World Medical Association. (1975). *Declaration of Helsinki and consent*. Helsinki, Finland: World Medical Association General Assembly.

World Medical Association. (2013). *The Helsinki Declaration: Ethical principles for medical research involving human subjects*. Fortaleza, Brazil: 64th World Medical Association General Assembly.

Zarb, G. (1992). On the road to Damascus: first steps towards changing the relations of disability research production. *Disability and Society, 7*, 125–138.

PART 3

Ethics, Leadership and Management in Healthcare

Ethical Leadership

LEARNING OUTCOMES

When you have read and worked through this chapter, you should be able to:

- Identify what is leadership
- Describe leadership theories, styles, virtues
- Identify nursing leadership and role of the nurse
- Think through cases on leadership
- Be aware of organisational leadership

Introduction

Revisiting the case of Mid Staffs, referred to in the first chapter, shows how complex ethical leadership is in healthcare. The case showed the absence of ethical leadership at several levels. Leadership at the head of the organisation was focused on the achievement of narrow targets. This led to a culture where many senior nurses ignored the imperatives of care to achieve the targets. For example, when the hospital administration prioritised the 4-hour waiting time targets, this led to ignoring ethical practice. Patients were discharged or moved to different treatment rooms despite not being assessed or given proper medication (Mastracci 2017) in order to achieve target time. In one case, this led to a patient's/client's death (Francis 2010, p. 207), in others, patients/clients left hospital in worse condition than when they arrived. In order to maintain records, the leadership of senior nurses encouraged junior doctors and nurses to alter and forge hospital notes (Francis 2010, p. 96). Some junior nurses attempted to exercise leadership by pushing back against the senior nurses, only to be met by bullying, from both co-workers and supervisors.

Across all sectors of healthcare there was failure of leadership. Incident reports were ignored, criticism was discouraged, staff and family complainants were bullied and bad practice was not addressed. The response of management and administration to nurse requests for more resources and staffing was ad hominem arguments – accusing staff of misrepresenting the situation and questioning their competence (Francis 2010, p. 199). The absence of sustained ethical leadership thus involved:

- No reference to professional values.
- No ethical modelling.
- A mutual lack of trust.
- Bullying and harassment of staff who resisted attempts to short cut or avoid ethical procedures.
- Significant changes, including budget cuts, implemented without consulting staff.

The result was corrosion of meaning, practice and relationships, and this chapter thus considers leadership and its relationship to ethics.

Understanding Leadership

Leadership involves setting the direction and tone of the organisation and ensuring that management will achieve this. Management and leadership are terms often used interchangeably, but there are clear distinctions between management and leadership. Management is seen as the attainment of organisational goals in an effective and efficient manner through planning, organising, staffing, directing and controlling organisational resources (Daft 2004). Leadership, on the other hand, is about action toward change, and establishing the vision (Daft 2004). In effect, management is about making things run well and stabilising them to work more efficiently by coping with complexity, creating order through systems fit for purpose, ensuring quality, planning budgets, organising staff and problem solving (Kotter 1990). Leadership then is about creating vision, inspiring and motivating, setting direction and planning for change (Kotter 1990). Although the two roles have a different focus, they are complementary and need to be held in tension. The leader has to have some form of management skills and the manager has to have some form of leadership skills (O'Leary 2016), involving three fundamental activities: leading (strategic aspects of the position); managing (working with others to get results) and doing (carrying out the task) regardless of the job title. Thereby, all healthcare professionals need time to think and plan for future organisational needs, together with the realities of today's technological change and complexity, along with the people who work with/for them. Leaders cannot achieve their role without leadership skills and enabling those they work with to engage with the vision and purpose, and, as indicated above, this falls within all healthcare professionals' roles.

8.1 PAUSE FOR THOUGHT

Identifying a Leader and Creating Time

Consider your practice and identify:
- A leader you have worked with who impressed you.
- What made them a good leader?

- What characteristics (personal and professional) made them a good leader?
- Your own leadership characteristics and compare them to that of a good leader.
- Do you use these characteristics in your practice?
- What percentage of your time is given to management activities?
- What percentage of your time is given to leadership activities?

Pye (2005) suggests that there are several hundred different definitions of leadership in academic literature. It is not surprising then that the concept of leadership is contested. Attempts have been made to narrow the term to ideas around the core actions of a leader, not least the simple idea that a leader gives direction. Fulop and Roberts (2015) and Covey (2002) argue for the macro, meso and micro aspects of leadership activity (Table 8.1).

All three levels of leadership involve change and enabling others to take responsibility for change (Rost 1991), and all three levels have to work together to make sense of the shared practice of healthcare.

8.2 PAUSE FOR THOUGHT

Demands and Limited Resources

Consider if you were in charge of a hospital:
- What would be your most important targets?
- Would they be to keep down expenditure, to cut down on waiting times, to keep wards clean, to maximise patient/client 'throughput', to increase the efficiency of staff? The list is endless, what would you add?
- How do your targets relate to the core vision of healthcare of enabling health and wellbeing?
  Considering that health and wellbeing are partly dependent on the communication of care and attendant qualities ('care and compassion are what matters most' National Health Service Constitution) National Health Service (2015) NHS Constitution: the NHS belongs to us all. Online available: https://www.gov.uk/government/publications/the-nhs-constitution-for-england:
- How can that square with cutting down staff contact time, or making staff focus on measurable targets, resulting in that attention to patients/clients becoming secondary?
  The issue is put starkly by the Parliamentary and Health Service Ombudsman's (2011) report about the care of the elderly in the NHS: 'I have collated this report because of the common experiences of the patients/clients concerned and the stark contrast between the reality of the care they received and the principles and values of the NHS' (report available at: https://www.ombudsman.org.uk/publications/care-and-compassion) Accessed 22 February 2020.

TABLE 8.1 ■ Macro-, Meso- and Micro-Contributions to the Quality of Healthcare

Macro (National Health Systems)	Meso (Hospitals)	Micro (Departments, Teams)
- Regulatory system - Finance - National priorities and policies - Accreditation	- Strategies - Systems - Processes - Cultures - Practices - Structures	- Relational issues - Communication - Professional work - Competence

From Fulop, N., & Robert, G. (2015). *Context for successful quality improvement*. London: Health Foundation.

Leadership has often been seen to be individualistic and based on the core traits and competencies of leaders which need to be developed (Yukl 1999). Western (2007) has argued that the NHS competency framework has, in the past, been focused on leadership as an individual role. However, this view has been increasingly challenged, built as it was on the myth of the 'great man' (sic!) who knows everything, and would cajole or inspire the workforce to follow. Responsibility for complex situations, then, was focused on a single person or group. However, as the Mid Staffs case showed, this can lead to the greater part of the organisation not taking responsibility for practice. Hence, the focus now is more on the development of distributed leadership, in which all members of the organisation take responsibility for leadership (Western 2007). Consistent across the literature are themes of leadership as:

1. a process
2. influencing others
3. focused on the better attainment of a mutually shared goal
4. focused on relationships (Bertocci 2009).

As a process, leadership is a methodical engagement that manages uncertainty and avoids disorder and chance (Northouse 2016; Robbins and Judge 2013; Kouzen and Posner 2012), and an interactive social engagement (Schermerhorn et al. 2020). It is based on influence in multidirectional ways that are non-compulsive and non-coercive between the leader and the collaborators (Yukl and Uppal 2017), dealing with how leaders inspire, motivate and enable followers or collaborators towards a purposeful action (Northouse 2016). This is less about leaders and followers and more about developing co-leaders and mutual purpose, sustained by good relationships (Northouse 2016; Robbins and Judge 2013; Kouzen and Posner 2012). In light of this, Ciulla (2005) and Eubanks et al. (2012) argue that ethics is at the heart of leadership. There is no value neutral view of leadership, and any approach or style is built upon values that have to be justified and may well be challenged. Leaders are a key source of the ethical guidance in social engagement as they set the ethical tone and define the ethical atmosphere of the organisation (Kar 2014). The desire for ethical leadership exists as, if effective, it offers a sense of meaning, morale, values, direction and assurance of common purpose and good (Alvesson and Spicer 2011). Leading is not a momentary activity; it develops over time, changing constantly in relation to the place, time, context and those involved. Ineffective and unethical leaders can cause problems for followers, organisations, stakeholders and society (Schyns and Schilling 2013). In general, divorcing ethics from leadership and interactive engagement has caused enormous damage to organisational wellbeing and the common good; studies have demonstrated a positive relationship between ethical leadership and employees' job satisfaction (Tu et al. 2017; Bedi et al. 2016; Okan and Akyüz 2015; Yang 2014).

THEORIES OF ETHICAL LEADERSHIP

The major values leadership theories (Ciulla 2005) have all been focused on the different ways in which values and principles can be developed in the workforce.

Transformational Leadership

Burns (1978) developed theory argues that the leader should guide followers to higher principles. He argues that the transformational leader should:

- Expand the followers' understanding and profile of needs,
- Transform the followers' view of self-interest. This will enable followers to see that concern for others is a key part of their own interest,
- Increase the confidence of the followers,
- Elevate the expectations of followers,
- Enable a fuller appreciation of the leader's intended outcomes,

- Enable behavioural change,
- Motivate followers to higher levels of personal achievement, seen in terms of Maslow's self-actualisation (see also Turner et al. 2002).

At the heart of this, the leader is enabling the members of the group to develop moral maturity (based on Kohlberg's stages of moral development; see Chapter 3). This, however, has led to critiques, that: the leader is seen as paternalistic; there is danger of manipulation of 'followers' (the wolf of the great man in sheep's clothing) and there is little room for genuine dialogue which engages followers' interests and perspectives of principle (Keeley 1995), or any consideration of the historical values narrative of the organisation and how it relates to core principles.

Transformational leadership has often been distinguished from transactional leadership (Rost 1991; Burns 1978). Transactional leadership focuses on a social system characterised by mutual feedback between leaders and followers (Rost 1991, p. 30), held in place by contracts. This is often falsely characterised as a battle between relationships focused on values which transcend self-interest and those focused on contracts of self-interest. In fact, both approaches reflect core ethical principles, not least autonomy and shared responsibility (Doody and Doody 2012; Judge and Piccolo 2004), requiring a marriage of both styles complementing and enhancing each other (Rolfe 2011). Healthcare leaders must understand the value and critical importance of delivering an emotionally and behaviourally intelligent style of leadership to ensure that their staff feel empowered and supported as they work through and implement the ongoing changes in healthcare (Delmatoff and Lazarus 2014).

Hence, Bass and Steidlemeier (2004) develop the idea of transformational leadership, distinguishing pseudo-transformational leadership from authentically transformational leadership (Table 8.2). Thus, transformational leaders make it safe for staff to risk and extend the boundaries of thinking and doing, creating ample conditions for energy, creativity and innovation to emerge (Porter-O'Grady 1997), where supportive environments of shared responsibility are created (Bally 2007).

Servant Leadership

Closely related to the transformational approach is that of servant leadership (Greenleaf 1977). Once again, this works against the heroic and individualistic view of leadership. Ciulla (2005) argues this is a simple but radical shift, because it questions the paradigm of leaders and followers, with leaders taking the function often associated with followers, that of servant. This has a strong religious background (see St. Mark's Gospel 8, vv. 27–30). A good example of servant leadership is the book Tolkien (1955) and film *Lord of the Rings* (Jackson 2004). Despite strong leaders such as Gandalf, Aragorn and Boromir, it is the insignificant hobbit Frodo who takes on the mantle of leadership, both in terms of holding the ring and finding the way to end its power.

TABLE 8.2 ■ Pseudo-Transformational Leadership From Authentically Transformational Leadership

Authentic Transformational Leaders	Pseudo-Transformational Leaders
• Have the charisma to get people to want to follow them and turn floundering companies into prosperous ones	• Have charisma and are successful at getting followers
• Drive towards long-term gains	• Tend to make short-term gains that ultimately result in long-term costs
• Are motivated by the good of the many, recognising that they succeed when the others around them succeed	• Are self-centred and motivated more by the desire for personal gain than by corporate success
• Empower and promote collaboration and autonomy	• Tend to promote competitiveness at the expense of collaboration
	• Tend to manipulate rather than empower their followers

TABLE 8.3 ■ **Qualities of Transformational Nurse Leaders**

Components
(From Bass 1985, 1998, 2005; Hall et al. 2002; Barbuto 2005)

Individualised consideration – identifying the needs of individual members of staff. Intellectual stimulation – question the status quo and present new ideas.	Inspirational motivation – present a vision in which people can achieve their personal goals through meeting the organisation's goals. Idealised influence – role model the behaviours.

Qualities

• Clear purpose, expressed simply • Value-driven • Strong role model • High expectations • Persistent • Self-knowing • Perpetual desire for learning • Love work • Lifelong learners • Identify themselves as change agents • Enthusiastic • Able to attract and inspire others • Able to deal with complexity, uncertainty and ambiguity	• Emotionally mature • Courageous • Risk-taker • Risk-sharing • Visionary • Unwilling to believe in failure • Sense of public need • Listens to all viewpoints to develop spirit of co-operation • Mentoring • Effective communicator • Considerate of the personal needs of employees • Strategic
	From Contino 2004.
From Sofarelli and Brown 1998.	

This model focuses on a change in mindset to 'an understanding and practice of leadership that places the good of those led, over the self-interest of the leader' (Laub 2004, p. 5). It moves away from a concern with organisational interests, and even the concern for the 'customers'. The concept of serving echoes that of care, and would seem to be a good basis for leadership in the health service. However, there are problems with this theory. First, feminist writers, (cf. Robinson 2008) note how, historically, women have been oppressed by models of unconditional service. Second, the focus on serving followers can take away from the need of the leadership to respond to core shared purpose and to the many different stakeholders, not least the patient/client (Polleys 2002). Nonetheless, in practice, servant leadership involves broader transformation of ethical culture. Hence, Laub (2004) sets out six key behaviours of servant leadership: valuing people; developing people; building community; displaying authenticity; providing leadership and sharing leadership. Greenleaf (1977) had previously identified 10 core characteristics of the servant leader: listening; empathy; healing; awareness; persuasion; conceptualisation (the capacity to develop a vision); foresight (the capacity to understand and learn from the past and apply these lessons to the present and future); stewardship; commitment to the growth of people and building community. It could be said there is a direct link to the components and qualities of transformational nurse leadership identified in Table 8.3.

Relational Leadership

Inevitably, this takes us away from a simple view of 'the leader' to a view of leadership that can hold together several different tensions. Collins (2001) highlights a tension of virtues, between iron will and humility. Hock (1999) identifies the need to maintain an appropriate balance between the functional tensions of chaos and order. A certain amount of chaos is needed for change, enterprise, energy and creativity, and a certain amount of order, structure and systematic, stable context is needed for the implementation of creative ideas, for working out the details of new ideas (Binney and Williams 1997). The plurality of purpose, identity and function, along with the different strengths required to keep these in tension, are focusing not simply on action but upon the development of meaning and worth in relation to the social environment. In all this, leadership ties into the social construction of meaning (Grint 2005), that we are continuously constructing and affirming our reality. We share our interpretations with others, and when our interpretation makes sense to others, they might choose to see the world, or an aspect of the world, according to our interpretation. In a complex internal and external environment, this requires the leader to facilitate an ongoing exploration through dialogue of the meaning all stakeholders see in their work. Hence, leadership is relational and holistic rather than a set of characteristics that are present or lacking in the individual leader or the technical capacity to develop transactions. Bass (2005) argues that the relational content of the interaction between people is the key aspect of leadership. Leadership is not simply about using certain techniques, but about the very being (ontology) of the leader as he or she develops relationships, and, with that, meaning and value.

Eco-Leadership Theory

Something of this is found in Western's (2007) eco-leadership. This takes account of the complex internal and external social and physical environment, arguing that leadership has to engage with those relationships. Focused on an interdependent and interconnected environment (local and global), it looks to enable the development of 'collective wisdom' to respond to that social environment. The stress on virtues such as wisdom is reinforced with Western's focus on formation, that is the personal and professional development of the individual, as well as the organisation. Western begins to deepen the question of meaning, noting four aspects of eco-leadership:

- Connectivity – Emphasising the interdependent social and physical environments and the emerging theme of the need for a holistic approach,
- Systemic ethics – The importance of some overall view of justice and care, centred around sustainability and the common good,
- Leadership spirit – Here, Western suggests a number of intangible aspects that radically affect meaning, including: logos and mythos (underlying value narratives and world views, such as stewardship, that give shared meaning), creativity and imagination (focused on empathy) and holistic consciousness,
- Organisational belonging – Belonging can relate to many relationships at once, and focuses on self and group worth.

This theory challenges accepted views of success and aims to unleash creativity. Strikingly, in his principles of eco-leadership formation, Western suggests that individual and organisational development (Senge 1990) must happen together, that leaders across the organisation should learn from each other, that it is an ongoing reflective process, and that leadership requires 'containing structures' that enable reflective, creative and developmental activity. Such a view of leadership presumes the development of organisations that will enable holistic thinking, such that meaning can be engaged at a deep level (Lips-Wiersma and Morris 2018). To keep together such engagement and the sustainability of the organisation requires dispersed leadership, sharing the responsibility of leadership. Alimo-Metcalfe and Alban-Metcalfe (2005) argue the need for strong virtues of leadership to ensure this tension together. In particular, they note six factors emerging from research with leaders in Health Care Trusts in the UK:

- Valuing individuals. This involves genuine concern for the wellbeing and development of others, based on inclusivity,
- Networking and achieving. This involves enterprise, developing networks inside and outside the organisation, and inspirational communication. This is based on a strong sense of connectedness,
- Enabling, through delegation and empowerment,
- Acting with integrity, involving honesty and openness,
- Being accessible. Behind this lies a sensitivity to the needs of others,
- Being decisive, and able to take risks.

Leadership Virtues

Leadership is not just about learning a set of skills or achieving outcomes. At its core is character: specifically, a character in harmony with its ethical responsibilities to others. The kind of character that, in regard to others, always tries to do the right thing, for the right reason. As noted in Chapter 3, a virtue is a habitual and firm disposition or capacity to do good which allows the person not only to perform good acts, but to give the best of themselves. Robinson and Smith (2014) propose leadership virtues under seven heads, each of which develops some aspect of responsibility:

- *Consciousness* of the complex environment (internal and external) in which the organisation exists. This includes awareness of thought, feeling and value which inform practice, and thus impact on the complex environment.
- *Connectivity*, appreciation (valuing) of relationship with the social and physical environment, involving a sense of belonging, solidarity.
- *Criticality*, involving a testing of different views and practice, and thus awareness of the complex and connected narratives which challenge our understanding, meaning-making and beliefs. It also works against the dominance of single narratives. Hence, plurality in the community is to be welcomed.
- *Commitment* to and care of person, purpose and project over time. Connectivity, criticality and commitment and care all contribute to consciousness. It is hard to be aware of the complexity of the other without being there for them, something which ties closely to the idea of shared and universal responsibility.
- *Community*, this is key to identity, which is in turn key to relationship and meaning. On the one hand, this means developing the disciplines of community which involved mutual support and shared responsibility. This requires a well worked out culture (system and discipline of meaning-making). On the other hand, this also requires working with difference both inside and outside the community, enabling learning and an associated sense of journey.
- *Character*, which is built up of one's strengths; the intellectual, moral, psychological and practical virtues (see Chapter 3). The practice of the virtues enables responsible action, including responsible leadership. Consciousness includes awareness of moral limitations, including dispositions which limit awareness and the capacity to respond to the social and physical environment.
- *Creativity*. The focus on character and community takes leadership away from the realm of simple technique to personal engagement, and expressing values in innovative practice; finding new ways to share responsibility in practice, across disciplines, sectors and so on. It is important in this context to recognise that leadership and management cannot be shackled to a single view of strategy. Focus on the complex social and physical environment demands thinking which responds to new discoveries and thus may not follow a rigid strategic design (Chia and Holt 2011).

These elements come together in leadership in healthcare, for example, in the model developed in the UK by the NHS Leadership Academy (NHS 2013). This model involves the following:

1. Inspiring shared purpose
2. Leading with care
3. Evaluating information
4. Connecting our service
5. Sharing the vision
6. Engaging the team
7. Holding to account
8. Developing capability
9. Influencing for results.

The stress on developing and working with the workforce, engaging stakeholders and ensuring communication is effectively handled and this involves four elements:

- Leadership as shared and occurring at all levels and across the board, with management, professional bodies and individual professionals sharing responsibility for the purpose of the organisation as a whole and for their area of practice in particular. Hence the stress in this model is on both self-regulation and focusing on the core purpose, with a culture not dominated by targets, rules, regulations or status hierarchies (Kings Fund 2015).
- The development of qualities which enable such leadership
- A focus on leadership practice, with a description of leadership in each of the nine headings which develops from essential to exemplary
- The consequences of good leadership as engaging employees, developing high quality care, patient/client satisfaction and a highly valued service.

The model is built on ethical values and virtues: shared purpose, leading with care, evaluating information, connecting our service, sharing the vision, engaging the team, holding to account, developing capability and influencing for results.

INSPIRING SHARED PURPOSE

The essential element of this is 'staying true to NHS principles and values'. Proficiency in this practice involves being able to hold to these principles and values under pressure. A strong perspective of this is taking risks to stand up for the shared purpose. The final exemplary element involves making courageous challenges for the benefit of the service. In effect, this aspect of leadership is about the virtue of *integrity*. This does not suggest integrity as ethical perfection. On the contrary, the four elements suggest integrity involving constant learning, in response to challenges to practice of the purpose. Robinson (2016) argues that integrity is focused on being true to personal, professional and social identity. The professional identifies with these principles and values, and so is being true not just to the values but also to him- or herself and his or her profession. This also involves the moral virtue of *courage* and the intellectual virtue of *phronesis* or practical wisdom (see Chapter 3). The focus on identity reinforces the idea of providing an example to others.

LEADING WITH CARE

It is important to remember that the focus of care is leadership *per se* and not healthcare as such. All leadership has to exercise care. The essential element is caring for the team, which demands awareness of the team dynamics and a willingness to address problems, understanding the underlying reasons for different behaviours and making connections between the health of the team and the quality of service. A strong example of this enabling the practice of mutual support in the team and exemplary practice involves enabling a caring environment across the service as a whole. The meaning of care is focused on the virtues of *empathy* and *kindness*. The Kings Fund report on Leadership in Healthcare (2015) notes that this also demands the principle of *fairness*, involving both equal respect and justice (Rawls 1971).

EVALUATING INFORMATION

This ties directly into the first three pillars of clinical governance, focusing on ensuring regular reflective data collection and feedback on practice, scanning widely to attend both to the complexity of the situation and the opportunities found; enhancing *creativity*. The core underlying virtues include *honesty* and *imagination*.

CONNECTING OUR SERVICE

This builds on evaluating information. The essential element involves recognising how one's particular area connects to other parts of the system or organisation. To appreciate those connections requires an understanding of the 'culture and politics across the organisation'. This in turn demands an awareness of the standards and demands across the organisation: professional, managerial and so on. The exemplary element of this involves working strategically across the system. This is partly about understanding the responsibilities and limitations of the different groups in the system and partly about sharing responsibility for the whole project and negotiating responsibility for particular actions. Lederach (2005) refers to this virtue as the moral imagination, holding together core principles and values and an awareness of possibilities, and how all involved can develop possibilities and new ideas.

SHARING THE VISION

As in the final section, this is focused on communication – helping to make clear the vision of the organisation and how individuals, teams and different groups contribute to that. Once again, it is about enabling all to take responsibility for that vison and how it is put into practice, developing trust and confidence and is focused on narratives that bring that vision alive.

ENGAGING THE TEAM

This involves appreciating the ideas and practice of the team, and enabling them to own purpose, plans and practice through creative participation. It stresses both cooperation and 'stretching the team' to deliver on shared purpose as well as individual targets. At the centre of this is building the value of self and mutual trust in and beyond the team.

HOLDING TO ACCOUNT

This focuses on responsibility in several ways. The essential element of this involves setting clear expectations and enabling the team to take responsibility for performance, with clear priorities which link to the organisational values and goals. Proficiency in this area of leadership involves managing and supporting performance: setting standards; challenging mindsets; giving feedback and showing how to manage poor performance. The balance is about developing both a supportive and challenging culture, moving to exemplary leadership which helps to create innovative and effective change. Leadership here encourages high expectations, sharing stories and symbols and taking pride in achievement focused on the ideals of the organisation. At its centre is *accountability*, that is the capacity to give a reasoned justification of thinking and practice.

DEVELOPING CAPABILITY

This aspect of leadership is precisely the pillar of governance around enabling staff development: building longer-term capability in individuals and enabling responsibility to be developed and passed on effectively. Key values to this aspect of leadership are the importance of individual agency and judgement, and with that, the importance of continuous learning focused on reflective practice. Once more, then, there is a stress on *phronesis*.

INFLUENCING FOR RESULTS

This aspect of leadership focuses on persuasion, enabling different groups to build consensus and work together, leading to exemplary leadership which builds sustainable commitments. The heart of this is clear, honest communication, involving respectful listening, effective dialogue with all stakeholders and the development of well-reasoned arguments. It also recognises the importance of narrative, both as an illustration which engages feeling and as the holistic focus for the core purpose of the organisation.

These factors apply to leadership in every aspect of professional practice in healthcare, from nurses to the organisational leadership. They link directly to the six Cs of Chapter 1 and to the core purpose of health services, care. This core idea of leading with care connects to compassionate leadership (NHS 2017) and to intelligent kindness as the basis of healthcare culture (Campling 2015). The latter is focused both on the idea of kin, involving unconditional acceptance of the other and the intellectual and practical aspects of professional practice. It is important to underline that neither of these terms involves a lack of critical thinking or practice. West and Bailey (2019) deal with the five myths about compassionate leadership, including the fear that such leadership will lead to loss of control and inability to challenge. Compassionate leadership involves an acceptance of the other and an 'epistemic' distance necessary if the professional is to remain focused on the core purpose, and the responsibility and needs of all the different relevant stakeholders (Campbell 1984). In Chapter 11, we examine this more closely, with a focus on care as the basis for normative ethics.

The Role of Nursing Leadership

Today, healthcare services are subject to ongoing changes focused on enhancing service quality, efficiency and patient/client satisfaction (Bahcecik and Öztürk 2003). A key method in promoting ethics in practice is for managers/leaders to role model ethical performance (Storch et al. 2013) and implement ethical leadership (Gallagher and Tschudin 2010), thereby playing a vital role in promoting patient/client safety (Kangasniemi et al. 2013), creating openness to discuss and act upon ethics in daily practice (Makaroff et al. 2014) and supporting ethical competence of their staff (Poikkeus et al. 2014). Nurse leaders are at the forefront of efforts to increase ethical thinking and discourse within the workplace. After identifying the need for resources to address ethical issues, it is possible to implement a successful ethics programme to promote better decision making and collaboration for the good of each patient/client. Failure to do so may result in increased rates of moral distress, noted in Chapter 6. As moral distress on a unit increases, so too does staff turnover and a loss of job satisfaction. A step taken toward more ethical practice by many nurse leaders is to select an ethics champion to facilitate the ethical decision-making process. These champions receive further training to broaden their understanding of ethics and the ethical challenges nurses face as part of their daily work. But nursing is an evidence-based practice, and evidence-based results can help pave the way toward a more ethical workplace. Beyond designating an ethics champion, nursing leadership needs to help other nurses evaluate ethical dilemmas by taking specific steps that promote ethical dialogue, including:

- Identifying common ethical problems occurring with regular frequency on the unit,
- Encouraging staff to seek out and utilise appropriate ethical resources within the facility, including the ethics champion, the organisation's ethics committee or the nurse leader themselves,
- Supporting a positive ethical environment by creating ethical policies, practices or guidelines,
- Providing further training and education to all staff members about ethics and ethical issues that may arise on the unit,
- Promoting open discussions among the entire healthcare team about specific ethical issues as they relate to patient/client care.

Leaders plays a vital role in creating a culture of care (Gustafsson and Stenberg 2017), and leadership ethics and confidence in one's leader are important constituents of a healthy work environment culture (Eneh and Kvist 2012; Gallagher and Tschudin 2010). In such work areas, where culture and confidence is present, staff are empowered to express their concerns and offer suggestions as to how their work environment and care provision can be improved (Bjarnason and LaSala 2015).

CASE 8.1 Ethics Related to Culture, Ethnic and Linguistic Diversity in Healthcare

Sakinah is a 63-year-old woman who presented to the emergency department at 4:00 a.m. with severe abdominal pain, chronic diarrhoea, weight loss and extreme fatigue. She has recently been diagnosed with advanced stages of colorectal cancer and is struggling to come to terms with her diagnosis. Following the oncology team assessment, Sakinah and her concerned family agreed to an admission to the medical assessment unit and were awaiting a bed. Sakinah, who is a practising Muslim, moved to Ireland with her husband (who was her cousin) from Pakistan over 22 years ago. Sakinah, who remained a stay-at-home mother, is very proud of the achievements of their two grown up daughters, Abir, who is 18 and currently in her first year of a business studies degree, and Aisha, who is 21 and studying accountancy.

At 2:00 p.m., Sakinah was transferred to the medical assessment unit. John Murphy was the nurse in charge of the ward and, following a brief handover from the emergency department nurse, he was taking responsibility for carrying out Sakinah's admission to the ward. Sakinah's family, who were accompanying her, had just left to get some refreshments, as they felt more relaxed now that she had been transferred to the ward. John who was born, brought up and educated in Ireland, always wanted to be a nurse and has worked on this ward for the last 5 years. John is educated to master's level and has over 17 years clinical nursing experience working in Irish acute healthcare settings. He is well respected by his colleagues who often describe him as the 'super nurse' for his upbeat personality and continued commitment to striving to provide 'high standards of care'.

When John enters the room to greet Sakinah and carry out the admission assessments and documentation, he notices that Sakinah appeared anxious and nervous. She appeared to have tears in her eyes, and he was concerned by her lack of eye contact with him. As John had been reading Sakinah's medical history, he felt this might be associated with her struggles to come to terms with her diagnosis. He empathised with this feeling, as he himself had undergone treatment for prostate cancer 5 years ago and recollected the uncertainties he experienced at that time. He introduced himself, welcomed her to the ward, sat down beside her and proceeded to inform her that he was the nurse looking after her today, and that 'she was in good hands'. He explained the process of the admission and assessments that he would carry out to get a baseline of her symptoms, whilst acknowledging the fears she may have. Sakinah continued to avoid eye contact and appeared withdrawn during their initial interaction. To reassure and comfort her, he pulled the curtains to protect her privacy, placed his hand (left hand as he was left-handed) on hers, continued to use eye contact and spoke clearly and slowly. He was surprised when Sakinah withdrew her hand without giving reasons for doing so. He could see she was upset, but was struggling to understand the cause of her lack of engagement.

John became more concerned when Sakinah did not respond to his general questions that formed the basis for his initial assessment and to help with completing the admission documentation. He decided that carrying out the admission and initial assessment with Sakina at this time might not be appropriate and wondered how he would overcome these problems. He decided to monitor her vital signs to, at the very least, gain a baseline and hoped she would relax and interact more with him afterwards. Although John felt that Sakinah was in pain, she was stating she had no pain and refused analgesia. This concerned John, as he could see that her non verbal communication indicated to him that she was in pain. She was prescribed a range of oral and intramuscular analgesics, which he felt she would benefit from, as he wanted to ensure her comfort, but was frustrated as she refused them. He decided he would go and talk to the doctor about her behaviour, which he felt was strange. He explained to Sakinah that he would come back later when she had settled in and explained that the doctor would be coming to see her soon.

It was lunch time, so John asked the catering team to provide Sakinah with some lunch, as he had checked her notes, and it stated that she could eat and drink. As Sakinah informed the catering team that she was not hungry, they felt they should bring her something light to eat, as they felt she looked frail and malnourished. The patients/clients on the ward had been saying that the bacon on the menu today was 'delicious', they decided that they would bring her in a small portion of bacon, cabbage and mashed potatoes, with white parsley sauce in a separate container, as they acknowledged that not everybody liked parsley sauce. They proceeded to leave the food on a table beside her bed in case she changed her mind.

When Sakinah's family returned, they demanded to speak with John and appeared angry at the care provided to Sakinah in their absence and proceeded to inform John of their reasons for being upset. John was saddened to hear that despite his intentions to reassure, empathise, comfort and provide compassionate care to Sakinah, he was culturally insensitive in his actions. Delivering quality care to patients/clients of the Muslim faith requires an understanding of similarities and differences in cultural and spiritual beliefs. Some important differences to consider include diet, ideas of modesty, privacy, touch restrictions and alcohol intake restrictions (Swihart and Martin 2019). John learned that health and social care professionals need to avoid eye contact and physical contact between a healthcare worker and patient/client when there are differences between sexes. Male health and social care professionals may need to communicate through a spouse or family member if the patient/client is female. It is important to the patient/client and their family that their body is not exposed unnecessarily, and being touched or examined by a male nurse may be frightening and insensitive. In relation to toileting practices, Muslims usually wash after toileting, both defecating and urinating, and disposable cups should be made available in bathrooms to facilitate this practice. The left hand tends to be used for any washing conducted after toileting, and John recalled how he used his left hand to comfort Sakinah earlier. Islamic rules prohibit pork, alcohol, non-halal meats and any animals that have not been slaughtered in line with Islamic custom. Halal food includes animals and poultry that have been ritually prepared and all seafood. Alternatively, food prepared to vegetarian standards will be suitable for Muslims provided that utensils used in preparation have not been used in preparing non-halal food or have been carefully washed.

8.3 PAUSE FOR THOUGHT

Cultural Sensitivity

- How do you show compassion in your own culture?
- How do you show compassion in other cultures?
- What practices and behaviours might be seen to be compassionate in your culture but offensive in other cultures?
- How can compassionate care in culturally appropriate ways be nurtured in your area of practice?
- How, as a whole, are organisations/leaders addressing ethical issues?
- How can organisations/leaders enable consciousness of the need to respond to cultural differences?

The importance of nurturing compassionate practices in culturally appropriate ways is widely recognised in healthcare services globally. This requires exploring the similarities and differences of how individuals interpret the meaning of compassion. What might be seen as providing compassionate care in one culture might be seen as insensitive in another. It is important for health and social care professionals to recognise that cultural, spiritual and religious values and beliefs vary not only among different cultures but also within different cultural groupings. This requires genuinely involving patients/clients in a dialogue about their experiences and desires for care, so that care is based on a mutually agreed and patient-/client-centred plan of care. This will also assist health and social care professionals to ascertain, rather than assume, that certain preferences and practices are of significance to individuals from diverse cultural, ethnic and linguistic backgrounds. Becoming more sensitive to the needs of individuals around you will assist in the development of knowledge and skills required to practice in a manner which is both compassionate and culturally competent.

All need to engage in the dialogue around what compassion looks like across cultures. Leadership carries responsibility for enabling colleagues to find the space to integrate this in practice. While it is less likely that decisions of management will directly harm individual patients/clients, responsible decision making on the part of hospital management is important if it is to be possible for all staff to integrate ethics into their daily work. Leadership bears responsibility to patients/clients who are being cared for in the hospital; the staff and the community that provides the funding to the organisation. These mirror the diverse interests which come together in the hospital: the interest of patients/clients to be treated adequately in the hospital; and the interest of hospital staff to work in an institution with appropriate ethical and social standards and the

CASE 8.2   Making a Reasonable Adjustment

A 20-year-old man, Paul, with autism and intellectual disability, has been admitted to the unit for investigative surgery. When the nurse enters his room to go through the admission process and upcoming procedure, she finds Paul lying on the floor and accompanied by his brother. The nurse asks Paul to come lie on the bed but the man shouts, 'NO'. Then Paul's brother approaches the nurse to say that Paul does not like beds and does not use one. Could she talk and examine Paul on the floor? The nurse presents a puzzled look to Paul's brother and says, 'Come on, Paul, hop up on the bed now'. Paul does not respond to the nurse but reacts by beginning to hum to himself. The nurse follows this up with, 'Come on Paul, you have to use the bed'. At this, Paul gets a little agitated, rushes to the bed, pulls off all the sheets, pulls the mattress down onto the floor and lies down on the mattress. The nurse seems startled by this and tries to coax Paul off the mattress. Paul's brother interjects to repeat, 'Paul will not use the bed, he does not like beds'. To which the nurse replies, 'What do you mean he does not use a bed? Where does he sleep?'. Paul's brother replies that, 'He will sleep on the floor, and at home, we put his mattress on the floor for him when he is going to bed'. The nurse replies, 'But he can't sleep on the floor; he is in hospital now', and she appears to be becoming a little anxious herself now and says, 'We have to get him onto the bed; he cannot sleep on the floor'. At this time, the unit manager comes into the room and says, 'Is there a problem?'. The nurse says that Paul will not use the bed, he prefers the floor. To which the manager replies, 'He cannot sleep there. What about infection control? They will not allow that. We should have known this. We cannot accommodate him here'.

This situation raises many issues for all concerned, and the question is what ethical aspects are at play here? Is Paul entitled to sleep on the floor? Is it the nurse's responsibility to support Paul and his family member/s and provide appropriate care? Is there any prejudice here when accommodation is denied? The fact of the matter is we are required to make reasonable adjustments which is a change to practice and processes which are implemented to prevent any disabled persons from being at a disadvantage. We identified in Chapter 5 the importance of rights, autonomy, decision making and the United Nations Convention on the Rights of Persons With Disability (2006). The question is were these principles adopted in the case above, and how can they be incorporated in the future? In this case, there was little evidence of engagement of the nurse with Paul and, when communication occurred, it was more with Paul's brother than directly with Paul himself. Although it may be acceptable for Paul's brother to speak up and advocate on his brother's behalf, that does not mean that Paul becomes redundant in the process, and that we do not need to listen to his voice and communicate directly with him. In the absence of such communication, it is impossible to build the aspect of trust as identified in Chapter 3 and later in this chapter. Failing to communicate and placing inappropriate demands on Paul was a source of stress and anxiety for him, and his non-verbal language clearly articulates this, such as when Paul began humming and pulled the sheets off the bed and the mattress to the floor. Even with this clear effort to communicate by Paul, the nurse remained focused on getting Paul onto the bed rather than being on the floor. This raises the questions about the principles of respect, autonomous choice, maleficence, and non-maleficence, as noted in Chapter 2.

At a practice level, then, each encounter has an ethical dimension and requires ethical competence. In this case, the manger confirms the nurse's perspective of seeing the problem rather than the person, situation or solutions. This raises the question of leadership on the unit and the influence of the leader on the practice of the staff. We need to consider if the nurse was operating to conform to the leaders thinking and practice, or were they practising independently and sharing a similar worldview as that of the management? Given that the healthcare environment caters for many people of diverse complexity, communication and cognitive ability, there is a need to be responsive but also proactive. In this case, the manager says, 'We should have known', and this could be a good proactive strategy, but only if to identify support and accommodation necessary to assist Paul for his admission, procedure and stay in hospital. However, in this case, we can question just what should have been known. Was that to avoid Paul's admission to the unit, postpone Paul's admission or identify that the unit could not accommodate his needs? If this is possibly the case, then we have to question, in any fellow professional, prejudice, discrimination, biases and fears of people with autism and/or intellectual disability.

This case highlights the need for adjustment prior to and during an individual's stay in hospital, with leadership ensuring an alert flag system that identifies that the person may require adjustments, and having someone following up on those adjustments prior to admission could assist. But regardless of the best laid plans, there is and will always be a need for adjustments during the stay, and this needs to be in all staff's mindset as it generally will be that adjustment is required in all care episodes. Although a one size fits all approach will not suffice, Blair et al. (2016) recommend the TEACH (Table 8.4) approach as a means to support care adjustment to meet the needs of a person, especially with more vulnerable patients/clients, such as those with a disability.

TABLE 8.4 ■ **TEACH Approach**

- Time – Take time to work with the person
- Environment – Alter the environment to meet the person's needs
- Attitude – Have a positive, solutions-orientated focus
- Communication – Find out the best way to communicate with the person and their family, carers and supporters, and communicate this to colleagues
- Help – Consider what help the person and their family, carers and supporters need, and how can you meet these needs.

From Blair, J., Busk, M., Goleniowska, H., et al. (2016). Through our eyes: what parents want for their children from health professionals. In S. Hardy, E. Chaplin, & P. Woodward (Eds.), *Supporting the physical health needs of people with learning disabilities* (pp. 197–212). Brighton: Pavilion Publishing and Media Ltd.

interest of society to have effective healthcare institutions. Leaders have an accountability to their patient/client, due to the particular nature of the relationship between patient/client and healthcare providers in the hospital setting, which is usually highly unequal, in terms of knowledge and authority.

Good nurse leadership can have a positive impact on both patient/client experience and outcomes, and nurse satisfaction and retention. Leadership needs to create a collective perception of autonomy and empowerment to create positive work environments. Leaders have to make sure the institutional mission statements and policies do not conflict with the professional ethical codes and encourage and promote initiatives from staff in the implementation of ethical guidelines in their daily work. However, the scarcity of resources, resource allocation and lack of staff and time may limit staff's engagement in activities that are ethically important, and leaders need to use their influence to reduce such issues and uphold ethical standards. In line with their community role of healthcare providers, leaders need to consider healthcare provision so as it adequately meets the needs of society, in order to fulfil their public functions. One means of improving the quality of healthcare and meeting societal needs would be in providing and supporting opportunities for staff to take part in continuing education which focuses on shared leadership and mutual challenge. This brings us to leadership in the organisation.

Organisational Leadership

Organisations are crucial instruments of growth, development and human flourishing (Morgan 2006). The organisation, formalised as an institution, structures political, economic and social interaction consisting of both informal constraints (sanctions, taboos, customs), formal rules (constitutions, laws) and developed to create order and reduce uncertainty in exchange (North 1991, p. 97). Institutions, such as the National Health, are organisations which add value to the larger society; as such, they come into existence due to social needs or pressure and are a part of a larger society or community. The characteristic features of an organisation are: (1) bureaucracy, which implies a rational and systematic process designed to enhance efficiency; (2) hierarchy of positions, which in some organisations is pyramidal; (3) rules and regulations that guide organisational operations; (4) technical competence – members are hired based on certain standards that can be monitored and evaluated; (5) impersonal and unbiased standard which allows that both customers and employees are treated alike and (6) formalised communication, which is a common phenomenon in organisations (Macionis 2012).

Organisations have three aspects – the rational system, the natural system and the open system (Scott and Davis 2007). The rational system definition focuses on normative structures of the organisations. As a natural system, organisations involve participants pursuing multiple interests, both disparate and common, but who recognise the value of perpetuating the organisation as an important resource. As open systems, organisations are congeries of interdependent flows and activities, linking shifting coalitions of participants embedded in wider material-resource and institutional environments (Scott and Davis 2007). Key to organisational leadership is engaging these complexities. Leadership of the organisation then is focused in the governance, which confirms and develops vision and purpose, and objectives and develops values, culture and communication which enables core practices in relation to context (Shafritz et al. 2011). We will examine that in more detail in the next chapter.

WELL-BEING AND WORKFORCE

In focusing on purpose and direction, leadership also affects the well-being of the workforce. Employees' job satisfaction is strategic in the attainment of organisational success (Robbins and Judge 2013). The employees are the backbone of organisational life and sustainability, and their job satisfaction influences organisational commitment, which in turn affects employee loyalty, retention and turnover (Robbins and Judge 2013; Mathis and Jackson 2011; Voon et al. 2011). Spector (1997) identifies nine aspects of job satisfaction: pay, promotion, supervision, benefits, contingent rewards, operating procedures, co-workers, nature of work and communication. Within nursing, Boamah et al. (2017) and Olu-Abiodun and Abiodun (2017) highlight that transformational leadership has a strong positive influence on workplace empowerment and is positively related to job satisfaction, job commitment and patient/client satisfaction with nursing services. Özden et al. (2017) and Benevene et al. (2018) highlight the effect of nurses' ethical leadership and ethical climate perceptions on their job satisfaction, noting that ethical leadership promoted ethical climate, which had a positive correlation with employees' job satisfaction and organisational commitment. In addition, a correlation exists between ethical climate and perceived nurses' support, organisational commitment, job satisfaction and turnover intention of nurses (Hashish 2017).

STRUGGLE

Today, healthcare organisations are subject to rapid and essential changes aimed at enhancing the quality of service, patient/client satisfaction and productivity. Parallel with these changes, nurses face challenges such as heavy workload, increased patient/client awareness, various problems related to staff skills, lack of resources, low occupational and life quality and workplace violence (Ulrich et al. 2007). Within practice, nurses are expected to treat patients/clients in an ethical manner, and that ethics is part of their professional performance. When the ethical climate of the institution is perceived as negative, this leads to a reduction in an individual's motivation, job performance, job satisfaction (Lemmenes et al. 2018; Wang and Hsieh 2012; Goldman and Tabak 2010), cooperation (Schulte 2002) and decreased organisational commitment (Martin and Cullen 2006).

This points to the genuine struggles between organisational leadership and the professions which, in the case of Mid Staffs, were not worked through. Nurse staffing levels, for instance, are closely related to the quality of the nursing practice environment, the care provided for patients/clients and patient/client outcomes (Squires et al. 2015). The international evidence identifies a significant association between staffing levels and lower mortality (Cho et al. 2015; Shekelle 2013; Kane et al. 2007). For every patient/client added to a nurse's workload, there is an associated 7% increase in risk-adjusted mortality following general surgery (Aiken et al. 2018). Increasing the number of nurses, meanwhile, results in greater labour costs. However, these costs are offset or even cause savings against the additional healthcare costs of low staffing rates, such as additional surgical procedures, diagnostic testing, drugs, days in intensive care and days in hospital, alongside the pain and suffering caused to patients/clients (Dall et al. 2009). Within the general hospital environment, hospitals with better nursing staff levels have been shown to have 30% fewer hospital acquired infections than hospitals with poor nurse staffing after taking into account patient/client risk factors and characteristics of hospitals such as size (Cimiotti et al. 2012).

Given this knowledge regarding staff ratios and its effect on care, how do we balance expectation against reality? For example, in the recent economic crisis, organisations were engaged in a policy of non-recruitment/replacing of staff. Was this justified given the economic climate or given the fact that we know staffing affects care outcomes? Should the health service continue to recruit no matter the economic climate? In addition, we know that health needs increase with age, and that there is a growing ageing population. In fact, by the year 2020, we will be in a situation that we will have more people over the age of 65 than under the age of 5 (Jeffrey 2016). This raises the question of how do we balance wanting to deliver a quality service against the overall needs of all, as there is limited economic wealth in a country and many services to deliver, for example health, education, social, transport.

Even if one is of the belief that health is the number one priority and finances are made available to employ an agreed ratio of nurse to patients/clients, this has to be considered in the context that it is estimated that a global shortage of about 9 million nurses/midwives will exist by 2030 (WHO 2016). Hence, there is need for more effective dialogue to understand how the institutions of care can attract and retain nurses within their profession. This suggests greater attention to working conditions and environment, opportunities for advancement and a progressive career pathway are needed, in addition to traditional cultures and systems resistant to change (or lack of support to change) need to be addressed. Addressing these factors is as much founded in ethical values as the caring identity of nursing. Today's organisations face ever-increasing change, which needs a more adaptive flexible leadership, this is becoming increasingly important in the 21st century (Doody and Doody 2012).

Ethical Leadership, Trust, Communication and Dialogue

8.4 PAUSE FOR THOUGHT

The Hospital Porter

The CEO of a major healthcare trust is informed on coming to work that one of the porters has been seen on CCTV the previous evening 'leaning into' a snack dispenser to take out a chocolate bar. This is theft. The organisation has a code of conduct which states that anyone found guilty of theft, of whatever value the object, will be dismissed. The CEO orders HR to dismiss the employee. His argument is that if rules are not followed, then this will lead to anarchy.

What would you have done and why?

The case above is adapted from an actual event. The CEO believed that he was doing the right ethical thing by reinforcing the ethical code. This involved a deterrence view of justice: 'if I let them off then no one will take the rules seriously'. Once that had been determined, there was no attempt from HR to push back and offer an alternative view. The whole incident in fact shows a lack of dialogue between leader, organisation, procedures and the member of staff who was fired. It presumes a view of justice that does not require dialogue, and view of leadership that has to be strong and assertive. As with most such decisions, the absence of dialogue in the initial phase of the event led to much more difficult problems emerging. Press interest was generated, leading to questions to board members about policy, not least because the record of the employee had been exemplary. Unions became involved, leading to a re-ignition of previous disputes, and so on. The leader in question had presumed that the incident was discrete, that is, not connected to other aspects of the organisation or beyond. He had also presumed that dialogue would weaken the ethical character of the organisation. The opposite was true. Lack of dialogue led to many more problems and a lack of clarity about how justice was understood and practised in the organisation. And, with that, there emerged questions about trust in the leadership, from board members to unions to press and clients.

Do you trust the leader of your organisation? If so, why? In the last two decades, many argue that there has been a crisis of leadership across all sectors. Edelmann's Trust Barometer (2015) suggested that doctors and priests are still trusted, in the sense of trust in them to tell the truth (https://www.kingsfund.org.uk/blog/2015/12/public-trust-doctors-nurses). Doctors top this survey, along with teachers, scientists and judges. Priests have slid down to fifth (around 40%), just above the police. Bankers, however, have a trust deficit, along with business leaders and trades union officials. The good news for bankers is that they are not the least trusted. That accolade falls to estate agents and politicians. These figures are a rough snap shot, but they suggest at least two things. First, despite the dire warnings from the media, key professions do, in practice, retain trust. As O'Neill argues (2000), if we are in trouble, we will still call the police or the doctor. Second, those who are trusted are trusted because they matter to personal and social well-being and because that focus makes them impartial. It is striking that those in trust deficit are perceived as partial and polarised, from trades union leaders to business leaders to politicians. If we drill further down in the barometer, another significant finding emerges. The general levels of trust have gone down, and this seems to be connected to change and the pace of change, chiming in with the finding of the Francis Report (2013).

Trust involves significant relations, and reliance upon others, in a variety of ways, 'to do something, to be something, to allow something, to complete, facilitate, or not impede something' (Colledge et al. 2014). It also involves something about the identity of the person in relation to the other person or organisation who they trust. The 'trustees' believe they are in a significant relationship in which they are valued. Simpson (2007) suggests that the interpersonal trust literature in psychology emphasises four core principles which speak to this value. Research around interpersonal trust is here taken to be applicable also to organisational trust. First, individuals determine the extent to which they can trust the other through evidence of 'proper transformation of motivation in trust-diagnostic situations' (Simpson 2007, p. 265). Most relationships, one-to-one or in the wider organisation, have points at which they are tested. Key to maintaining trust in these situations is whether the other makes a decision which goes against self-interest and supports the best interest of the individual or the relationship.

The second finding was that 'trust-diagnostic situations often occur naturally and unintentionally during the ebb and flow of everyday life' (Simpson 2007, p. 265). Trust diagnosis often depends on circumstances. Moments of transition (Bridges 1980) involve challenges about individual and organisational identity, which inevitably involve questions about purpose, worth, values and relationships. The third finding was that individual differences in attachment orientations, self-esteem or self-differentiation (working models of self and others in relationship) will influence the development or decline of trust. Those who have a secure sense of self-worth, and of their distinctiveness in relationships, would be more likely to experience and practice mature trust, as well as develop trust over time. Simpson's final point is that understanding the degree and direction of trust also depends on awareness of the 'dispositions and actions' of both people in the relationship. This demands an awareness of the virtues and motivations of the other. Such evidence suggests that mature trust is not absolute but is tied to ongoing testing, confirmation and assurance that the other is focused on the wellbeing of the person. Much of this kind of leadership is focused on authentic persuasion, that is rhetoric. Rhetoric is often seen as rabble rousing. Aristotle (1991), however, argues that it is based on ethical attitude and has three elements:

Logos, clear rational arguments (avoiding the fallacies noted in Chapter 2). This also includes empirical evidence.

Pathos, attention to relationships and associated feelings. This involves both the feelings of the leader and of the members of the organisation. Many leaders claim an empathy which connects to these feelings without actually checking these feelings. Much populist leadership goes further, to try to evoke feelings based in fear. In effect, such leadership tries to use feelings to avoid the use of logos, and thus avoiding appreciation of complex truth.

Ethos, evidence of a credible character. Aristotle suggests three aspects of *ethos*: character (*arete*), practical wisdom (*phronesis*) and benevolence (*eunoia*). This deepens the understanding of the basis of trust because it looks beyond simple benevolence, and commitment of the leader to the workforce, to a focus on the good. Hence, the trust is not based purely on the interest of the relationship but on wider values and meaning – the core purpose of the organisation. This includes evidence of relational values such as justice and respect. Both of these confer a sense of worth that is acknowledged in the workplace. Hence, some philosophers argue that trust, and our assessment of trust, is not simply about the expressed care of the other and its confirmation or otherwise, it is also 'truth-directed' and 'end-directed' (Akker et al. 2009; Baker 1987; de Sousa 1987). I trust a nurse to help me partly because of the wider shared view of purpose that is expressed in the professional body. Similarly, I trust the leader of a healthcare provider because they are publicly focused on the same purpose and values.

In addition to a focus on shared values and purpose, trust requires that an account of this is given in the organisation, reflected in the structures and procedures. The procedures provide another buttress to trust, demonstrating procedural integrity focused on purpose and values. These will be examined more closely in the next chapter about governance. The three elements of rhetoric form the basis for trusting leadership, and critical to all three is dialogue. Only through dialogue can trust be tested and diagnosed. Importantly, such dialogue has to be more than a series of rehearsed talking points. Unrehearsed dialogue tests rational thinking in real time. Can the leader provide a rational justification for actions, without having to spend time working it out? It also tests motivation and feeling. If a leader focuses only on targets, can he or she really be trusted with the well-being of the members of the organisation?

Mature trust of leaders, then, focuses on dialogue which is:

- Mutual. Mutuality does not require that all parties are equal. On the contrary, any organisation has inequalities, not least of power (focused on authority). Hence, dialogue has to develop asymmetrical mutuality which acknowledges both different and shared identity.
- Enabling. Mutuality is characterised by the practice of giving trust to the other, that is enabling the other to take responsibility, by accepting trust from the other and by mutual trust expressed in the practice of shared responsibility. Maitland (2008) argues that trusting employees through cutting back on intense monitoring of their performance also enables the practice of the virtues. Hence, 'low levels of legal contract enforcement crowd *in* trustworthiness' (Osterloh and Frey 2004, p. 203).

It is important to note that whilst giving trust is a risky venture, the focus on shared values, purpose and procedures, and being open to account, provides the procedural framework to enable this. Once more, a counselling perspective on trust is instructive. If the therapist and patient/client agree on a contract (procedural framework), involving shared expectations about the meaning and practice of the therapy, then when the therapist does not fulfil the contract in some way, this allows the patient/client to challenge the therapist, and thus hold him or her to account (Robinson 2008). The therapist, by allowing the challenge and acknowledging it, confirms that the relationship is based in the meaning, value and purpose of therapy, involving respect for autonomy, mutuality and care, not dominance or self-interest. The dialogue is both cognitive and affective. By showing a measured response to the patient's/client's expression of feeling, not least anger, the therapist precisely communicates that he does not view such a challenge as a threat, but rather part of the ongoing dialogue. This enables the patient/client to develop trust based in mutuality and not in dominating relationships which have been part cause of the client's problems in the first place (Kohut 1982). In this exchange, they begin to experience mutuality, and with that, mature trust. Hence, trust becomes a part of learning experience (Colledge et al. 2014), always being tested, learned and developed, often in different contexts, with different stakeholders. In effect, trust is the value of faith and leads to the virtues of faithfulness (see Chapter 3), the capacity to engender trust in others and to trust others and the self. Important to enabling such trust in organisations is the kind of culture we spell out in Chapter 9, involving clear procedures embodying dialogue, including external arbitration.

Dialogue and Ethical Leadership

MacNamara's Reference not linked like other ones (2015) research suggests that many leaders believe they communicate through listening and dialogue, but that the vast majority of communication in organisations is in fact one-way transmission. This raises the question why one might imagine that dialogue is happing when it is not. Often, this is because it is replaced by ideas such as 'consultation'. A consultancy firm is brought in to effect, for instance, the development of an ethical policy or the 'brand' of an organisation. How this is used can raise major problems in relation to ethical leadership. It sets up some dialogue in small groups, but often does not extend that more widely, and can, without careful attention, entirely circumvent dialogue between leadership and the broader workforce. In those situations, leaders simply receive the summaries of dialogue, with no opportunity for clarification or challenge. The result is that responsibility of the different parties is not engaged, and accountability only narrowly practised.

An even simpler explanation of the leaders' self-perception is that there is a lack of understanding about the nature of listening. MacNamara (2015) suggests that listening involves: recognition of others' rights and views; acknowledgement; paying attention; interpreting what is said to gain understanding of others' views; giving consideration to what is said and an appropriate response. Much of this comes from Rogerian counselling theory (Robinson 2008; Rogers 1983), which focuses on enabling the counselee to develop their own story and thus develop their self-identity. The core conditions for this are:

- *Congruence* – the willingness to transparently relate to clients without hiding behind a professional or personal facade,
- *Unconditional positive regard* – offering an acceptance and prizing for the other as an end in themselves, without conveying disapproving feelings, actions or characteristics and demonstrating a willingness to attentively listen without interruption, judgement or giving advice,
- *Empathy* – communicating the desire to understand and appreciate their client's perspective.

Isaacs (1999) notes four practices in dialogic leadership: listening, respecting, suspending and voicing:

- *Listening as a participant.* Too often the leader feels themselve above the fray and thus does not listen to others. Isaac argues that listening together to the different narratives in the organisation breaks down this barrier and enables learning about the other and the broader purpose and practice. 'Following' then is focused on the emergent meaning and not the leader.
- *Respecting* the coherence of others' views. Such respect encourages people to look for the sense in what others are saying and thinking. This searches for the coherence in their views, even when we find what they are saying unacceptable. This in turn clarifies the views of leader and workforce to each other and to themselves. This enables genuine enquiry and learning.
- *Suspending* one's certainties and assumptions (affective and cognitive). This provides a psychological space to better hear the different narratives, and avoid the serial monologues of many leaders.
- *Voicing*–speaking one's true voice and encouraging others to do the same. This requires ensuring formal and informal space where the different narratives of the workforce can be articulated. This underlines the authenticity of the leadership. Algera and Lips-Wiersma (2012)

argue for a radical view of authenticity, focused on existentialism. Heidegger's (2010) term *Eigentlichkeit* is more literally translated as 'ownedness', or 'being owned'. It involves taking responsibility for meaning and practice. Hence, any action, and its authenticity, is truly an embodiment of the self and related meaning (Ladkin and Taylor 2010), emerging over time through deliberation and deliberative action (Taylor 1989). Authenticity, as noted above, is seen at its most intense when the questioning of dialogue is unrehearsed (Sparrowe 2005). Rehearsed dialogue involves no surprises and no genuine listening. Unrehearsed dialogue is focused on openness to personal encounter (Bakhtin 1984), not simply to rational ideas, suggesting that such dialogue does not attempt to change or control the other.

Such leadership enhances collective wisdom, encouraging different groups to take up the different aspects of leadership. This might, for instance, involve strengthening those with opposing views, if they are unsure, or reinforcing those who have become bystanders, if they have information but have withheld it. Genuinely making room for someone who wants to challenge makes it more possible for others to hear what they have to say. This can also address the problem of ambiguity in leadership. Leadership communication is often uncertain or ambiguous. As Eisenberg (1984) notes, this can be intentional (strategic), with the leader leaving others to decide what is meant. This can have good effects, leading to diversity of response and innovation. It can also be a means of avoiding leadership responsibility, with the leader able to blame them for any failure to understand. Dialogue tests ambiguity, enabling shared responsibility.

This view of dialogic leadership is not simply about making effective or efficient decisions. It is built on ethical principles, involves the practice of virtues and responsibility and is holistic. The core principles are respect and justice. The autonomy and agency of all the players are respected and empowered. This enables mutuality even in a situation where power is unequal. It enables the practice of responsibility through the focus on agency amongst all stakeholders, focused on shared deliberation (April 1999). Dialogue also enables all involved to give an account of their values and actions, thus developing mutual accountability. Dialogue also enables stakeholders to become involved in positive responsibility, generating imaginative possibilities and becoming co-creators (Van Loon 2017). This applies in the case of the hospital porter above. In the original event, the CEO fired him. The logic was that not to do so would weaken the Code of Conduct. However, there were several stakeholders in that situation, from the unions and the porter himself, to the HR team (responsible for dealing with staff), to other employees for whom this action said something about the values and attitude of the leadership, to the other professions who work with the leadership, to the wider community who have an interest in the ethical tone of such an important organisation. The narrow view of justice precisely precluded any dialogue with such stakeholders, either direct or through reference to previous dialogues, around the Code.

Leadership in healthcare institutions then can be summed up as:

- Distributed leadership. By definition, such leadership and management is not about directives or targets sent down from high, but about shared ownership of meaning and practice
- Involving dialogue around the meaning of values, and professional practice, and the relationship to the organisation
- Engaging a complex identity and context, with many different groups within any health service
- Enabling different levels of responsibility, including shared positive responsibility.

Interactive Leadership

Ethical identity is often focused on particular professions. Hence, we speak of medical ethics, nursing ethics, leadership ethics, governance ethics and so on. However, as noted in Chapters 1 and 2, a profession such as nursing relates to all stakeholders in healthcare. By definition then, ethics is inter-professional, with all professions, including administration, management and leadership, focusing on the practice of core modes of responsibility and understanding, and standing up for the core purpose, value and principles of the profession, opening themselves up for genuine accountability and working with other professions to share responsibility for good and creative practice. A good example of this in management is the ICAEW (Institute of Chartered Accountancy in England and Wales) Report Reporting With Integrity (ICAEW 2007). Practising accountancy with integrity is, in the Report's judgement, essential if the financial market is to maintain the trust of society. In this sense, by taking responsibility for professional practice, the profession itself provides leadership, for the members of its profession, for wider professions involved in this area of work, for the institutions that employ the accountant, and for wider society. In healthcare, this interactive, inter-professional leadership is increasingly developing. A good example of this is the duty of candour, which we examined in the last chapter from a nursing perspective. This applies also to organisational leadership.

DUTY OF CANDOUR AND ORGANISATIONAL APOLOGY

Just as it is important for professionals to demonstrate leadership through the practice of candour, it is also important for the organisation as a whole to demonstrate this integrity. There have been several models developed which focus on both the communication of failure and on the redevelopment of trust after an organisational crisis, and we will refer to two. The first is the reintegration model (Pfarrer et al. 2008). This is a four-stage model which aims to increase the speed and likelihood of restoring 'legitimacy with stakeholders following a transgression'. This involves following four complex actions in sequence which are designed to address the concerns of stakeholders (Pfarrer et al. 2008, p. 731):

- An open investigation of the facts, in co-operation with stakeholders
- Clear presentation of the cause of the crisis. This includes acknowledgement of the nature of the transgressions, accepting responsibility and the expression of remorse
- Acceptance of penance and punishment
- Reforming the organisations' procedures, relationships and its external image.

Pfarrer et al. (2008) tie in the process to stakeholder management (Mitchell et al. 1997), focusing on power, legitimacy or urgency of stakeholder claims. They argue that focus on elite and active stakeholders will lead to dialogue which serves to prompt key questions and demands, shape perceptions leading to concurrence, 'a generally shared opinion amongst stakeholders regarding the transgression and the appropriateness of the organisation's actions' (2008, p. 733). Concurrence does not have to be complete so long as a general threshold agreement is reached, that is an agreement which allows the firm to move through the threshold of each stage. The second model, the organisation-level trust repair model, from Gillespie and Dietz (2009), is again a four-stage approach for responding to failure. Such a failure is defined as an incident, or series of incidents, that threatens the legitimacy of the organisation, questioning its trustworthiness. Gillespie and Dietz argue that organisational trustworthiness is generated internally in four ways: leadership and management practices; culture and climate; strategy and sub-strategies and systems, policies and processes. Each of these provides signals and cues for significant meaning in practice. Trustworthiness is also shaped through two external elements: governance mechanisms, involving regulation and legislation, and the organisation's public reputation.

Such trustworthiness requires consistent promotion over time and is focused on 'behaviours and verbal responses that actively demonstrate ability, benevolence and integrity' (Gillespie and Dietz 2009, p. 134; Baier 1991). The first of these involves competence, which enables reliability in meeting goals and responsibilities, whereas benevolence involves respect and care for stakeholders. Integrity is described as consistent adherence to moral principles, such as honesty and fairness (Gillespie and Dietz 2009, p. 128). Consistent displays of such trustworthiness will reassure stakeholders of the likelihood of good conduct and acceptable actions in the future, enabling trust to be restored. Underpinning this has to be procedures that will demonstrate reliability in avoiding recurrence of failure (Gillespie and Dietz 2009, p. 134). To achieve this Gillespie and Dietz (2009) argue for a four-stage process:

- an immediate response, acknowledging the problem, expressing sincere regret and announcing a thorough investigation, leading to
- a credible explanation, the expression of apology and an acknowledgment of responsibility,
- system-wide reforms, built from the investigation and focused on the four areas above, and demonstrating renewed trustworthiness
- an accurate, transparent and systematic 'evaluation' of the reforms to enable ongoing learning.

Both models are focused on the development of an organisational culture of learning, based on candour and dialogue, and the dynamics of apology are critical. An authentic apology focuses on taking responsibility. It should come from the leader representing the board/firm. Whilst there may be other members of the firm who were the immediate cause, this recognises that the board is ultimately responsible for the direction, culture and practice of the organisation. An apology should not diminish or deny the event or its consequences. It should focus not simply on publicly recognising the feelings of different parties or that anger, confusion, disbelief are all proper responses to the event, but on the meaning of the perceived breach. Leaders and managers who focus on control see the expressions of emotions as a threat to their authority, and so focus on the problem of the person or the person as problem. The relationship, however, cannot be addressed without focusing on perceived experience of injustice or betrayal. Being able to handle anger in an organisational context is a mark of being trustworthy, revealing a capacity to handle ambiguity and conflict and still stay focused on the persons and issues. This is a little more profound than demonstrating that the other has the person's interests at heart rather than his or her own. It involves rather the exercise of respect for the autonomy and identity of the other, an expression of commitment towards the other and a concern for justice. *Finally, as noted above, in the light of a shared appreciation of justice and in the development of positive responsibility, shared commitment and creative action affirm genuine change. The authenticity of the change is confirmed in the practice of taking responsibility for meaning and practice in relationships.*

Conclusion

This chapter has examined leadership, noting the same basis for leadership, as both transformational and dialogical, in the nursing profession and in organisational leadership. The focus on dialogue takes into the detail of how such leadership can be established through the development of ethical governance, to which we now turn.

References

Aiken, L. H., Cerón, C., Simonetti, M., Lake, E. T., Galiano, A., Garbarini, A., et al. (2018). Hospital nurse staffing and patient outcomes. *Revista Médica Clínica Las Condes, 29*(3), 322–327.

Akker, L., Heres, L., Lasthuizen, K., & Six, F. (2009). Ethical leadership and trust: it's all about meeting expectations. *International Journal of Leadership Studies, 5*(2), 103–122.

Algera, P. M., & Lips-Wiersma, M. (2012). Radical authentic leadership: co-creating the conditions under which all members of the organization can be authentic. *The Leadership Quarterly, 23*(1), 118–131.

Alimo-Metcalfe, B., & Alban-Metcalfe, J. (2005). Leadership: time for a new direction. *Leadership, 1*(1), 51–71.

Alvesson, M., & Spicer, A. (2011). *Metaphors we lead by: understanding leadership in the real World*. London: Routledge.

April, K. (1999). Leading through communication, conversation and dialogue. *Leadership and Organizational Development Journal, 20*(5), 231–241.

Aristotle. (1991). *The art of rhetoric*. London: Penguin.

Bahcecik, N., & Ozturk, H. (2003). The hospital ethical climate survey in Turkey. *JONA's Healthcare Law, Ethics, and Regulation, 5*(4), 94–99.

Baier, A. (1991). Trust and its vulnerabilities and sustaining trust. *Tanner Lectures on Human Values, 13*, 107–174.

Baker, J. (1987). Trust and rationality. *Pacific Philosophical Quarterly, 68*, 1–13.

Bakhtin, M. (1984). *The dialogic imagination.* Austin: The University of Texas Press.

Bally, J. M. (2007). The role of nursing leadership in creating a mentoring culture in acute care environments. *Nursing Economics, 25*(3), 143–148.

Barbuto, J. E. (2005). Motivation and transactional, charismatic and transformational leadership: a test of antecedents. *Journal of Leadership and Organizational Studies, 11*(4), 26–40.

Bass, B. (2005). *Transformational leadership.* New York: Erlbaum.

Bass, B., & Steidlmeier, E. (2004). Ethics, character and authentic transformational leadership. In J. Ciulla (Ed.), *Ethics the heart of leadership* (pp. 175–196). Westport: Praeger.

Bass, B. M. (1985). *Leadership and performance beyond expectations.* New York: The Free Press.

Bass, B. M. (1998). *Transformational leadership: industry, military and educational impact.* Mahwah, New Jersey: Lawrence Erlbaum Associates.

Bedi, A., Alpaslan, C. M., & Green, S. (2016). A meta-analytic review of ethical leadership outcomes and moderators. *Journal of Business Ethics, 139*(3), 517–536.

Benevene, P., Corso, L., De Carlo, A., Falco, A., Carluccio, F., & Vecina, M. (2018). Ethical leadership as antecedent of job satisfaction, affective organizational commitment and intention to stay among volunteers of non-profit organization. *Frontiers in Psychology, 9*, 2069. doi:10.3389/fpsyg.2018.02069.

Bertocci, D. (2009). *Leadership in organizations.* New York: UPA.

Binney, G., & Williams, L. (1997). *Leaning into the future.* London: Nicholas Brealey Publishing.

Bjarnason, D., & LaSala, C. (2015). Moral leadership in nursing. *Journal of Radiology Nursing, 30*(1), 18–24.

Blair, J., Busk, M., Goleniowska, H., Hawtrey-Woore, S., Morris, S., Newbold, Y., et al. (2016). Through our eyes: what parents want for their children from health professionals. In S. Hardy, E. Chaplin, & P. Woodward (Eds.), *Supporting the physical health needs of people with learning disabilities* (pp. 197–212). Brighton: Pavilion Publishing and Media Ltd.

Boamah, S. A., Laschinger, H. K. S., Wong, C., & Clarke, S. (2017). Effect of transformational leadership on job satisfaction and patient safety outcomes. *Nursing Outlook, 66*(2), 180–189.

Bridges, W. (1980). *Transitions: making sense of life.* Reading: Addison Wesley.

Burns, J. (1978). *Leadership.* New York: Harper and Row.

Campbell, A. (1984). *Moderated love.* London: Society for Promoting Christian Knowledge – SPCK.

Campling, P. (2015). Reforming the culture of healthcare: the case for intelligent kindness. *BJPsych Bulletin, 39*(1), 1–5.

Chia, R., & Holt, R. (2011). *Strategy without design.* Cambridge: Cambridge University Press.

Cho, E., Sloane, D. M., Kim, E. Y., Kim, S., Choi, M., Yoo, I. Y., et al. (2015). Effects of nurse staffing, work environments, and education on patient mortality. an observational study. *International Journal of Nursing Studies, 52*(2), 535–542.

Cimiotti, J. P., Aiken, L. H., Sloane, D. M., & Wu, E. S. (2012). Nurse staffing, burnout, and health care–associated infection. *American Journal of Infection Control, 40*(6), 486–490.

Ciulla, J. (2005). *Ethics the heart of leadership.* Westport: Praeger.

Colledge, B., Morgan, J., & Tench, R. (2014). The concept(s) of trust in late modernity, the relevance of realist social theory. *Journal for the Theory of Social Behaviour, 44*(4), 481–503.

Collins, J. (2001). *Good to great: why some companies make the leap . . . and some don't.* New York: Harper Collins.

Contino, D. S. (2004). Leadership competencies: knowledge, skills, and aptitudes nurses need to lead organizations effectively. *Critical Care Nurse, 24*(3), 52–64.

Covey, S. (2002). *Principle centred leadership.* London: Simon and Schuster.

Daft, R. (2004). *The Leadership Experience.* London: Thompson.

Dall, T. M., Chen, Y. J., Seifert, R. F., Maddox, P. J., & Hogan, P. F. (2009). The economic value of professional nursing. *Medical Care, 47*(1), 97–104.

de Sousa, R. (1987). *The Rationality of emotion.* Cambridge: MIT Press.

Delmatoff, J., & Lazarus, I. R. (2014). The most effective leadership style for the new landscape of healthcare. *Journal of Healthcare Management, 59*(4), 245–249.

Doody, O., & Doody, C. M. (2012). Transformational leadership in nursing practice. *British Journal of Nursing*, *21*(20), 1212–1218.

Edelmann's Trust Barometer. (2015). *2015 Edelman Trust Barometer*. Edelman Trust. Online available: http://www.edelman.com/insights/intellectual-property/2015-edelman-trust-barometer/.

Eisenberg, E. (1984). Ambiguity as strategy in organizational communication. *Communication Monographs*, *51*(3), 227–242.

Eneh, V., & Kvist, T. (2012). Nursing leadership practices as perceived by Finnish nursing staff: high ethics, less feedback and rewards. *Journal of Nursing Management*, *20*(2), 159–169.

Eubanks, D. L., Brown, A. D., & Ybema, S. (2012). Leadership, identity, and ethics. *Journal of Business Ethics*, *107*(1), 1–3.

Francis (2013). *Report of the Mid Staffordshire NHS Foundation Trust Public Inquiry*. London: The Stationery Office. Online available: https://www.gov.uk/government/publications/report-of-the-mid-staffordshire-nhs-foundation-trust-public-inquiry.

Francis, R. (2010). *Robert Francis Inquiry report into Mid-Staffordshire*. NHS Foundation Trust. Online available: https://webarchive.nationalarchives.gov.uk/20130104234315/http://www.dh.gov.uk/en/Publicationsandstatistics/Publications/PublicationsPolicyAndGuidance/DH_113018.

Fulop, N., & Robert, G. (2015). *Context for successful quality improvement*. London: Health Foundation.

Gallagher, A., & Tschudin, V. (2010). Educating for ethical leadership. *Nurse Education Today*, *30*(3), 224–227.

Gillespie, N., & Dietz, G. (2009). Trust repair after an organization-level failure. *Academy of Management Review*, *34*(1), 127–145.

Goldman, A., & Tabak, N. (2010). Perception of ethical climate and its relationship to nurses' demographic characteristics and job satisfaction. *Nursing Ethics*, *17*(2), 233–246.

Greenleaf, R. (1977). *The servant as leader: a journey into the nature of legitimate power and greatness*. New York: Paulist Press.

Grint, K. (2005). *Leadership: limits and possibilities*. Basingstoke: Palgrave Macmillan.

Gustafsson, L., & Stenberg, M. (2017). Crucial contextual attributes of nursing leadership towards a care ethics. *Nursing Ethics*, *24*(4), 419–429.

Hall, J., Johnson, S., Wysocki, A., & Kepner, K. (2002). *Transformational leadership: the transformation of managers and associates*. Florida: Institute of Food and Agricultural Sciences, University of Florida. Online available: http://edis.ifas.ufl.edu/pdffiles/HR/HR02000.pdf.

Hashish, E. (2017). Relationship between ethical work climate and nurses' perception of organizational support, commitment, job satisfaction and turnover intent. *Nursing Ethics*, *24*(2), 151–166.

Heidegger, M. (2010). *Being and time*. Syracuse, NY: SUNY Press.

Hock, D. (1999). *Birth of the Chaordic Age*. San Francisco: Berrett-Koehler Publishers, Inc.

Institute of Chartered Accountancy in England and Wales. (2007). *Reporting with integrity*. London: Institute of Chartered Accountancy in England and Wales.

Isaacs, W. (1999). Dialogic leadership. *The Systems Thinker*, *10*(1), 1–5.

Jackson, P. (2001–2003). *The Lord of the Rings*. New Line Cinema.

Jeffrey, T. P. (2016). First time in human history: people 65 and older will outnumber children under 5. Reston: CNS News. March 31, 2016. Online available: https://cnsnews.com/news/article/terence-p-jeffrey/first-time-human-history-global-population-over-65-poised-pass.

Judge, T. A., & Piccolo, R. F. (2004). Transformational and transactional leadership: a meta-analytic test of their validity. *Journal of Applied Psychology*, *89*(5), 755–768.

Kane, R. L., Shamliyan, T. A., Mueller, C., Duval, S., & Wilt, T. J. (2007). The association of registered nurse staffing levels and patient outcomes: systematic review and meta-analysis. *Medical Care*, *45*(12), 1195–1204.

Kangasniemi, M., Vaismoradi, M., Jasper, M., & Turunen, H. (2013). Ethical issues in patient safety: implications for nursing management. *Nursing Ethics*, *20*(8), 904–916.

Kar, S. (2014). Ethical leadership: best practice for success. *IOSR Journal of Business and Management*, *1*(14), 112–116.

Keeley, M. (1995). The trouble with transformational leadership: toward a federalist ethic for organizations. *Business Ethics Quarterly*, *5*(1), 67–96.

Kings Fund (2015). *Leadership and leadership development in health care: the evidence base*. London: Kings Fund. Online available: https://www.kingsfund.org.uk/sites/default/files/field/field_publication_summary/leadership-in-health-care-apr15.pdf.

Kohut, H. (1982). Introspection, empathy and the semi-circle of mental health. *International Journal of Psychoanalysis*, *63*, 395–407.

Kotter, J. (1990). *A force for change: how leadership differs from management*. London: McMillan.

Kouzen, J., & Posner, B. (2012). *The leadership challenge: how to make extraordinary things happen in organizations*. London: John Willey.

Ladkin, D., & Taylor, S. (2010). Enacting the true self: towards a theory of embodied authentic leadership. *The Leadership Quarterly*, *21*(1), 1–6.

Laub, J. (2004). Defining servant leadership: a recommended typology for servant leadership studies. In *EBT Proceedings of the 2004 Servant Leadership Research Roundtable*. Virginia Beach, Virginia: Regent University.

Lederach, J. P. (2005). *The moral imagination*. Oxford: Oxford University Press.

Lemmenes, D., Valentine, P., Gwizdalski, P., Vincent, C., & Liao, C. (2018). Nurses' perception of ethical climate at a large academic medical center. *Nursing Ethics*, *25*(6), 724–733.

Lips-Wiersma, M., & Morris, L. (2018). *The map of meaning: a guide to sustaining our humanity in the world of work* (2nd ed.). Abingdon, Oxon: Routledge.

Macionis, J. J. (2012). *Sociology*. Boston: Pearson Educational.

MacNamara, J. (2015). *Creating an architecture of listening in organizations*. Sydney: UTS Press.

Maitland, I. (2008). Virtue or control in the governance of the firm. In *Society for Business Ethics Annual Meeting 2008*. Society for Business Ethics.

Makaroff, K., Storch, J., Pauly, B., & Newton, L. (2014). Searching for ethical leadership in nursing. *Nursing Ethics*, *21*(6), 642–658.

Martin, K. D., & Cullen, J. B. (2006). Continuities and extensions of ethical climate theory: a meta-analytic review. *Journal of Business Ethics*, *69*(2), 175–194.

Mastracci, S. (2017). Beginning nurses' perceptions of ethical leadership in the shadow of Mid Staffs. *Public Integrity*, *19*, 250–264.

Mathis, R. L., & Jackson, J. H. (2011). *Human resource management*. South-Western: Thomson.

Mitchell, R., Agle, B., & Wood, D. (1997). Toward a theory of stakeholder identification and salience: defining the principle of who and what really counts. *The Academy of Management Review*, *22*(4), 853–886.

Morgan, G. (2006). *Images of organization*. Thousand Oaks, CA: Sage Publications.

National Health Service. (2013). *Leadership model*. London: National Health Service. Online available: https://www.leadershipacademy.nhs.uk/wp-content/uploads/2014/10/NHSLeadership-Leadership-Model-colour.pdf.

National Health Service. (2017). Leading with compassion: a 'how to' guide for all NHS organisation. London: National Health Service. Online available: http://www.nhscompassion.org/compassion/wp-content/uploads/2017/11/HowToGuide.pdf.

North, D. (1991). Institutions. *The Journal of Economic Perspectives*, *5*(1), 97–112.

Northouse, P. (2016). *Leadership: theory and practice*. London: Sage Publications.

O'Leary, K. (2016). The effects of safety culture and ethical leadership on safety performance. *Dissertations and Theses, 201* Online available. https://commons.erau.edu/edt/201.

O'Neill, O. (2000). *A question of trust*. Cambridge: Cambridge University Press.

Okan, T., & Akyüz, A. (2015). Exploring the relationship between ethical leadership and job satisfaction with the mediating role of the level of loyalty to supervisor. *Business and Economics Research Journal*, *6*(4), 155–177.

Olu-Abiodun, O., & Abiodun, O. (2017). Perception of transformational leadership behaviour among general hospital nurses in Ogun State. *Nigeria. International Journal of Africa Nursing Sciences*, *6*, 22–27.

Osterloh, M., & Frey, B. (2004). Corporate governance for crooks: the case for corporate virtue. In A. Grandori (Ed.), *Corporate governance and firm organization: microfoundations and structural forms* (pp. 191–211). Oxford: Oxford University Press.

Özden, D., Arslan, G., & Ertuğrul, B. (2017). The effect of nurses' ethical leadership and ethical climate perceptions on job satisfaction. *Nursing Ethics*, *26*(4), 1211–1225.

Parliamentary and Health Service Ombudsman. (2011). *Care and compassion: report of the Health Service Ombudsman on ten investigations into NHS care of older people*. London: The Stationery Office. Online available: https://www.ombudsman.org.uk/publications/care-and-compassion.

Pfarrer, M., DeCelles, K., Smith, K., & Taylor, M. (2008). After the fall: reintegrating the corrupt organization. *Academy of Management Review*, *33*(3), 730–749.

Poikkeus, T., Numminen, O., Suhonen, R., & Leino-Kilpi, H. (2014). A mixed-method systematic review: support for ethical competence of nurses. *Journal of Advanced Nursing*, *70*(2), 256–271.

Polleys, M. S. (2002). One university's response to the anti-leadership vaccine: developing servant leaders. *Journal of Leadership Studies*, *8*(3), 117–130.

Porter-O'Grady, T. (1997). Process leadership and the death of management. *Nursing Economics*, *15*(6), 286–293.

Pye, A. (2005). Leadership and organising: sense making in action. *Leadership*, *1*(1), 31–49.

Rawls, R. (1971). *A theory of justice*. Cambridge, MA: Harvard University Press.

Robbins, S. P., & Judge, T. A. (2013). *Organisational behaviour* (15th ed.). Boston: Pearson.

Robinson, S. (2008). *Spirituality, ethics and care*. London: Jessica Kingsley.

Robinson, S. (2016). *The practice of integrity in business*. London: Palgrave.

Robinson, S., & Smith, J. (2014). *Co-charismatic leadership*. Oxford: Peter Lang.

Rogers, C. (1983). *The freedom to learn*. Columbus: Merrill.

Rolfe, P. (2011). Transformational leadership theory: what every leader needs to know. *Nurse Leader*, *9*(2), 54–57.

Rost, J. (1991). *Leadership in the twenty-first century*. New York: Praeger.

Schermerhorn Jr, J. R., Bachrach, D. G., & Wright, B. (2020). *Management* (Fifth Edition). Toronto, Canada: John Wiley and Sons.

Schulte, L. E. (2002). A comparison of cohort and non-cohort graduate student perceptions of the ethical climate and its importance in retention. *Journal of College Student Retention: Research, Theory and Practice*, *4*(1), 29–38.

Schyns, B., & Schilling, J. (2013). How bad are the effects of bad leaders: a meta-analysis of destructive leadership and its outcomes. *Leadership Quarterly*, *24*(1), 138–158.

Scott, W., & Davis, G. (2007). *Organizations and organizing: rational, natural, and open system perspectives*. Boston: Pearson Prentice Hall.

Senge, P. M. (1990). *The fifth discipline: the art and practice of the learning organization*. New York: Doubleday/Currency.

Shafritz, J. M., Russell, E. W., Borick, C. P., & Hyde, A. C. (2011). *Introducing public administration*. London: Taylor and Francis.

Shekelle, P. G. (2013). Nurse–patient ratios as a patient safety strategy: a systematic review. *Annals of Internal Medicine*, *158*(5 Part 2), 404–409.

Simpson, J. (2007). Psychological foundations of trust. *Current Directions in Psychological Science*, *16*(5), 264–268.

Sofarelli, D., & Brown, D. (1998). The need for nursing leadership in uncertain times. *Journal of Nursing Management*, *6*(4), 201–207.

Sparrowe, R. T. (2005). Authentic leadership and the narrative self. *The Leadership Quarterly*, *16*(3), 419–439.

Spector, P. (1997). *Job satisfaction*. Thousand Oaks, CA: Sage Publications.

Squires, A., White, J., & Sermeus, W. (2015). *Quantity, quality and relevance of the nursing workforce to patient outcomes*. ICN Policy Brief. Geneva, Switzerland: International Council of Nurses.

Storch, J., Makaroff, K., Pauly, B., & Newton, L. (2013). Take me to my leader: the importance of ethical leadership among formal nurse leaders. *Nursing Ethics*, *20*(2), 150–157.

Swihart, D., & Martin, R. (2019). Cultural religious competence in clinical practice. *StatPearls*. Online available: https://www.statpearls.com/sp/rn/199/41244/.

Taylor, C. (1989). *Sources of the self*. Cambridge: Cambridge University Press.

Tolkien, J. R. R. (1955). The Lord of the Rings: Being the Third Part of The Lord of the Rings. The Return of the King. New South Wales, Australia: Allen and Unwin.

Tu, Y., Lu, X., & Yu, Y. (2017). Supervisors' ethical leadership and employee job satisfaction: a social cognitive perspective. *Journal of Happiness Studies*, *18*(1), 229–245.

Turner, N., Barling, J., Epitropaki, O., Butcher, V., & Milner, C. (2002). Transformational leadership and moral reasoning. *Journal of applied Psychology*, *87*(2), 304–311.

Ulrich, C., O'Donnell, P., Taylor, C., Farrar, A., Danis, M., & Grady, C. (2007). Ethical climate, ethics stress, and the job satisfaction of nurses and social workers in the United States. *Social Science and Medicine*, *65*(8), 1708–1719.

United Nations. (2006) United Nations Convention on the Rights of Persons With Disability. Available online: https://www.un.org/disabilities/documents/convention/convention_accessible_pdf.pdf.

Van Loon, R. (2017). *Creating organizational value through dialogical leadership: boiling rice in still water*. Geneva: Springer.

Voon, M. L., Lo, M. C., Ngui, K. S., & Ayob, N. B. (2011). The influence of leadership styles on employees' job satisfaction in public sector organizations in Malaysia. *International Journal of Business Management and Social Sciences, 2*(1), 24–32.

Wang, Y. D., & Hsieh, H. H. (2012). Toward a better understanding of the link between ethical climate and job satisfaction: a multi-level analysis. *Journal of Business Ethics, 105*(4), 535–545.

West, M., & Bailey, S. (2019). *The five myths about compassionate leadership*. London: Kings Fund.

Western, S. (2007). *Leadership: a critical text*. London: Sage.

World Health Organisation. (2016). *Global strategy on human resources for health: Workforce 2030*. Geneva, Switzerland: World Health Organisation.

Yang, Y. F. (2014). Transformational leadership in the consumer service workgroup: competing models of job satisfactions, change commitment, and cooperative conflict resolution. *Psychological Reports, 114*(1), 33–49.

Yukl, G. (1999). An evaluative essay on current conceptions of effective leadership. *European Journal of Work and Organisational Psychology, 8*(1), 33–48.

Yukl, G., & Uppal, N. (2017). *Leadership in organizations* (8th ed.). London: Pearson.

Ethical Governance

When you have read and worked through this chapter, you should be able to consider:

- The remuneration of Healthcare CEOs as part of governance in healthcare
- The history of the development of governance
- Theories of ethical governance
- King III and IV and the ethical underpinning of governance
- The virtues of governance, what relational governance looks like
- Clinical governance, and the pillars of governance
- Developing an ethical culture in healthcare
- Anchor points of an ethical organisation, leading to listening and learning organisation
- Whistleblowing

Introduction

Our understanding of ethical meaning in the practice within an organisation is central to this chapter. Personal, professional and organizational ethics can be seen as distinct but relate directly to each other in practice and dialogue needs to occur between them. The ethical culture of an organisation is based on its values framework and needs to foster reflection which is central to ethical and strategic thinking. The interplay between ethically questionable practice is considered in this chapter, with staff often feeling that it is the responsibility of the leader or identifying that they had no choice: 'my boss told me to do it'. Thereby this chapter challenges all persons working in the health system to accept responsibility for testing ideas and values.

Fat Cats and Dirty Rats?

One of the most contentious areas of management and governance in the last 20 years has been how much we pay leaders. Debates about inflated salaries and the like have now hit healthcare in the UK, as the following article by Laura Donnelly shows.

9.1 PAUSE FOR THOUGHT

Healthcare CEO Remuneration

NHS hospital chief executives have been handed pay rises of up to £35,000, with the highest annual earnings reaching a record £340,000, a Daily Telegraph investigation has found. Despite government pledges that the most senior NHS managers would have their pay frozen, 40% of trusts increased executives' wages by at least £5,000 during 2014–15. Some managers' earnings rose by almost a quarter, the findings from more than 200 NHS trust boards show. Patients/clients groups accused the NHS of "scandalous excesses" at a time when the health service is facing the greatest financial crisis in its history.

The head of the Royal College of Nursing said it was "immensely demoralising" to find that some executives had been awarded rises larger than a full year's salary for the average nurse. The highest individual increase of £35,000 went to Sir Andrew Morris, at Frimley Health NHS Foundation Trust in Surrey, taking his earnings to £215,000. The 19% rise followed a takeover of another nearby NHS trust. The finance director, Martin Sykes, also received a 19%, or

£25,000, increase in his earnings taking them to £155,000. Nicola Ranger, the director of nursing, enjoyed a 23% boost, taking her earnings to £135,000. Simon Barber, chief executive of 5 Boroughs Partnership trust in the North West, was paid £200,000 during 2014–15 – a rise of £25,000 thanks to a pay bonus.

In total, 40% of boards made at least one pay rise of between £5,000 and £15,000. At least 10 senior managers received rises of at least £20,000, according to the analysis by the Telegraph. The highest overall package went to Dr Tracey Batten, the chief executive of Imperial College Healthcare, who was paid £290,000 plus a £50,000 relocation payment to move from Australia. Several of those with the highest earnings left the NHS in recent months. The second highest earner overall was Peter Morris, the chief executive of Barts Health trust, on £275,000 until he resigned in February amid a growing financial crisis. The trust is now facing a deficit of £135 million, the largest any trust has ever had.

Tim Smart, who earned £255,000 a year as chief executive of Kings College Hospital Foundation Trust, announced his retirement in April, just after an inspection which later saw the trust rated as "requiring improvement". Katherine Murphy, the chief executive of the Patients Association, said she was concerned that the NHS had developed a culture of "rewards for failure" with many of the highest salaries paid to chief executives who had left as serious problems emerged. In March 2014, the Treasury promised most public sector workers a rise of 1% in 2014–15, but said the most senior managers would see pay frozen, amid efforts to put the nation's finances on a sustainable footing.

The NHS is facing the worst financial crisis in its history, with three quarters of trusts forecasting deficits, which are expected to reach £2.2 billion across the service by March. Janet Davies, chief executive of the Royal College of Nursing, said: "Nursing staff have been repeatedly told that there isn't enough money to improve their pay, even after years of pay restraint. To learn that many senior NHS staff are enjoying pay rises and bonuses while nurses struggle to make ends meet is immensely demoralising". The trusts with the most highly paid chief executives defended the sums paid, saying they were among the largest trusts in the country, with rates in line with those for similar roles in other NHS organisations. A spokesman for Frimley Health said: "Recent salary adjustments in executive pay at Frimley Health were a reflection of the added responsibility associated with the acquisition of Heatherwood and Wexham Park Hospitals NHS Foundation Trust. These were independently assessed by the Hay Group and set by a committee of non-executive directors".

The 5 Boroughs Partnership NHS Foundation Trust said its chief executive had received a 1% pay increase, plus a performance-related bonus which recognised that the trust had achieved quality and financial targets. A spokesman for the Royal Free said it became one of the largest trusts in the country after taking over Barnet and Chase Farm hospitals in July 2014. It said pay was agreed by a committee of non-executive directors based on value for money.

Excerpts from an article by Laura Donnelly, Health Editor, Daily Telegraph 02 Jan 2016.

It is the job of the board of a healthcare trust to set the remuneration for chief executive officers (CEOs), and we can see there is real debate, mirroring the debate in corporate governance (Kolb 2005). Is the debate significant or are there ethical issues at its centre, and, if so, how is the deliberation handled? Donnelly's reporting suggests that there are key ethical principles at stake, the most obvious being justice. The representatives of the trusts come up with two aspects of justice. First, the CEO should be rewarded for being responsible for leading increasingly complex organisations. This is reinforced by the argument that the job is highly stressful, requiring adequate compensation. Second, reward should be tied to success – justice as desert.

Behind the arguments is also something about context and also about the nature of leadership. The marketplace for CEOs, it is argued, is limited, with few leaders capable of fulfilling the core positions. Therefore, there needs to be a compensation package that will attract the best, and retain them, not just in the organisation but in the country (Griffiths 2009). Hence, in some cases trust CEOs have been brought from Australia. Hovering behind this argument is one about consequences. If we do not offer adequate remuneration, we lose the 'best people' to other countries; again, reflected in the corporate debate. Against this is the argument that this approach has a negative impact on other staff, especially nurses. The references to nurses being demoralised suggests that justice is not simply about the rational calculation of rewards. It is about how people are valued in an organisation and beyond. This raises questions as to why the measurement of value should be largely financial. The ethical spotlight here is on equal respect and how we show it in organisations.

The response to such arguments is often an appeal to procedural justice. This goes something like: 'we have in place a remuneration sub-committee made up of non-executive directors (members of the board who have experience of governance). This is a largely disinterested group who will do what is in the best interest of the Trust.' This mirrors corporate governance practice (Financial Reporting Council (FRC) 2018), and sometimes is reinforced by independent organisational consultancies. However, like many corporate governance approaches (Kolb 2005), much of this debate reads like recitations of dogma rather than effective dialogue about core principles and values.

INCENTIVES

The empirical evidence about financial incentives actually motivating good performance or alignment with the goals of the organisation is not promising. Several studies across different sectors show little connection between high compensation and improved firm performance (Mishra et al. 2000). Some work even suggests that high compensation decreases firm performance, and a tendency for firms to focus on the individual performer rather than the organisation (Blasi and Kruse 2003). Other research suggests that over a certain level of financial reward is not effective. Key motivators rather include opportunities to practice mastery, the practice of autonomous judgement and tying into a significant purpose (Pink 2011), something critical to clinical governance. Genuine reward is important, but the principle of justice remains unfocused if financial reward is the only player. Worse still, it loses credibility when reward remains for poor performance.

THE LEADERSHIP MARKET

The idea that a limited leadership market should form the basis for an ethical argument about high levels of remuneration is another form of an argument that seeks to use a supposed empirical truth to take away the responsibility of thinking through ethical reasons. This is how the market works, so this is what we must do, goes the argument. In fact, none of this has been substantiated. Research suggests that openings for CEOs are scarce (Kolb 2005). There is little evidence of many better jobs that would attract leaders away, and some evidence of available leaders who would take the job for considerably less pay (Kolb 2005). Conger (2005) argues that behind this is an inflated view of the leader that again brings us back to the romantic, almost mystical, view of the charismatic leader, with everything dependent upon the one person.

IMPARTIAL PROCEDURE

Underlying the concern for an independent process (procedural justice), there are two strands – the freedom of the organisation to determine its own practice, and the disinterested framework used for decisions about remuneration. In the first of these, it is not clear what ethical force freedom has. Other stakeholders have an interest, including patients/clients, the general public, employees and government, all of whom have a view of what the criteria of justice look like. The disinterested framework assumes an independent and rational approach to all these relationships. But what does impartiality look like in this case? Is an external consultancy impartial simply because they are external? Is a remuneration committee impartial because it has external members who have experience of governance?

For the remuneration committee to demonstrate impartiality, it would require engagement with all the different stakeholders to test the coherence of a view of justice – one that all can accept as impartial. At one level, this takes us back to convincing leadership which focuses on *logos*, *pathos* and *ethos*. Part of that would involve dialogue about justice. The corporate codes advice includes 'levels of remuneration should be sufficient to attract, retain and motivate directors of the quality required to run the company successfully, but a company should avoid paying more than is necessary for this purpose' (FRC 2018).

This guidance is important but does not really tell us much. Is finance the only basis for attraction, motivation and retention? What do we mean by success? And why, we might add, is lack of success often rewarded? What counts as necessary? What counts as justice? As we noted in Chapter 2, there are several different views of justice, and justice is not simply about rational calculation but also good and healthy relationships. If governance is to be ethical, these questions, and others around ensuring the sustainability of the organisation and the wider healthcare project, need to be genuinely open to accountability.

JUSTICE AND COMPENSATION PHILOSOPHY

Developing a convincing practice of justice for CEO remuneration requires more effective dialogue. It is a mark of organisational integrity that an issue such as justice, a core value, be opened up to dialogue and testing, leading to a shared philosophy of justice (i.e. understanding of what is meant by justice) and clear, stated criteria that all can support. The development of a compensation philosophy (Evans and Dalik 2011) allows an organisation to work through all the issues noted above, examining shared values around rewards beyond the economic. It also provides an ongoing basis for transparent critical dialogue about leadership and justice. Such a philosophy could also involve reflection on rewards for all in the workplace. Inevitably, this takes compensation away from narrow economic criteria and into the broader culture and ethos of the organisation. This allows for reflection on the worth and purpose of the organisation and of the different areas and roles within the organisation. Bloom's (2004) research confirms that the work force is concerned about the basis of any view of fairness (cf. Rawls 1971). Any procedure and view about fairness can represent the attitude of the firm, the leaders and the workforce. Shared understanding, values and culture act as a focus to commitment and effort, something confirmed by research on the importance of organisational justice for understanding the non-economic effects of compensation systems (Greenberg and Cropanzano 2001; Rousseau 1995), suggesting that fairness is central to employment relationships. It should not be a surprise that issues of justice are central to trust. In recent years, there has been increased focus on democracy in the workplace and beyond (Norman 2015; King 2009) and stress on stakeholder dialogue as the basis for a less legalistic view of regulation. A philosophy of compensation aims, then, to articulate all this, feeding in different narratives around organisational justice, including different philosophies of justice, that go towards establishing criteria for judgement (desert, fairness, motivation, restorative), and different aspects of justice such as interactional (relational) and procedural (the practice). These precisely reflect the rational (philosophies of justice), affective (to do with relationships) and somatic (to do with embodiment) aspects of holistic meaning, and all are a part of the critical dialogue that tests values. All can see what it means to be just in that organisation, and all can critique any aspects of that justice.

Salaries could then be determined by several different criteria agreed across the organisation and beyond, focused on the achievement of the core purpose, as well as more conventional criteria such as hours spent at work; the skills and capacities that are needed for the job; or the difficulty, stress, danger, or unpleasantness. This would allow transparent comparison of the proposed remuneration with not just similar CEOs but also other leaders and members of the organisation, enabling a sense of mutual value, with principles driving this and the other aspects of governance.

Governance

The term 'governance' comes from the Latin verb *gubernare*, (Greek *kubernaein*), meaning to steer. Governance in the context of the health service, then, is about determining the direction of the organisation, and ensuring that the rules, practices and processes are in place to steer the organisation in that direction. Hence, governance of an organisation is a function of leadership. Governance is the responsibility of the governing body, which is usually the board. Governance is, by definition, difficult because any board has to steer an organisation through complex and challenging waters, summed up in the acronym VUCA: volatility, uncertainty, complexity and ambiguity. This involves holding together the tensions in management, not least between ensuring the survival of the overall project and related organisations and maintaining their social identity and role, focused on vision and values. In the corporate sector, the concern for governance was focused on the many crises, culminating in the credit crisis of 2007/8 (Sun et al. 2010), and over time involved the development of codes of governance (see, for instance, FRC 2018; King IV 2017; King III 2009). Regulation and responsibility are at the heart of all of these codes, with the US Codes focusing on legal regulation of governance, and others, such as the UK, focusing on the organisation taking responsibility for regulating itself.

Governance Theories

There is debate about whether the corporate governance and clinical governance are fundamentally opposed. Corporate governance is often seen as focused on the so-called *agency theory*. This focuses on the self-interest of the firm and the CEO, and financial incentives. However, the focus on financial capital is too narrow, even in business theories. The International Integrated Reporting Council (IIRC 2013), for instance, argues that there are six capitals (broadly, areas of value in which any organisation has to work):

- Financial, focused on personal, national and global economy
- Manufacturing, focused on the purpose and products (in a broad sense) of an organisation
- Human, the psychological environment involving affective as well as cognitive understanding
- Social and relational, the social environment in all its complexity
- Intellectual, the rational environment
- Natural, the physical environment.

Adams (2013) argues that natural capital provides 'the environment within which the other capitals sit' (p. 3). In other words, sustainability transcends the other capitals, demanding that we look at all of the other capitals together. We would argue that this has to involve both social and natural capitals, that is that inclusive respect for humanity also provides a moral basis for governance that includes all of these capitals. Ethical thinking about corporate governance is thus much wider, exemplified by two other theories: stewardship and stakeholder.

Stewardship theory focuses on shared purpose and responsibility. The leader and board agree on the core purpose of the organisation and work together to achieve it. The steward, then, is seen as acting on behalf of a corporation, whose values and purpose he or she believes in. The downside of this theory can be uncritical acceptance of the CEO.

Stakeholder theory of governance maintains stakeholders should be involved in some way. This suggests that there are other indications of good performance than shareholder value and takes account of the social and environmental context. The major limitations of this theory to governance are questions of how it handles conflicts between stakeholders, both in terms of their needs and responsibilities. Nonetheless, the stakeholder model is increasingly the focus for governance. Perhaps the strongest example of this is the emergence of the King Reports in South Africa.

The King Reports

Alongside, and partly influenced by, the UK Code of Governance is the third King Report (King III 2009), based in South Africa. This accepts the need for organisations to take responsibility for their governance, but systematically ties governance to ethics and begins to show how ethical awareness and decision making should and can become central to governance.

ETHICS CENTRED

King III suggests a six-stage process of governing ethical performance that consists of:
- Identifying, through stakeholder engagement, the perceptions and expectations that stakeholders have of the ethical performance of a company
- Determining the ethical values and standards of the company and codifying it in a code of ethics
- Institutionalising the values and code of ethics of a company on both the strategic and systems levels
- Monitoring and evaluating compliance to the code of ethics
- Accounting and auditing ethical performance according to emerging global standards on ethical accounting and auditing
- Disclosing ethical performance to relevant stakeholders.

The third stage emphasises the need to take organisations beyond implementing the code of ethics in order to make a significant difference to company culture and performance. Examples of how this can be achieved include regular ethical risk assessment, confidential reporting systems through which unethical or suspicious behaviour could be reported, the integration of ethical performance into existing performance appraisal systems and integrity assessment as part of selection and promotion procedures. We will explore such approaches shortly.

King III focuses on the responsibility of the board for the underlying purpose and philosophy, and accountability to stakeholders, working against a non-thinking use of rules (King III, p. 3). In contrast, he argues that the board should take responsibility for working through what the ground principles of governance mean in practice. This looks to build ethical thinking into the culture of the board, such that members take responsibility in all senses of the word: defining and continually re-evaluating the purpose, aims and values of the organisation; being accountable to stakeholders and embodying the shared responsibility for the social and physical environment.

PHILOSOPHY

The philosophy of King III revolves around leadership, sustainability and corporate citizenship.

Leadership is characterised in terms of the core ethical values of *responsibility, accountability, fairness* and *transparency*. These concepts are not analysed in depth by the report, but echo the main meanings of responsibility noted in Chapter 2. There is a clear stress on taking responsibility for meaning and practice and on being accountable to all stakeholders.

The report goes further, in arguing that these are 'based on moral duties that find expression in the concept of "*Ubuntu*". *Ubuntu* is a pan-African communitarian worldview stressing the interdependent nature of humanity – 'I am because you are'. It stresses empathy, understanding, reciprocity, harmony and cooperation. Moreover, as Andreasson (2011) notes, 'it provides a guiding principle for determining how to organise African societies and measure wellbeing'. Happiness or well-being has always been key to ethics. The utilitarians (see Chapter 11) wanted to maximise happiness, and Aristotle (2004) thought the aim of ethics was happiness or well-being. For the South African situation, this provided an important bridge between business and society. This includes awareness of social development issues and also of the continuing culture of reconciliation post-apartheid. This sense of business contributing to the healing of the nation leads King III to stress the use of alternative dispute resolution (ADR) not only as an action of mediation, but also as part of ongoing governance. This is confirmed with the stress on sustainability and corporate citizenship.

Sustainability

Sustainability is seen by King III as the primary ethical and economic imperative of the 21st century. It is at the heart of opportunities and risks for all organisations. The interconnections of nature, society and business, therefore, demand governance that genuinely integrates all of these aspects both in reporting and development. Inclusivity of stakeholders must also be taken into account in decision making and strategy. Hence, values such as *innovation, fairness and collaboration* are key aspects of any transition to sustainability. The integration of sustainability and social transformation in a strategic and coherent manner will, argues King III (p. 13), lead to 'greater opportunities, efficiencies, and benefits, for both the company and society'. In light of this, the company is a corporate citizen, of which is required the exercise of responsibility.

In short, then, the King Reports bring together all the key elements of responsibility demanding an awareness of meaning, purpose and role in society; clear integrated accounting of practice and shared response to the needs of the social and physical environment. Because of this integrated and holistic approach to governance, King III and IV argue there is no dichotomy between corporate governance and social (including clinical) governance. Any organisation has to keep the enterprise on the road as well as fulfil its core social role. In this sense, prudent management is as much an ethical imperative as broader sustainability of purpose and of the environment. Key to any governance is stakeholder dialogue about purpose and strategy, focusing on the moral imagination, continued learning and development of possibilities (Lederach 2005). Dialogue is thus at the heart of good governance, and offers a critical balance to any regulation, political or professional. Regulation of governance then also becomes a stakeholder function, with stakeholders in continued dialogue, holding each other to account.

Clinical Governance

Clinical governance was first introduced into the NHS in 1997 and was defined in terms of quality, 'a framework through which NHS organisations are accountable for continuously improving the quality of their services and safeguarding high standards of care by creating an environment in which excellence in clinical care can flourish' (NHS Executive 1999; Scally and Donaldson 1998). Key to this definition are: high standards of care which are recognised by all; responsibility for these standards; accountability to key stakeholders and a dynamic of constant reflection and improvement.

In the UK, until 1999, clinical governance responsibilities were clearly divided. National Health Service Trust Boards were responsible for the proper financial management of the organisation and patient/client safety. The quality of care was seen as the responsibility of the different clinical professions. In 1999, the Trust Board was given the legal responsibility for developing and maintaining the overall quality of care alongside their other statutory duties. Now responsibility for care and the care services was shared with all the different groups within the service and beyond. Like the UK Corporate Governance Code (FRC 2018), there was no prescription of any particular structure, system or process. It is the responsibility of the Board to develop clinical governance in the most effective way and to give an account of this practice in an Annual Review of Clinical Governance. This was a clear statement of accountability. Key to this responsibility is the interpretation of the principles of clinical governance into locally appropriate structures, processes, roles and responsibilities.

It is not the Board's task to do all the management tasks but rather to ensure that leadership and management is in place to achieve quality standards. Clinical governance is about the quality and safety of patient/client care. It is everything we do as individuals and as an organisation to achieve high standards of clinical care.

The Seven Pillars of Clinical Governance

Views of the pillars of clinical governance have varied over the last decade. However, perhaps the strongest view involves seven pillars or areas of activity which are used to ensure the highest quality health care to service users and represent the integration of the different aspects of quality:

- Service user, carer and public involvement
- Risk management
- Clinical audit
- Education and training
- Clinical effectiveness
- Clinical information
- Staffing and staff management.

SERVICE USER, CARER AND PUBLIC INVOLVEMENT

This partly involves initiatives which improve communication with stakeholders, including:

- Local patient/client feedback questionnaires
- The development of the Patient Advice and Liaison Service (PALS) in handling issues with patients/clients and patient/client reference groups to enhance awareness and decision making
- National patient/client surveys organised by the Healthcare Commission, which then feed into Trusts' rankings
- Local Involvement Networks (LINks), to enable Communities to influence healthcare services at a local level (formerly 'Patient forums')
- Ensuring that some Trust Board of Governors are elected by members of the local community and have a say on who runs a hospital and how it should be run, including the services it provides.

At one level, this is about improving the everyday practice of the service, such that it reflects the needs and concerns of the patient/client. As such, this focuses on the ethical principles of openness and transparency. However, the focus on dialogue takes this beyond simply individual concerns, improving services to ethical principles of justice and the practice of responsibility across all stakeholders, including patients/clients. The focus on responsibility takes this ethically beyond simply refining a service, and more to the sense of patients/clients and 'service providers' as partners in care, sharing responsibility for health. This stress is most obviously in the NHS Constitution, with its reference to shared ownership of the NHS and setting out patient/client as well as service provider responsibilities. We will examine this in more detail in the next chapter. A key part of patient-/client-centred care is enabling people to engage in their own health and help design health systems. This includes service design, process design, feedback/feedforward and participatory health and patient/client activation.

Service Design

It is possible to involve patients/clients in the designing of the service, thereby empowering them through the exercise of shared responsibility. Such co-designing radically affects the experience of the service, focusing on improved dignity and the agency of the patient/client (Royal Brompton and Harefield 2008).

Process Design

Patient/client dialogue can focus on the review of processes such as drug rounds, mealtimes and home visits. A good example of this is how nurses fill in lengthy forms before surgery. There is a danger of a focus on filling in the form leading to lack of engagement with the patient, in some cases involving the nurse sitting to the side or just behind the patient, unable to make eye contact.

Feedback/Feedforward

Any system requires continuous feedback to ensure that it remains focused on the core purpose. Some hospitals have developed apps which enable speedy anonymous comments to be fed through to the manager in charge. This is a good example of King's stakeholder regulation, ensuring accountability as a regular practice focused on the development of shared positive responsibility, rather than regulation which is focused on blame and possible punishment.

Participatory Health and Patient/Client Activation

This involves patient/client provider partnership focused on mutual respect and acknowledgement of mutual expertise. It focuses on the agency of the patient/client, hence the knowledge, skills and confidence developed in managing one's own health (Hibberd and Gilbert 2014). Such approaches enable a better understanding of the priorities and concerns of those who use our services. This goes beyond the idea that the service is 'separate' from the patient/client, with the patient/client being included in that service. Rather, as the NHS Constitution (2019) suggests, the patient/client is already involved and, through ongoing dialogue, is empowered fully to be responsible, with carers, for health.

RISK MANAGEMENT

Risk management demands ensuring that effective systems are in place to understand, monitor and minimise risks to patients/clients by:

- Complying with protocols that reduce risk, such as handwashing, identifying patients/clients correctly
- Identifying what can and does go wrong during care
- Understanding the factors that influence this
- Learning lessons from any adverse events
- Ensuring action is taken to prevent recurrence
- Ensuring that systems are reviewed and questioned.

This is focused on the ethical principle of non-maleficence. It demands practice which goes beyond the unthinking following of rules, and the development of a learning culture. In turn, this means the constant practice of the key virtues noted in Chapter 3. Increasingly, risk management developments go beyond protocols to the quality of the professional relationships, including the capacity to raise critical challenge becoming a core aspect of professionalism. This demands the development of a culture focused on positive responsibility rather than the avoidance of blame. Two aspects of this are the duty of candour (both to fellow professionals and to patients/clients, see Chapter 8) and whistleblowing (see below). Risk management also involves consideration of the risks to professionals and to the organisation.

Risks to Practitioners

This includes ensuring that healthcare professionals are appropriately immunised and have a safe environment, including a culture which is anti-harassment.

Risks to the Organisation

The sustainability of the organisation is often seen as secondary. It is, however, critical to maintaining care and commitment. This forms the basis of reputation and, with that, trust. Hence, poor quality in the broadest sense is risk. Part of reducing that risk is to ensure high quality employment practice (including locum procedures and reviews of individual and team performance), a safe environment (including estates and privacy) and well-designed policies on public involvement.

Fischer and Ferlie (2013) argue that clinical care involves first-order risks and organisational reputation are second-order risks, and that the two can lead to contradictions, with more concern for image than the substance of care. However, first, the reputation of the organisation is more than simply image. It involves the identity and purpose of the organisation and thus is critical to the very meaning of healthcare. Risk, then, is focused on both care and organisational sustainability in the core purpose and value of healthcare, demanding the practice of *phronesis* at all levels of the service.

CLINICAL AUDIT

The aim of the audit process is to ensure that clinical practice is continuously monitored and that deficiencies in relation to set standards of care are remedied. Clinical audit is basically reflective practice, the capacity to reflect on practice and develop it in response to critical assessment. Developing the cycle of reflective practice occurs at all levels of the service, from professional practice in trust and primary care to a cyclical process of improving the quality of clinical care. The broader view of quality seeks to integrate both the development of care and the overall governance of care. If national audits are included, such as the National Confidential Enquiry into Patient Outcome and Death and the Healthcare Commission's National Audit Programme, there are many that any trust might participate in, and this raises questions about how these different mechanisms are integrated into the reflective narrative. This process, then, presupposes corporate and individual commitment to evidence-based reflective practice, including effective collection and communication of relevant information and data for this purpose. This includes commitment to the organisation as essentially a 'learning organisation' (Senge 2002).

EDUCATION AND TRAINING

Like a clinical audit, this assumes a commitment to continued learning and training. At one level, this is about the development of competency and related skills – involving life-long learning. In practice, this involves all the different professions:

- Attending courses and conferences (CPD – Continuous Professional Development)
- Taking relevant examinations
- Having regular assessment, ensuring appropriate training
- Having appraisals (identifying and discussing weaknesses, strengths and opportunities for personal development).

The case of the Mid Staffs Hospital Trust suggests that this development is not value neutral. On the contrary, it demands, first, reflection on the core purpose, and thus the practice of *phronesis*, at individual, professional and corporate levels. Because our choice of values determines the means we adopt to achieve short- and long-term goals, it is also crucial that in any organisation there is clarity about the values that operate within it, at the corporate management professional, and individual levels. It is also important that employers and employees not only have insight into the competing (and sometimes conflicting) values which operate in any moral community, but also have the necessary skills to deal with and resolve serious conflicts of values. This process also enables people to understand how the fundamental principles and values should influence decision making and policy setting in the organisation. This also requires broader ethical decision-making skills and virtues. Such skills are not confined to skilled application of problem-solving methods by individuals in making personal ethical decisions. In any organisation, hospital, business or government department, most decision making is an activity of committees or teams and requires complex skills in analysis and negotiation to explore the interests of concerned stakeholders. At a corporate level, CEOs and senior managers are involved in the complex diplomacy and politics of negotiations with government and in inter-agency consultation and collaboration. Devising means to consult with and involve relevant external stakeholders in the process, and suitable methods for taking account of different agencies' policies and procedures, makes ethical decision making at these levels even more complex, and we need training and skills to do it properly. The virtues related to this practice are those of the mean, such as justice, patience and courage. These enable proper time to be spent on shared reflection and effective mutual challenge.

CLINICAL EFFECTIVENESS AND RESEARCH

Clinical effectiveness means ensuring that everything you do is designed to provide the best outcomes for patients/clients, that is that you do 'the right thing to the right person at the right time in the right place'. In practice, this means:

- Adopting an evidence-based approach in the management of patients/clients
- Changing your practice, developing new protocols or guidelines based on experience and evidence if current practice is shown inadequate
- Implementing National Institute for Clinical Excellence (NICE) guidelines, National Service Frameworks and other national standards to ensure optimal care (when they are not superseded by more recent and more effective treatments)
- Conducting research to develop the body of evidence available and therefore enhancing the level of care provided to patients/clients on an ongoing basis
- Ensuring research is carried out ethically and is focused on the core purpose.

Clinical effectiveness is very much focused on measuring how any intervention works, which is important for developing a practice for patients/clients. The danger of this is if it narrows an appreciation of purpose, and therefore has to be developed in the light of a core purpose which is concerned not just for improving clinical outcomes but also for improving care where there can be no successful outcomes. Alongside that has to be a concern for value for money. Again, however, this is not a simple economic calculus. It involves reflection on justice, and how limited resources can be properly shared, and, most importantly, how this can be justified. Chapter 10 will examine this in more detail. To ensure comprehensive and continuous quality improvement, the systematic use of methods of strategic planning is necessary. The strategic planning process or cycle involves, at a macro level, the familiar stages applicable to most types of problem-solving methods, namely:

- Clarification and definition of the problem/s or strategic issues to be addressed
- Collection and assessment of relevant evidence, based on present and past performance, and estimates of resource inputs required
- Developing relevant action plans to deal with identified problems, with clear and achievable objectives and anticipated outputs
- Managing the implementation of action plans, setting standards for performance assessment and monitoring the overall process

■ Evaluating the outputs and outcomes of strategic actions in the light of pre-established objectives and performance measures

■ Feeding back information to the management team to identify areas for quality improvement and for ongoing review.

CLINICAL INFORMATION

This aspect of clinical governance is about ensuring that:
■ Patient/client data are accurate, secure and up-to-date
■ Confidentiality of patient/client data is respected
■ Full and appropriate use of the data is made to measure quality of outcomes (e.g. through audits) and to define priorities and develop appropriate services innovative solutions.

Clinical information, then, is focused on the work of the Trust and ensuring good reflective practice and deliberation. Separate questions, such as the confidentiality of patient/client data are part of the principles of respect for the patient/client.

STAFFING AND STAFF MANAGEMENT

This involves the need for:
■ Appropriate recruitment and management of staff
■ Ensuring that underperformance is identified and addressed
■ Encouraging staff retention by motivating and developing staff
■ Providing good working conditions.

Again, some of these aspects are involved in the other pillars. The focus on staff, however, has deeper elements to it. In one respect, it involves building a community of practice, such that all take responsibility for care. This kind of meaning and focus on core value and purpose is as much about well-being in the workplace as any staff support facilities. It involves core questions about motivation and developing the ethical identity of the organisation.

Integrated Governance

The integration of these different pillars of governance is focused on:
■ Careful deliberation and critical reflective practice
■ Determination both of clear lines of responsibility for areas of practice and for shared responsibility for the project of healthcare. In England, the chief executives of the NHS Trusts and Primary Care Trusts have overall responsibility for the quality of services and are required to appoint appropriate senior officers to ensure that quality standards set nationally in the National Service Frameworks and by NICE are achieved if possible. They are also required to ensure formal reporting arrangements are in place through clinical governance committees.
■ Transparency, such that all involved in healthcare are accountable
■ Shared concern for innovative and imaginative pathways to delivering effective healthcare
■ The integration of core principles and values that connect principles of competency (such as the capacity to learn, good communication and effective team work) and principles of ethics (such as respect, justice and non-maleficence)
■ The integration of moral, psychological, intellectual and practical virtues (see Chapter 3), focused on staff development.

Central to this integration is the practice of narrative development, focusing on identity, and dialogue, focusing on the practice of shared responsibility. This enables the practice of governance to hold together the several tensions implicit in managing an organisation's human, financial and material resources, and thus to ensure that:

- The organisation and its stakeholders flourish, as defined by its mission, vision and values
- The organisation achieves both its short- and long-term objectives
- The organisation achieves its optimum potential, in terms of its purpose, patient and staff satisfaction and cost-effective use of resources.

At its heart is the embodiment of care, the core purpose, something which eludes simplistic measurement. The quality of the care is found as much in the culture of the organisation as in any metrics.

The Development of an Ethical Culture

Culture in healthcare can be defined as the beliefs, traditions, values and narratives that are shared in an organisation and shape the identity of that organisation and its members (Trevino and Nelson 2008; Paine 1984; MacIntyre 1981). The danger of governance is to focus on compliance, with reliance on systems rather than the development of a culture which enables individual and shared responsibility. If we get the system right, then all we have to do is follow it, without the need for persons in that system to take responsibility for their thoughts or actions.

T.S. Eliot's poem 'The Rock' sums up this reliance on system thinking:

They constantly try to escape
From the darkness outside and within
By dreaming of systems so perfect that no one will need to be good.

(Eliot 1942)

Ethical governance suggests the opposite. Goodpaster (2007) suggests there are three phases in developing a culture of responsibility:

- Orienting, involving leadership setting the course of the organisation
- Institutionalising, making the company's values part of its operating consciousness
- Sustaining the culture.

His view focuses on the transmission of the core values in practice over time and is based on a socio-cultural view of conscience as a function of the community as well as the individual – ethical deliberation as shared.

9.2 PAUSE FOR THOUGHT

Conscience and the Organisation

Conscience is one of the words that we all use but often don't consider what it means. Most people view it as a personal thing. It is often also seen as an internal voice of feeling that makes one uneasy at the prospect of doing the wrong thing, or after doing the wrong thing. It is even referred to as the voice of a feeling.

Hence, the last place you might think is the home of conscience is an organisation. However, there is no reason to see conscience as simply affective or purely personal. Aquinas, for instance, defines 'conscience' as the 'application of knowledge to activity' (*Summa Theologiae*, I-II, I). This knowledge is partly reason and partly the natural disposition of the human mind to apprehend general principles of behaviour.

Goodpaster (2007) argues that conscience was originally a cultural attribute, not simply personal. Hence, it is possible to speak of the cultural development of ethics as the development of corporate conscience.

Orienting

Orienting involves providing the ethical direction of the board (King III 2009), including:

- Developing the vision and values of the organisation
- Ensuring the use of ethics expertise, either through appointments to the board or through consultancy

- Ensuring that ethical objectives and benchmarks are an integral part of the firm's central objectives. This should show ethical meaning and values as core to the identity and purpose of the firm
- Establishing how things are done, for example confirming that strategic decision making requires careful consideration of consequences to all stakeholders
- Ensuring that ethics is articulated as a normal part of company policies, procedures, practices, conduct and business agendas, and that all decisions are preceded by deliberation on ethical issues
- Communicating a clear message that ethical objectives are critical to the success of the firm and failure to address these could affect the success of the firm
- Ensuring that a member of the board is responsible for developing the ethical culture and that resources are in place to operationalise the programmes
- Demonstrating the core virtues in the board's practice. The leadership has to embody the core values, demonstrating their practice of the key virtues of practical wisdom, empathy, justice, courage and integrity.

This demands attention to the practice of the board, to vision and to values.

THE BOARD

King III (2009) argues that the function of the board should include: developing the vision and values of the organisation; ensuring ongoing dialogue; the use of ethics expertise, either through appointments to the board or through consultancy and ensuring that ethical objectives and bench-marks are an integral part of the firm's central objectives. This should show ethical meaning and values as core to the identity and purpose of the organisation and to all decision making, ensuring that a member of the board is responsible for developing the ethical culture and that resources are in place to operationalise related programmes. This begins to demonstrate the practice of responsibility and core virtues in the board practice. A board focused on critical dialogue is one which reflects different perspectives and is thus able to practice effective deliberation (Sonnenfeld 2002).

Ensuring this requires minimally that:

- The board should be effective and collectively responsible
- The chairman's/CEO's roles and responsibilities should be divided
- There should be a balance of executive and non-executive directors on the board
- Appointment of directors should involve formal, rigorous and transparent procedures
- There should be a formal board performance review annually, with planned training, board refreshment and regular elections
- Boards should be ready to enter into dialogue with major shareholders based on a mutual understanding of objectives.

The division of roles of chair and CEO is aimed precisely at ensuring a critical relationship where no leader dominates or excludes dialogue. All of this looks to build integrity into the culture of the board itself, such that all members take responsibility in all senses of the word, defining and continually re-evaluating the purpose, aims and values of the organisation (King III 2009); being accountable to stakeholders and embodying awareness and shared responsibility for the social and physical environment. This can involve complex responsibilities which the chair has to handle. For instance, the finance director is responsible to the CEO and also to the board and for the wider healthcare project. This could lead to disagreements in board meetings which endanger professional relationships. The chair has to ensure that all voices are heard and appreciated and differences worked through. It is precisely the diversity of perspectives that would enable clarity and transparency of the oversight. In effect, all this enables dispersed leadership, a sense of shared responsibility and clear negotiation of responsibility. The board would then begin to reflect wider discourse amongst stakeholders and in the wider community. Ultimately, the chair would be responsible for ensuring the practice of dispersed leadership.

These principles, which balance organisational sustainability with social and environmental sustainability, require much more focused processes and structures acting as buttresses, possibly including:

- A professional watchdog to ensure an external perspective that fully enables critical reflection
- Sharpening of the annual board review, possibly with the provision of ongoing board and board member coaching. This can also reflect on the power dynamics in the board dialogue practice. Another reflective mechanism is the values audit applied to the board. This involves guided reflection with board members around the core values and how they relate to the deliberative practice of the board (cf. Gregory and Willis 2013). This could be connected to an annual review of directors' performance, developing their accountability.
- Non-executive directors who reflect the range of stakeholders. In some cases, this might mean involving non-governmental organizations (see the next chapter).
- Developing ways of opening dialogues between the board and different stakeholders. This might include: more frequent meetings with stakeholders, for instance, focusing on the core vision and values; board members going out to develop dialogue with internal and external stakeholders; setting up dialogues between the board and stakeholders as to be part of the annual general meeting (AGM) and developing social media both around decisions taken and ongoing dialogue.
- The development of formal reflection in board meetings on how the agenda relates to the core purpose or values, and on how critical deliberation can be improved.

Developing such structures for boards provides holding moments (Western 2007) for reflection and planning which bridge belief, value, virtues and practice. All of this sets the tone as one of both seriousness and support in developing ethical meaning. It establishes how things are done, confirming, for instance, that strategic decision making requires careful consideration of consequences to all stakeholders. It ensures that ethics is articulated as a normal part of company policies, procedures, practices, conduct and business agendas; and that all decisions should be preceded by deliberation on ethical issues. It communicates a clear message that ethical objectives are critical to the success of the organisation.

An effectively structured board, focused on vision, meaning and values, can begin the orientation, through developing critical dialogue amongst the workforce, towards the visions and values of the organisation. Ethical leadership then involves enabling the group and group members to critique their own and the group's myths – the big stories that give value and identity to the group – not least through engaging other narratives that provide a challenge (Western 2007). Hence, critical dialogue has to be part of that process. All this demands development in the board of more creative, non-linear thinking. Linear thinking increasingly fails to engage possibilities in a complex social context (Heifetz et al. 2009; Welbourn 2015). A key element of this is paradoxical thinking (Lederach 2005). This is characterised by being open to difference and the challenges that different perspectives bring to the board. Often, differences are seen in boards as potential points of conflict, leading to chairs avoiding conflict or pushing through undigested action. Hence, Paul Polman, former CEO of Unilever suggests that the chair of the board should 'cook' conflict (Welbourn 2015), that is, enable real differences to emerge and be addressed. This will lead both to clearer ethical focus and more effective creativity. Polman continues, 'we must find and create tensions, force people into different space for thinking, this is not just a performance issue but a survival issue, because managing paradox helps foster creativity and high performance' (cited in Welbourn 2015, p. 1). Some writers even argue against attempts to solve conflict situations too quickly, precisely because this enables different perspectives, with their affect aspects, to inform thinking (Heifetz et al. 2009). This demands practice of care in board deliberation, including the explicit referencing and testing of purpose and values (Gregory and Willis 2013).

9.3 PAUSE FOR THOUGHT

Responsibility and the Board

The first mode of responsibility (see Chapter 2) includes responsibility for knowing what you are doing. It cannot be assumed that board members in any organisation all know what they are doing (Sonnenfeld 2002). In the credit crisis of 2007/8, the HBOS board (banking) followed the corporate governance code, but the majority of the board were from retail backgrounds and had no experience of banking. The result was that they had no understanding of the nature of the risks they were taking, no awareness or appreciation of the wider industry or social environment and how they connected to the banks activity, little appreciation of the meaning of banking in relation to society as a whole and the different stakeholders and no understanding of the different narratives that might test their views. Hence, the board lacked effective deliberation and thus any practice of the first mode of responsibility, genuine agency and understanding of purpose and context.

The consequences are summed up in the title of the report for the Parliamentary Commission on Banking Standards (2013) *'An accident waiting to happen' the failure of HBOS.*

VISION

Developing a vision can too often be left to a consultancy, with the effect of developing an anodyne, generalised vision. The focus can often be on image or brand rather than the core purpose and value which brings substance to the practice of the organisation. Hence, vision has to connect to the different narratives in the organisation's history (local and national). The narratives embody the purpose and value and enable the stakeholders to identify with these. The focus on narrative and dialogue enables individual responsibility to lock into meaning, recognising not simply the worth of the organisation but the membership as co-authors of the ongoing narrative. It thus enables shared meaning and identity to develop.

Leading through dialogue is the same for any organisation. The vision may emerge from the history of the organisation, something hinted at by the NHS Constitution but not fully developed (see Chapter 10). It may emerge from the nature of the service, in this case, inclusive care. It might emerge in the context of a wider ethical debate, such as the morality of the marketplace in healthcare (see Chapter 10). The task of such a vision, then, needs to begin with the mindset of having a larger purpose that is bigger than simply making ends meet. This involves exploring how healthcare is contributing to the common or greater good. The relationships may be local and immediate or wide and over time. Establishing such a vision, based on engagement with all the narratives, including those of the workforce, sets the value and tone of the organisation and the basis of its integrity. This demands all stakeholders are involved in the debate and dialogue about vision. This effectively does two things: ownership of the overall vision (not authentically possible without critical engagement) and clarity about the different perspectives, roles and value of the stakeholders, inside and outside the organisation. Vision is not focused exclusively on the future but on value over time, the historical narrative of the organisation. Only from that base is the focus for pathways into the future, fuelled by the imagination. Even this is focused on dialogue, enabling different possibilities for the future to be envisaged. Critical to this is dialogue which enables the different stakeholders to test the vision and values and to establish shared responsibility.

9.4 PAUSE FOR THOUGHT

In Dreams Begins Responsibility

One of the greatest examples of envisioning is Martin Luther King's Dream Speech. Examine the speech and explore what makes it so powerful (https://www.archives.gov/files/press/exhibits/dream-speech.pdf).

The dream of the future is rooted in the values of the past, we hold these truths to be self-evident, that all men are created equal (King 1963, p. 4). It is focused on shared identity (the US Declaration of Independence) and in the ethical principle of equality.

> ...and so even though we face the difficulties of today and tomorrow, I still have a dream. It is a dream deeply rooted in the American dream. I have a dream that one day this nation will rise up and live out the true meaning of its creed.

It then locks into different narratives, political and religious, that all sides would recognise, not least the Gettysburg Address, which quotes the Declaration, and deepens the narrative to include the value of democracy and the fight to end slavery, engaging identity, values, worth and thus feelings.

Only in the light of that narrative, focused on Lincoln, whose memorial he was standing in front of, does he imagine the future, 'I have a dream that my four little children will one day live in a nation where they will not be judged by the colour of their skin but by the content of their character, I have a dream'.

Yeats, in *Responsiblities* (1916), suggests that dreams form the basis of action, 'In dreams begins responsibility' (iii). Quite literally, King's dream enables the development of responsibility, reflecting on meaning, value, purpose, worth, narrative and so on, but also giving a public account of that and one that responds to the different contextual and relational dialogues. With the engagement of imagination, then, come the possibilities for the future.

VALUES AND PRINCIPLES

Establishing the values of an organisation has often been problematic. If the organisation has begun to focus on vision, then the development of values emerges from that, not least because vision work focuses on worth and common good, and, in effect, the corporate practice of *phronesis*. This can be contrasted with the practice of value clarification (Raths et al. 1978), a more anodyne process which sets out values, attempts to identify a hierarchy and then establish commitment to these from employees. The underlying assumption is that differences in views about values should be avoided. This leads to standard expressions of general values such as respect or justice, with no critical assessment and understanding of the values. This reflects a lack of genuine engagement from members of the institution, with no context-specific examples of how these values are embodied in relationships.

However, first, as noted above, values are related to vision and purpose. Justice and respect, for instance, are not simply general principles of relating, but are focused on the community of practice. In health or education organisations, for example, this reinforces that the goods of health or education are inclusive, and that justice is integral to the experience of learning or healing (just assessment procedures, equal access to care and so on). The same can be said of responsibility, with focus on the patient/client or learner taking responsibility as part of the community of practice for good in their life. Hence, they are not simply customers, but are actually part of the community of practice. In other words, dialogue begins to affect the identity of the different stakeholders. Second, there is a need to subject values development to critical dialogue. The dialogue at this point is about seeing what is meant in everyday practice. Does respect mean: being polite to staff, giving them choices, including them in decision making, keeping them informed, about good or bad news? What does one mean by justice? How does the organisation practice justice? What procedures are in place? Organisational justice, as we noted above with remuneration, is enabled through good governance.

Key to developing principles and values is, once more, dialogue with stakeholders inside and outside the organisation, whether it is in the review, planning, assessment or feedback processes, or in undertaking shared responsibility for monitoring and evaluating progress and achieving an organisation's objectives.

STAKEHOLDERS

Whilst some authorities have argued that in any organisation, managers are primarily responsible to the organisation's 'shareholders', others have argued that many other parties have a real stake in the success or failure of a business or public service organisation, for example, employees, customers or clients, suppliers, the community and both local and state government. Some argue that it is necessary for practical purposes to establish distinctions between those with immediate interests and more remote interests in the performance of the organisation (Arnold et al. 2019), suggesting various methods of stakeholder analysis can be used to ensure that the appropriate stakeholders are involved. These include:

- Brainstorming a comprehensive list of the stakeholders
- Clarifying the rights and duties of the various stakeholders in the organisation relative to management and patients/clients
- Ranking/ordering these on the basis of objective criteria for their relative importance to the organisation
- Determining which 'stakeholders' it is essential, or desirable, to involve directly in the process of strategic planning, and, alternatively, deciding who should be consulted, in order to ensure understanding of the organisation's mission and objectives, and to gain endorsement and support for implementation of its strategic plan.

Application of these approaches to healthcare is not straightforward. First, there is a sense in which all persons are stakeholders with regards to health – health is everyone's interest. Human life is vulnerable and the nature of human health is contingent on many things outside any individual's control. In this sense, we are all potential patients/clients. Second, the concept of stakeholders as those who have an interest in an organisation is limited. Stakeholders in relation to health clearly also have a responsibility, something spelled out in the NHS Constitution (see Chapter 10). Hence, the model is more aligned in healthcare to the concept of partnership or even a cooperative. The third point about stakeholders is that they most often do not represent a single relationship to an organisation. Stakeholders of healthcare, for instance, are also stakeholders in family, work, education and so on, and each of these environments reflect shared concern for health. Equally, those responsible for these environments share responsibility for health in these environments. Hence, business, educational institutions and local authorities becomes key stakeholders in healthcare.

In this light, the final point about stakeholders (engagement with them) is not simply about aligning interests but about developing shared responsibility for healthcare and contributing ideas and practice to the healthcare innovation. A good example of this is the work on childhood obesity in Amsterdam, which we examine in detail in Chapter 10. Involving stakeholders, as well as staff and actual patients/clients, in the processes of healthcare development is costly in terms of time and resources, but it has been repeatedly shown that the investment required is worthwhile if it ensures that representative stakeholders from across the whole organisation are enabled to participate meaningfully in the processes involved. The evidence is that it more than pays off in terms of public support, improved staff commitment and organisational productivity and efficiency (George and Weimerskirch 1994).

Biennial reviews of the values and vision of the organisation, focusing on the NHS Constitution can enable reflection (see Chapter 10). These could provide anchor points for stakeholders to come together and hear the different voices within the organisation. Do the different groups accept the board's views? Do they see these ideas actually being put into practice, and so on? There is great benefit to bringing stakeholders from different perspectives and interests together in one place, so that the listening becomes part of ongoing dialogue. This is where the attention of the leadership can actually be tested and real trust developed (O'Neill 2002). Such anchor points could be extended regionally to include higher education institutes and business. This could involve groups such the institute of directors, chambers of commerce and trades unions building dialogue platforms with external stakeholders around the health issues of the region. The environment of work is key to the health of most people. Health dialogues could provide different perspectives and pathways about healthy lifestyle.

Institutionalising

Following the direction, then, structure and processes are put into place. This may involve including codes of ethics and ethics committees.

CODE OF ETHICS

If the vision statement is the compass for direction, then codes of ethics provide the ethical map (see Chapter 3). Developing a code of ethics or conduct is not a once-off exercise, but an ongoing process, subject to regular reflection. This may involve an annual review of the code or more regular reflection. The code then becomes part of the development of a learning organisation (Senge 1990), exemplifying ongoing critical dialogue and the practice of integrity. In establishing the code of ethics, then, care must be taken to see them as guides to ethical judgement and dialogue. To get this right, the purpose of the code needs to be established. Initially, it will be a function of the board to identify this in consultation with experts and stakeholders. Kaptein (2008) argues that the code should link to: the mission and vision of the corporation; the company's relationship to the wider social and physical environment, so that ethical vision is reflected in the performance vision and the core values. Hence, the code should link to the value narrative of the organisation.

A code may be intended to prevent unethical behaviour (with a prescriptive stress), or to promote and encourage ethical behaviour (focusing on the practice of responsibility and how dialogue about that can be engaged). Corporations tend to combine both elements. The first tends to focus on typical ethical issues of dilemmas in that area, such as how to deal with conflicts of interest, respectful treatment of stakeholders or the company judgement on receiving gifts. The second focuses on broad responsibilities, encouraging thought about how they will be managed. The code may have several focuses. It may be intended primarily for leaders, managers and employees, or may include external stakeholders, such as in the supply chain (see the next chapter), or in partnerships. Any worker or company, then, may be subject to several different codes – industry codes (e.g. the alcohol industry), professional codes, codes of governance, or codes to do with specific areas such as advertising (see the Advertising Standards Agency). Hence, far from a single code dominating, they may reflect the different narratives in any organisation. Kaptein (2008) suggests that codes can link into relation to disciplines and stakeholders, including strategy, quality, human resources, security, communication, law, finance, environment and community. Working with codes, therefore, locks into both dialogue with different narratives and the development of identity. Familiarity with the core principles and values of the different codes can help inter-professional working and leads often to joint guidance, reaffirming shared identity (see Chapters 6 and 8 on the duty of candour).

9.5 PAUSE FOR THOUGHT

Johnson and Johnson

Johnson and Johnson are famous for their credo. It forms the basis of their culture (https://www.jnj.com/sites/default/files/pdf/our-credo.pdf).

The credo focuses on:

Responsibilities. It clearly asserts plural responsibilities and carefully shows how these affect practice. Hence, for instance, the primary responsibility is to the health industry, health professions and patients/clients. This leads to an objective of affordable pricing. The many different responsibilities mean that the firm will aim for a fair return to shareholders (stockholders).

Virtues and values. Implicit in the credo are core virtues of integrity, maintaining core values such as respect in all operations; justice (in the concern for fair return and fair treatment) and empathy in the need to be aware of all the aspects of their ethical environment.

Ongoing reflection. In the 1980s, Johnson and Johnson reacted rapidly and effectively when faced by poison found in one of their products, Tylenol. They withdrew all stocks, and faced up to the safety issue, leading the way in developing tamper proof seals. It was assumed that the company credo was the key to this strong ethical response. In fact, the CEO noted that it was not so much the credo, as the regular session held in the firm to reflect on, review and challenge what the meaning of the credo was in practice, that led to that response. In effect, this was the practice of *phronesis*.

None of this means that things will not go wrong. Nonetheless, such codes provide the basis of thinking, practice and learning in the face of crises (see the US opioid crisis, McGreal 2019).

ETHICS COMMITTEE

Key to the operation of a code would be the equivalent of an ethics committee with an ethics officer, and an independent chair. Such a committee might include advisory and arbitration roles, ethics training roles, integration roles, focusing ethics on dialogue and responsibility. An ethics officer would report to the board and operationalise the ethical programme. This might include developing a good communication strategy, training, structures for action and auditing. In relation to strategy development, an ethics risk and opportunity profile might be developed, identifying its ethics risks through a process of engagement with its stakeholders, helping to clarify the risks and opportunities (not least to reputation and trust) incurred through ethical and unethical behaviour. An ethics committee can be focused both internally and externally. The internal focus enables it to help reflection on the meaning and practice of ethics, with members of the organisation bringing to them issues and feeding into training. The external focus builds trust with stakeholders but also feeds into media relations. The communication strategy is key to such a committee. Often, the very best of values are not communicated well, so that, for instance, employees do not feel that they are being listened to, do not sense the concern for justice and do not see the way in which the organisation is practising *phronesis*. Transparency in the organisation involves opening out these practices.

Sustaining

TRAINING, STAFF DEVELOPMENT AND A CARING CULTURE

The importance of training to the development of an ethical culture is critical. Effective training of students, which focuses as much on the core virtues and how these might be practiced, as well as on clinical skills, including immersive learning and reflection on practice, will begin to enable student nurses to engage power relations effectively. Effective inductions for new employees will involve rehearsal of core purpose and related values, and the narratives that embody these. MacIntyre (1981) notes the importance of narrative in showing what virtues look like in practice.

Justice and equity in access to training, and opportunities for self-improvement in general, also foster a sense of being valued by all staff. Ethics is fundamentally about human beings, about valuing human beings, and making human resources management critical to developing a caring culture based on justice and respect is a priority in any firm. The time invested in training personnel in interpersonal skills, in group work and communication skills, in effective support and supervision of others, in skills in developing their potential, pays off not only in better understanding, trust and cooperation, but in effective teamwork and higher productivity (Campling 2015).

ANNUAL MEETING

For large organisations, frequently the only opportunity to reflect on action and create dialogue is the annual meeting. In a narrow context, this has a critical function in the practice of accountability, but it does not usually engage in wider dialogue. Indeed, in the corporate world, the communication at annual meetings has often been designed to limit dialogue and ensure that a narrow agenda is presented. However, an annual meeting could be developed on a more dialogic footing, making accountability much more rigorous. This might involve an extended annual event, with the annual meeting as part of a one- or two-day conference. This would set the tone of: dialogue, with board members open to questioning or working with groups around aspects of meaning and practice; and plurality, inviting different shareholder groups to share their narrative from inside and outside the organisation. In one event, the tone of vertical and horizontal dialogue can then be set, focusing both on celebration of value (expressed through successes, relationships and so on) and the development of value expressed by dialogue. Such a meeting would model mutual nonjudgemental dialogue between board members and different levels through the organisation.

Key to this process would also be critical reflective practice reporting at individual professional levels and at an organisational level. Hence, staff development could link into annual reviews and include reflection on core principles and values and how they are embodied in the achievement of targets. This can be extended to everyday practice, with business meetings and staff development inductions shaped in dialogue, or different perspectives collected through local community forums. Dialogue can also be extended to the social media. One healthcare trust, for instance, uses twitter to generate dialogue, and even feeds into board meetings, so that discussions and decisions are communicated as they happen.

REPORTING

Sustaining the ethical culture involves developing a learning organisation (Senge 1990). Having worked through vision, values, responsibilities and practice, this leads to reflection on the practice and how far practice and purpose are developing. A good example of this is integrated reporting noted in the last chapter. Effective integrated reports bring together narrative and measurement which focus on the values of all the different capitals (financial, manufacturing, human, social, intellectual and natural). None of the value represented in these six capitals can be simply assumed. For them to be maintained, they have to be articulated as part of regular reflection so that all stakeholders can both hear and contribute to them. The first two are about the sustainability of the purpose and practice of healthcare. The term manufacture has, of course, a corporate feel to it. It refers to the value of what is created, which, in health terms, is the creation of a service focused on health and well-being for all. Financial capital refers to the resources needed to maintain it. Sustaining these two core elements demands continued open dialogue which reinforces the identity and value of the organisation and all involved. Human capital is at the heart of the health service precisely because it is focused on the quality of care. Hence, the importance of stories which show care embodied in imaginative and innovative ways. Social capital takes the service not just to 'users' of the service but the mutual responsibility of all to be involved in the practice of care, for the self and others. Intellectual capital is focused on scientific and social research which adds to the learning process and provides evidence-based practice. Natural capital looks at wider sustainability and our dependence on the natural environment.

All this links to dialogue which reflects on narrative, purpose, value and relationships. It is worth reminding ourselves that the root meaning of audit is to hear (*audire*). Original audits were presented orally. This focus on voice reinforces the notion of narrative and giving an account, something less about measurement and more about the quality of the engagement. Part of any reporting will involve measurement, for example in relation to the environment. However, integrity cannot be measured, partly because it involves focus on core values and principles and how they can be embodied in practice. This requires the development of shared narrative.

ETHICS AUDIT

An internal ethics audit might also be set up, as part of an ethics committee's work, involving assessment of the ethical culture of the company, including reporting on:

- The ongoing development of the codes, and allied risk assessments
- All ethics related policies and procedures – gifts and entertainment policy, declaration of interest policy
- Feedback from training sessions, with training sessions that could be developed as part of the communication system
- Steps taken to combat misconduct
- Any other ethics interventions or initiatives
- Weaknesses in formal and informal systems and processes.

Such audits can test the gaps noted by Argyris (1964) between different narratives. This would form the basis for reflecting on and developing the ethical culture.

EXPLICIT VALUES LANGUAGE

In all this, ethics and broader value language has to be explicit. Trevino and Brown (2004) note that if the use of language can obscure the ethical issues, it can also influence moral awareness. For example, if the words 'stealing' music (rather than downloading) or 'forging' documents (rather than signing) were used, the individual would be more likely to think about these issues in ethical terms. In some cases, practices have been redefined. In the second Gulf War, for instance, the White House legal advisor listed over 20 acts of 'aggressive interrogation' that were deemed acceptable (Robinson 2011). Later court appeals confirmed that these were all examples of torture. Once you have a new, non-value language, this can lead to other professions accepting this practice. Again, in the Gulf War, this led to medical and healthcare professionals being used to check the health of victims, to ensure that the 'interrogation' could be completed. Technical language, then, can also be used to obscure ethical reality. A remarkable example of this is the engineering memo of Willy Just about refining the Nazi gas trucks on the Eastern front in the Second World War (cited in Bauman 1989, p. 197). The memo refers to the 'cargo', "thick and thin fluids" created in the operation, and focuses on the technical problems in achieving the right balance and incline of the vehicle floor to make the operation more efficient.

ETHICAL CULTURE, NARRATIVE, SYMBOL AND SPACE

Developing a culture of value demands the use of time and space to remind all stakeholders about central stories, national and local, which form a part of the identity of the organisation. This might include an annual event that brings together different cultures, professions, businesses and religions around health in the region. It might include: the use of photos and pictures in corridors and eating areas; symbols which focus on local identity and medical history and reminders of the core purpose in foyers, in meetings and so on.

REWARDING ETHICAL BEHAVIOUR

Rewarding ethical behaviour and disciplinary actions taken against unethical behaviour make common sense. We know that reward, in general, reinforces behaviour, good or bad. In the Mid Staffs case, many staff were rewarded (albeit unintentionally) for bad behaviour. A reward system is more than a means to an end. It is the embodiment of the end, core ethical values, and as such, key to demonstrating integrity and justice. This can be part of a long-term commitment, with, for instance, a review of ethical behaviour included in annual evaluations, making it one amongst other criteria for promotion and compensation decisions. Of course, there is the danger of employees simply aping what they think the organisation wants to hear, and of colleagues competing to be ethical, thus missing the point. Hence, any review would have to be part of a critical conversation that reflects on the meaning of the key values and how the virtues can be evidenced, such as the concern for justice.

9.6 PAUSE FOR THOUGHT

Reflect on the Ethical Culture of the Organisation That You Work for or Are Part of

Does it express integrity? If so, how?
Does it express a sense of justice?
Do you feel that it is concerned with justice and fairness?
Does it express a sense of empathy? If so, how does it model that empathy?
Does it express practical wisdom? Is it open to rigorous reflection on purpose?
Does it give you a voice?
Can you challenge your leadership?
If you were in a leadership position, how would you improve the practice?

SAFE SPACE

The culture should include safe spaces, integrated into everyday clinical practice, which can allow members of the organisation to work through struggles with values and practice. One example is Schwartz Rounds, which offer a safe space for staff to come together and reflect upon the experiences and challenges they face at work. Maben et al (2018) found a statistically significant improvement in staff psychological well-being, increased empathy and compassion for patients/clients and colleagues and positive changes in practice connected to these events.

VIRTUES

The stress in integrity on responsibility and dialogue means that practice of the virtues is key to any governance system. Moore (2012) refers to governance systems which crowd out virtues, with compliance viewed as more important than taking responsibility for judgement. Moore (2012), Osterloh and Frey (2004), and Maitland (2008) work through how virtues can be developed in governance procedures across all levels of the organisation, not least *phronesis* in board deliberation (Osterloh and Frey 2004, pp. 206–207). Critical to this development is attention to the power and authority noted above. The power imbalance within a board can be striking, with psychological and intellectual power being asserted through dominant CEOs. Hence, part of any board code of practice needs to explicitly address the issue of power, to ensure that the views and desires of particular constituencies are not privileged. This also would require explicit attention to the virtues board members would bring to enabling dialogue when appointing them to the board. All this requires carefully designed systems of participation and self-governance (Norman 2015) which enable the practice of responsibility and the virtues. The latest UK Corporate Governance Code (FRC 2018) begins to move the board in this direction but still has a top down perspective and does not include stakeholders effectively in the dialogue.

WHISTLEBLOWING

Developing a whistleblowing procedure is a critical function of governance. It is the backstop for making sure that the organisation really does look at itself, its meaning, and its practices. Often this is where the shadow side (Fawkes 2014) of the organisation is revealed. Anyone who works in the NHS or for an organisation that provides services for the NHS is encouraged to raise concerns about risk, malpractice or wrongdoing in the service, including: unsafe patient/client care or working conditions; inadequate induction or training for staff; inadequate response to a reported patient/client safety incident or a bullying culture (across a team or the Trust rather than individual instances). The NHS policy on whistleblowing (https://improvement.nhs.uk/resources/freedom-to-speak-up-whistleblowing-policy-for-the-nhs/ accessed 21 Feb 2020) seeks to ensure:

- Organisations will each appoint their own whistleblowing guardian, an independent and impartial source of advice to staff at any stage of raising a concern
- Any concerns not resolved quickly through line managers are investigated
- Investigations will be evidence-based and led by someone suitably independent in the organisation, producing a report which focuses on learning lessons and improving care
- Whistleblowers will be kept informed of the investigation's progress
- High-level findings are provided to the organisation's board, and the policy will be annually reviewed and improved.

These have been developed from the Francis Review (2015) *Freedom to Speak Up*, itself emerging from the Francis Reports. Such a culture has to be developed by the board and the *Guidance for boards on Freedom to Speak Up in NHS trusts and NHS foundation trust*s (England NHS and NHS Improvement 2018) confirms this. It states that executive directors should:

- Be able to articulate both the importance of workers feeling able to speak up and the Trust's own vision to achieve this
- Speak up, listen and constructively challenge one another during board meetings
- Be visible and approachable and welcome approaches from workers
- Have insight into how their power could silence truth
- Thank workers who speak up
- Demonstrate that they have heard when workers speak up by providing feedback
- Seek feedback from peers and workers and reflect on how effectively they demonstrate the Trust's values and behaviours
- Accept challenging feedback constructively, publicly acknowledging mistakes made.

Executive directors, then, have to embody the key virtues of whistleblowing not least:

- Courage to articulate problems
- Temperance in deliberation and in listening carefully to all complaints
- Care in feeding back and ensuring support for whistleblowers and all colleagues
- Practical wisdom, in focusing on core shared purpose and value.

However, there are issues with the idea and practice of whistleblowing in the NHS. First, it is less about ongoing critical discourse and more about *post hoc* revelation. By definition, it is reporting about activity which has already gone too far. Second, it demands that the individual take responsibility for the whole organisation. It is hardly surprising that few would want to take responsibility for that, and for the very detailed data gathering required or the problems that any action might create for the person's future prospects (Borrie and Denn 2002). Third, whistleblowing can quickly move into an adversarial dynamic, with the organisation as a whole and with particular colleagues. The NHS has a bad history around whistleblowing (Cleary and Doyle 2016), frequently involving retribution from management. Fourth, Edgar and Pattison (2011) argue that care should be taken not to assume that whistleblowers are always right. They suggest that some might be motivated by a sense of their own heroism. This underlines the importance of focusing the procedure on forensic justice, that is the impartial testing of all perception and evidence.

Miceli and Near (1984) and Cleary and Doyle (2016) argue that whistleblowing has to be part of a wider culture which normalises both trust and challenge. Without that, any procedures will be less effective. One survey (NHS 2014), focusing on leadership and whistleblowing, noted that 94% of directors thought that staff could raise concerns compared to only 57% of nurses. More concerning was that 90% of directors believed that such concerns would be handled appropriately, but only 26% of nurses agreed. This points to classic organisational disjunction (Argyris and Schoen 1978), where individuals and groups within organisations continue to operate with different perceptions of what is happening in the organisation.

Such different perspectives lead to the 'deaf effect' (Mannion and Davies 2015), where individuals and groups within the organisations are unable to hear what the other groups say. They are perceived as threats and therefore any evidence is discounted. The threat itself comes from a defensive view of a narrow identity, based partly on narrow measurement of success, exemplified once more in the Mid Staffs case. There, whistleblowers were from the staff and patients'/clients' families and suffered the additional dynamic of being accused of endangering the service. Hence, protection for the whistleblower has to be as robust as any examination of the facts. For whistleblowing to be effective, then, there has to be a culture that accepts challenge as a positive good, and thus rewards it. One aspect of this is to acknowledge that all organisations have a shadow side (Fawkes 2014), and that ongoing self and organisational reflection, holding members, each other, to account, is critical. In that light, the voice of the whistleblower is not isolated but rather speaks for the whole organisation.

Key to effective whistleblowing procedures is a combination of disinterestedness and care. The first ensures that there is a distance (not taking sides, at any point in the process) which is necessary for the effective practice of justice. Care ensures that all parties are respected, and thus given the support necessary for working through the issues. Alongside justice and respect is the need for genuine transparency, such that the organisation and all stakeholders can clearly see the embedment of justice and respect.

Conclusions

At the heart of this chapter has been the development of ethical meaning in the practice of an organisation. Several things can crowd out such meaning, from modern management techniques to excessive and plural quality control and regulation (Thompson and Bevan 2013). Rozuel (2011) notes how this adds to the dynamic of compartmentalisation, with personal, professional and institutional ethics viewed separately and not focused on responsibility or identity. This crowds out both the individual and the organisational voice (Verhezen 2010; Gentile 2010). With that, the practice of the virtues, individually and corporately, is also crowded out. The voice of the individual and the organisation has to be worked out in dialogue. As this is worked through, both individual and organisation can give a clearer account of shared ethical principles, in particular, justice and non-maleficence.

Working through the meaning and practice of justice thus become an anchor for the practice of integrity in the organisation, providing the confidence of a shared ethical value. The broader culture provides other key anchor points, some in the organisation, some in the wider industry, profession or community, contributing to the development of shared narrative. The development of an ethical culture based on a values framework does several other things. It establishes a discipline of reflection in which ethics is central to ongoing strategic thinking, not seen as merely a necessity for dealing with corruption or fraud – a positive rather than a negative responsibility. It recognises that individuals take their ethical cue from the surrounding culture. This is at its most problematic when unethical behaviour is associated with success. Nearly a third of respondents from one survey (Trevino and Brown 2004) said that colleagues condoned the ethically questionable practice of leaders who achieved success. In other contexts, typically if a junior member of a work team raises an ethical issue, then the leader will reframe the issue, focusing on the 'needs' of policy, saying that this is the leader's responsibility (Trevino and Brown 2004). When asked why they engaged in unethical conduct, employees will often say, 'I had no choice' or 'My boss told me to do it' (Hinrich 2007; Trevino and Brown 2004). The assumption of the follower is that the leadership is responsible for any values held and any decisions based on those values, and they do not accept responsibility for testing ideas and values.

References

Adams, C. (2013). *Capitals: background paper for IR*. London: International Integrated Reporting Council. Online available: http://integratedreporting.org/wp-content/uploads/2013/03/IR-Background-Paper-Capitals.pdf accessed 02 Feb 2020.

Andreasson, S. (2011). Understanding corporate governance reform in South Africa: Anglo-American divergence, the King Reports, and hybridization. *Business and Society*, 50(4), 647–673.

Aquinas T. (1981) *Summa Theologica*. New York: Resources for Christian Living.

Argyris, C. (1964). *Integrating the individual and the organization*. New York: Wiley.

Argyris, C., & Schön, D. (1978). *Organizational learning: a theory of action perspective*. Reading, MA: Addison Wesley.

Aristotle. (2004). *Nicomachean ethics*. London: Penguin.

Arnold, D., Beauchamp, T. and Bowie, N. (2019) *Ethical Theory and Business*. Tenth edition. Cambridge: Cambridge University Press.

Bauman, Z. (1989). *Modernity and the Holocaust*. London: Polity.

Blasi, J., & Kruse, D. (2003). *In the company of owners: the truth about stock options*. New York: Basic Books.

Bloom, M. (2004). The ethics of compensation systems. *Journal of Business Ethics*, 52(2), 149–152.

Borrie, G., & Denn, G. (2002). Whistle blowing the new perspective. In C. Megone, & S. Robinson (Eds.), *Case histories in business ethics* (pp. 96–105). London: Routledge.

Campling, P. (2015). Reforming the culture of healthcare: the case for intelligent kindness. *BJPsych Bulletin*, 39(1), 1–5.

Cleary, S., & Doyle, K. (2016). Whistleblowing need not occur if internal voices are heard: from deaf effect to hearer courage. *International Journal of Health Policy Management*, 5(1), 59–61.

Conger, J. (2005). Oh Lord won't you buy me a Mercedes Benz: How compensation practices are undermining the credibility of executive leaders. In J. Ciulla, T. Price, & S. Murphy (Eds.), *The quest for moral leaders: essays on leadership ethics* (pp. 80–98). Cheltenham: Edward Elgar.

Edgar, A., & Pattison, S. (2011). Integrity and the moral complexity of professional practice. *Nursing Philosophy*, 12(2), 94–106.

Eliot, T. S. (2004). *The rock, the complete poems and plays*. London: Faber and Faber.

Evans, G., & Dalik, A. (2011). *The Wynford Group*. Canada: HR Reporter.

Fawkes, J. (2014). *Public relations ethics and professionalism*. London: Routledge.

Fischer, M., & Ferlie, E. (2013). Resisting hybridisation between modes of clinical risk management: contradiction, contest, and the production of intractable conflict. *Accounting, Organizations and Society*, 38(1), 30–49.

Francis Review. (2015). *Freedom to speak up*. Online available: http://freedomtospeakup.org.uk/wp-content/uploads/2014/07/F2SU_Executive-summary.pdf accessed 15 Jan 2020.

Financial Reporting Council. (2018). *UK Corporate Governance Code*. London: Financial Reporting Council.

Gentile, M. (2010). *Giving voice to values: how to speak your mind when you know what's right*. New Haven, CT: Yale University Press.

Goodpaster, K. (2007). *Conscience and corporate culture*. London: Blackwell.

Greenberg, J., & Cropanzano, R. (2001). *Advances in organizational justice*. Stanford, CA: Stanford University Press.

Griffiths, B. (2009). *Public must learn to 'tolerate the inequality' of bonuses, says Goldman Sachs vice-chairman*. London: The Guardian. Online available: http://www.guardian.co.uk/business/2009/oct/21/executive-pay-bonuses-goldmansachs accessed 10 Feb 2020.

George, S., & Weimerskirch, A. (1994). *Total quality management.* London: John Wiley.

Gregory, A., & Willis, P. (2013). *Strategic public relations.* London: Routledge.

Heifetz, R., Grashow, A., & Linsky, M. (2009). *The practice of adaptive leadership: tools and tactics for changing your organization and the world.* Cambridge, MA: Harvard Business Press.

Hibberd, J., & Gilbert, H. (2014). *Supporting people to manage their health.* London: King Fund.

Hinrich, K. (2007). Follower propensity to commit crimes of obedience. *Journal of Leadership and Organizational Studies, 14*(1), 69–76.

International Integrated Reporting Council (2013) *Integrated Reporting.* London: International Integrated Reporting Council.

King III. (2009). *King III report on corporate governance.* Johannesburg: Institute of Directors in Southern Africa.

King IV. (2017). *King IV report on corporate governance.* Johannesburg: Institute of Directors in Southern Africa.

King, M. L. (1963). *I have a dream: speech by the Rev. Martin Luther King at the march on Washington.* Online available: https://www.archives.gov/press/exhibits/dream-speech.pdf accessed 18 Jan 2020.

Kaptein, M. (2008). *The living code.* Sheffield: Greenleaf.

Kolb, R. W. (2005). *The ethics of executive compensation.* Oxford: Blackwell.

Lederach, J. P. (2005). *The moral imagination.* Oxford: Oxford University Press.

MacIntyre, A. (1981). *After virtue.* London: Duckworth.

McGreal, C. (2019). *Johnson and Johnson signals climbdown ahead of major opioids crisis test case.* London: The Guardian. Online available: https://www.theguardian.com/us-news/2019/oct/02/johnson-johnson-settlement-ohio-case accessed 14 Feb 2020.

Maben, J., Taylor, C., Dawson, J., Leamy, M., McCarthy, I., Reynolds, E., et al. (2018). A realist informed mixed-methods evaluation of Schwartz Center Rounds® in England. *Health Services and Delivery Research, 6*(37), 1–260.

Maitland, I. (2008). Virtue or control in the governance of the firm. In *Society for Business Ethics Annual Meeting 2008.* Society for Business Ethics.

Mannion, R., & Davies, H. T. (2015). Cultures of silence and cultures of voice: the role of whistleblowing in healthcare organisations. *International Journal of Health Policy and Management, 4*(8), 503.

Miceli, M., & Near, J. (1984). The relationships among beliefs, organizational position, and whistle-blowing status: a discriminant analysis. *Academy of Management Journal, 27*(4), 687–705.

Mishra, C., McConaughy, D., & Gobeli, D. (2000). Effectiveness of CEO pay-for performance. *Review of Financial Economics, 9*(1), 1–13.

Moore, G. (2012). The virtue of governance, the governance of virtue. *Business Ethics Quarterly, 22*(2), 293–318.

National Health Service Executive. (1999). *Clinical governance; quality in the new NHS.* London: HMSO.

National Health Service Improvement. (2018). *Freedom to speak up: guidance for NHS trust and NHS foundation trust boards.* Available online: https://improvement.nhs.uk/resources/freedom-speak-guidance-nhs-trust-and-nhs-foundation-trust-boards/ accessed 21 Feb 2020.

National Health Service. (2014). *Building and strengthening leadership: leading with compassion* London: HMSO. Online available: https://www.england.nhs.uk/wp-content/uploads/2014/12/london-nursing-accessible.pdf accessed 10 Fen 2020.

National Health Service. (2019). *National Health Service Constitution.* London: HMSO. Online available: https://www.gov.uk/government/publications/supplements-to-the-nhs-constitution-for-england accessed 10 Mar 2020.

Norman, W. (2015). Rawls and corporate governance. *Business Ethics Quarterly, 25*(1), 29–64.

O'Neill, O. (2002). *A question of trust.* Cambridge: Cambridge University Press.

Osterloh, M., & Frey, B. (2004). Corporate governance for crooks: the case for corporate virtue. In A. Grandori (Ed.), *Corporate governance and firm organization: microfoundations and structural forms* (pp. 191–211). Oxford: Oxford University Press.

Paine, L. S. (1984). Managing organizational integrity. *Harvard Business Review, 72*(2), 106–117.

Parliamentary Commission on Banking Standards. (2013). *An accident waiting to happen: the failure of HBOS. Fourth Report of Session 2012–13.* London: The Stationery Office Limited.

Pink, D. (2011). *Drive.* London: Canongate.

Raths, L., Harmin, M., & Simon, S. (1978). *Values and teaching* (2nd ed.). Columbus, OH: Charles E. Merrill.

Rawls, J. (1971). *A theory of justice.* Oxford: Clarendon Press.

Robinson, S. (2011). *Leadership responsibility.* Oxford: Peter Lang.

Rousseau, D. (1995). *Psychological contracts in organizations.* Thousand Oaks: Sage Publications.

Royal Brompton and Harefield. (2008). *Annual performance review and accounts 07/08: inspiring, improving, investing.* Online available: https://www.rbht.nhs.uk/sites/nhs/files/Publications/Annual%20report%20 and%20accounts%20including%20quality%20reports/Annual%20performance%20review%20and%20 accounts%202007-2008.pdf accessed 10 Mar 2020.

Rozuel, C. (2011). The moral threat of compartmentalization: self, roles and responsibility. *Journal of Business Ethics, 102*(4), 685–697.

Scally, G., & Donaldson, L. J. (1998). Clinical governance and the drive for quality improvement in the new NHS in England. *British Medical Journal, 317*(7150), 61–65.

Senge, P. (2002) *The Fifth Discipline: The Art and Practice of A Learning Organization.* New York: Doubleday.

Senge, P. (1990). *The fifth discipline: the art and practice of a learning organization.* New York: Doubleday.

Sonnenfeld, J. (2002). What makes great boards great. *Harvard Business Review, 80*(9), 106–113.

Sun, W., Stewart, J., & Pollard, D. (2010). Reframing corporate social responsibility. In W. Sun, J. Stewart, & D. Pollard (Eds.), *Reframing corporate social responsibility: Lessons from the global financial crisis* (pp. 3–19). Bingley, UK: Emerald Publishing Limited.

Thompson, M., & Bevan, D. (2013). *Wise management in organisational complexity.* London: Palgrave.

Trevino, L., & Nelson, K. (2008). *Managing business ethics: straight talk about how to do it right.* London: John Wiley.

Trevino, L. K., & Brown, M. E. (2004). Managing to be ethical: debunking five business ethics myths. *Academy of Management Executive, 18*(2), 69–81.

Verhezen, P. (2010). Giving voice in a culture of silence: from a culture of compliance to a culture of integrity. *Journal of Business Ethics, 96*(2), 187–206.

Welbourn, D. (2015). *Leadership in a contested space: a review of literature and research.* London: Virtual Staff College.

Western, S. (2007). *Leadership: a critical text.* London: Sage.

Yeats, W. B. (1916). *Responsiblities.* New York: MacMillan.

CHAPTER 10

Public Health Ethics and the Social and Political Ethics of Healthcare

LEARNING OUTCOMES

When you have read and worked through this chapter, you should be able to:
- Critically examine public health ethics focusing on the example of obesity
- Critically examine different views of paternalism
- Explore stigma, shame and responsibility
- Outline a community healthcare which practises shared responsibility in the community
- Critically examine different approaches to social ethics and healthcare
- Explore the ethical tensions of morality and the marketplace, focusing on the case of the UK Health and Social Care Act 2012

Introduction

In this chapter, you might say that healthcare ethics goes public. This is so in two senses. First part of the chapter, we will examine the values and practice of public health, in the sense of how we promote health. At the heart of this practice are questions about paternalism, freedom to determine one's own lifestyle and responsibility for health. We will once more focus on the key ethical element of dialogue, involving all stakeholders (and a social view of health), and how dialogue relates to motivation. We will focus on childhood obesity as a key example in public health and will include a scenario about nursing practice, a case about promoting awareness of the link between cancer and obesity and a case study about an integrated response to the problem in a European city. The case will make some reference to identity ethics or politics. We will invite you to work through the underlying debate about such ethics. In the second part of the chapter, we will examine the public or social ethics of managing the distribution of health and social care nationally, and to some degree, globally. We will examine the different approaches to the distribution of health and use the narrative of the UK. Ethical tensions similar to that of public health will be explored, the central issue being care, morality and the marketplace.

CASE 10.1   Obesity

Jean and her 5-year-old daughter come into the health centre to get inoculations for travel to Nigeria and a repeat prescription for asthma inhalers for both. Both are short of breath, look very uncomfortable in the heat and are clearly overweight or possibly obese. As the nurse is working out what inoculations will be needed, she wonders whether she should raise the question of weight, and at least frame the beginning of a conversation about this. Would you mention the issue of weight, and if so, why and how? Are there any considerations against raising this issue with these patients?

The Health Survey for England 2016 estimated that 28.7% of adults in England were obese (body mass index (BMI) 30 or above), with a further 35.2% overweight (BMI between 25 and 30). Men are more likely to be overweight or obese (66% of men, 57% of women). Levels of both are highest among those aged 45–74 (https://researchbriefings.parliament.uk/ResearchBriefing/Summary/SN03336).

In children, 9.6% of reception age children (age 4–5) were obese and 13.0% overweight. At age 10–11 (year 6), 20.0% are obese and 14.3% overweight. There are variations amongst different regions in childhood figures, with children from deprived areas, for instance, more likely to be obese. At age 10–11, 12.8% of children in the least deprived areas are obese, compared with 26.2% in the most deprived areas. This gap has increased over the last decade. There is evidence of related medical conditions, including type 2 diabetes, coronary heart disease, some types of cancer including endometrial, breast, ovarian, prostate, liver, gallbladder, kidney and colon cancer, stroke and related psychological problems. Apart from the individual suffering experienced, it is estimated that by 2050 the annual cost to the NHS of treating obesity and related complications will be £9.7 billion. Wider social costs are estimated at £49.9 billion. Such a problem is confirmed globally (WHO 2017).

The mother and daughter in the scenario above are part of a very complex phenomenon, one which illustrates the issues for public health. It involves several different stakeholders, including: the state, whose problem it is to ensure that medical provision is equitable, and that a major personal and societal problem is engaged; medical and healthcare professionals, who are both agents of the state and representatives of their professions; individuals who have become overweight or obese and their families; intermediate institutions who can affoot weight control and a positive attitude to food, such as schools and local councils; the food industry who market and supply food that contributes to the obesity crisis and non-governmental organisations (NGOs), local or global, who focus on obesity.

There are several ethical issues at play in this situation, including respect for self-determination, the promotion of the common good, questions of responsibility, for example, parents to children or the food industry to stakeholders and justice. All of these fall into the area of public health. The Wanless Report (Wanless 2004, p. 3) defines public health as 'the science and art of preventing disease, prolonging life and promoting health through the organised efforts and informed choices of society, organisations, public and private, communities and individuals'.

This definition leaves little place to hide. Health, both in negative and positive terms, that is the prevention of illness and the promotion of health, has to involve everyone, from the individual to the government. The key ethical issues are first whether it is ethical to intervene to promote a person's health, either for their good or for the wider common good, and second, how is responsibility to be worked out amongst the different stakeholders. This is true for interventions at an individual, professional or family level, as much as interventions from government through the law.

It is tempting to see this as a simple debate between liberals (in the sense of thinkers who want to protect the freedom of the individual to determine their own health choices) and communitarians (whose focus is the good of the community as a whole). The first focuses on individual liberty, seen as freedom from interference of coercion (Berlin 1969). The second focus is on the needs of the community and our responsibility to that community, or, in other words, to each other. The liberal position has an underlying world view of the individual as existing apart from society, whereas the communitarians see the individual as part of and in a mutual relationship with society (Chapter 2). This polarised position assumes a view of personal agency which is limited. It sees autonomy as essentially a right to choose, one that has to be protected. Autonomy, however (see Chapter 2), is focused on the capacity to deliberate, and this involves more than simply the right to make a choice (though including that). Effective deliberation involves developing awareness of the self and the social situation which enable the person to see not just the consequences of different decisions in terms of out outcomes, but also how these outcomes might affect the person and people and institutions connected to that person. This suggests the importance of providing a framework that will enable dialogue and reflection and the development of awareness and learning. Empowerment in this is not simply about giving the person the relevant information, but rather enabling agency and the development of responsibility.

Paternalism

In this debate, paternalism is often seen as taking away our freedoms, that is, 'the Nanny State'. There are in fact different kinds of paternalism. MacDonald (2015) notes the difference between democratic communitarians and a more assertive communitarianism. The democratic communitarian approach focuses on dialogue (Habermas 1992), bringing together individual choice and societal good. Hence, Häyry (1991) suggests a distinction between three different forms of paternalism: hard paternalism, soft paternalism and maternalism. Hard paternalism involves direct coercion, soft paternalism involves giving unasked for information or foreclosing some options for action and maternalism involves control by psychological means such as targeting a sense of guilt.

Hard paternalism is most often applied by the law, such as ensuring that all car travellers wear seat belts. This demands very strong evidence that demonstrates that the action in question is focused on both individual responsibility and the common good. Soft paternalism and maternalism both focus on democratic communitarianism. A good example which combines both is the nurse informing pregnant women that they are potentially harming their babies if they drink alcohol during pregnancy. This does not take away choice but enables better choice focused on responsibility.

Hence, the nurse faced by mother and daughter in the case above would be engaging in hard paternalism if she told the patients that she would not give them their vaccination unless they signed up to a weight loss class in the practice. Softer paternalism would involve noting how uncomfortable they were in the heat and engaging in a conversation about how weight loss might help their well-being. Maternalism would begin to examine the duty of the mother. Which approach would you take and why?

There is detailed guidance from the National Institute for Health and Care Excellence (NICE 2014) (www.nice.org.uk/guidance/cg189/chapter/1-Recommendations). The guidance includes details of the information that could be passed on to the patient, including about:

- being overweight and obesity in general, including related health risks
- realistic targets for weight loss; for adults, please see the NICE guideline on managing overweight and obesity in adults
- the distinction between losing weight and maintaining weight loss, and the importance of developing skills for both; advise them that the change from losing weight to maintenance typically happens after 6–9 months of treatment
- realistic targets for outcomes other than weight loss, such as increased physical activity and healthier eating
- healthy eating in general
- self-care
- voluntary organisations and support groups and how to contact them.

The advice suggests that adequate time should be provided to build up such dialogue and also suggests different strategies for enabling the dialogue, and empowering the person. Behind such a professional framework is the relational foundation which enables dialogue about obesity to emerge. Hence, the guidance urges nurses who are working with children to 'use tact and diplomacy to find out if the family and the child or young person accepts that the child or young person is overweight' (Recommendation 8).

In the case at the beginning of this chapter, then, the dialogue might begin to emerge by enabling the mother and child to begin a narrative about how they feel in the heat. This focuses on a sense of well-being or distress, and on where they want to be rather than on the issue of weight. The stress is on affect, the feeling of the patient and on self-reflection. This is where agency begins for the patient, enabling them to reflect on what they want, and how they want to be. As Habermas (1992) argues, rational reflection is not simply about examining information at arms-length but about how that information makes sense in relation to the person and his or her identity. In this the patient can begin to develop an understanding of the significance of what is being shared. In other words, there is a relational element which looks at the person's particular situation. In effect, this process enables deliberation (see Chapter 2), moving through to possibilities in action and the use of the imagination.

The Public Context

The same ethical dynamic is there in the national context of public health. This can be seen in the public debate, questions about stigma and issues of responsibility.

THE PUBLIC DEBATE

In the public context, the dialogue is perhaps more complex. Swierstra (2011) notes at least three discourses in play in relation to obesity, for instance:
- The behaviour discourse. Obesity is the result of individual choices
- The body discourse. Obesity is genetically or metabolically determined
- The environment discourse. Obesity is determined by the social and physical environment.

All play some part in the development of obesity, and each is a complex phenomenon. The obesogenic environment, for instance, involves several different elements, including:
- The physical environment, such as the layout of a shopping centre which makes it difficult to get to stairs, discouraging exercise
- The social environment, including practices that encourage sedentary activity (such as social media, or the work environment)
- The market environment. This involves marketing goods with high sugar content.

Responding to any of these environments involves questions about principles. How, for instance, can we persuade people to use the stairs? The market environment has involved several ethical issues:
- Building physical and psychological dependency on sugar
- Misleading adverts which suggest that certain products are healthier when they still contain high sugar levels
- Advertising which focuses on children, with the aim of them becoming agents in making their parents buy certain goods
- Focusing adverts on narratives (often humorous) which either connect to good feelings or values that the buyer might identify with
- Strategic placement of foods, close to the check out in supermarkets.

Hence, the field of dialogue is often not even, with powerful forces focusing on the non-rational aspects of identity. This includes locking into guilt with, for instance, parents feeling guilty about not buying their children's favourite cereal. It should come as no surprise that the market communication has evolved its own form of maternalism.

It is precisely because of this that debate about public health has to be public and is inevitably long term. The public nature of it enables the testing of different narratives about health. A good example of an ongoing debate is smoking (Chadwick and Gallagher 2013). The banning of smoking was the result of a long public debate, in which different positions were tested. This allowed debate about empirical data (which, over time, the tobacco industry had to accept). It allowed debate about core values. In this, the tobacco industry argued that it had a concern for the common good in defending freedom of choice, and that the responsibility for smoking was with the smoker. None of these arguments were set out in the context of an interest-free or emotion-free rational debate. On the contrary, the tobacco industry worked hard at associating the product, at times, with strong personal values, such as resilience and independence (Hafez and Ling 2005). Only over a long period of time, where all the different narratives, including the fallacies, were tested, did things change, not least because the evidence of passive smoking demonstrated that this was not an individual but a social issue. Developing the public debate about obesity remains complex, exemplified by the stigma of obesity.

STIGMA AND OBESITY

One of the major complications of public health, especially in relation to the issue of obesity, is the associated stigma. How can we even raise the issue of obesity when this runs the danger of shaming the person or persons? Shaming another is deemed to be morally wrong because:

- It focuses on the person rather than the condition, making them feel bad about their body image and sense of self
- In turn, this has led to an exacerbation of the condition itself. In other words, far from empowering the person, it has led to a lack of motivation to change
- It leads to a broader sense of exclusion based on body image. Hence, it is argued that it is more important to enable overweight people to be accepting of their body image.

A good example of this debate was when Cancer Research UK (2019) instituted a campaign to raise awareness of the connection between obesity, smoking and cancer. A letter from a number of health care professionals (Thomas 2019) raised several objections, including:

- The causal connection between cancer and obesity is not clear
- The campaign reinforced the public assumption that obesity is a 'lifestyle choice'. This contradicts evidence that 'over 100 complex and interacting factors including genetics, the built environment, and a vast array of psychological and social factors' determine obesity.
- The campaign reinforced obesity stigma: 'This is particularly concerning in relation to cancer; women report weight stigma as a reason for delaying or avoiding cervical, breast, and colorectal cancer screenings, citing disrespectful treatment, embarrassment at being weighed, negative attitudes of providers, and unsolicited advice to lose weight as the main barriers. In addition, weight stigma has been identified as a barrier to accessing treatment in women with endometrial cancer'.
- Implying that individuals are largely in control of and responsible for their body size (and therefore cancer) supports a culture of blame and plays into prejudices and negative stereotypes.

The letter ends by urging Cancer Research UK to change focus to empowering people to make health-promoting changes, regardless of their BMI. The response of CRUK involved several elements:

- The campaign was to raise awareness of the issues generally, and this contributes to the public debate about obesity. The aim was to work against the incessant advertising and price promotions for junk food that nudge us towards eating unhealthily (Plummer 2019).

- It was specifically aimed at government, in attempting to help them reach their targets for reducing obesity levels.
- It was simply making information available and does not involve any image or words that would constitute 'fat shaming'.

This debate amply sums up some of the major ethical issues about public health, but perhaps raises more questions than answers. Here we have two groups, both of whom are perceived as the 'good guys', trying to focus on public health and behaviour change. One argues that you cannot focus on the issue of obesity as lifestyle change because this puts too much emphasis on the responsibility of the individual. The other group wants to raise awareness and develop debate and dialogue to show how obesity is not a discrete phenomenon.

How does the phenomenon of obesity stigma relate to the issue of freedom and personal responsibility? The argument seems to suggest that raising the issue of obesity will tend to disempower rather than empower. Does this mean that the 'patient' has neither freedom (actions are determined by the experience of stigma) nor personal responsibility? ten Have et al. (2011, p. 1) provide a formidable list of physical and psychological determinants that work against responsibility, including: 'uncertainty, fears and concerns, blaming and stigmatisation and unjust discrimination; inequalities are aggravated; inadequate information is distributed; the social and cultural value of eating is disregarded; people's privacy is disrespected; the complexity of responsibilities regarding overweight is disregarded; and interventions infringe upon personal freedom regarding lifestyle choices and raising children, regarding freedom of private enterprise or regarding policy choices by schools and other organisations'.

If that is so, then how is the person to develop agency in this situation? Against this, it could be argued that stigma is simply another social narrative, albeit negative and powerful, and along with the other discourses, the development of agency needs to empower the person to push back at such narratives, be they about body shape, individualist narratives, parental identity and so on.

RESPONSIBILITY

Beneath the different narratives referred to above are critical questions about responsibility. At one level, it seems obvious that individuals are responsible for the consequences of their choices and behaviour. This adds to the notion that obese people are responsible for their condition. There is no doubt also that, at some point, successful therapy is dependent upon individuals taking responsibility for their own selves and therefore their bodies. This applies to alcohol and drug addiction (Robinson and Kenyon 2009), both of which have been medicalised. Part of some approaches to therapy in these areas is a recognition of the negative effects of these behaviours on the self and others, and the re-establishment of a relationship with all who have been affected. In achieving this, such individuals become accountable to others for their actions.

The problem is when individual responsibility is seen as the only responsibility, that is, ignoring the obesogenic environment and the responsibility of different players in that environment. Once responsibility is narrowly individualised, this sets up the dynamic of negative responsibility and the assumption that the individual is to blame (MacDonald 2015; Ricoeur 2000). However, this does not mean that individual responsibility should be ignored. On the contrary, person-centred care recognises exactly its importance. In the midst of such complexity, how can public health begin to engage the responsibility of all stakeholders and effectively address the different but connected issues?

Public Health and the Moral Imagination

We have noted the different stakeholders involved in the issue of obesity and how each of those can partly own responsibility. To achieve this requires both dialogue and coordination, with all parties looking to be involved. It also requires a disciplined framework which enables all stakeholders to remain focused on purpose. It moves beyond the simple idea of provider and consumer to one where all stakeholders are empowered to identify and practice individual and shared responsibility. This also takes us beyond the simple idea of a discrete healthcare provider. Health and well-being become the responsibility of individuals, families, NGOs, intermediate organisations such as schools and colleges, local and national government, businesses and so on. With all of these sharing and negotiating responsibility, the moral imagination can focus on possibilities. We will return to this in the second part of this chapter. At this point, we will give a good example of how a public health initiative can bring together the different stakeholders around deliberation, dialogue and learning.

CASE 10.2	AAGG Amsterdam Healthy Weight Programme (Amsterdamse Aanpak Gezond Gewicht)

In 2013, the AAGG (https://www.amsterdam.nl/sociaaldomein/blijven-wij-gezond/amsterdam-healthy/#h66c45d7e-bfca-4788-8511-7f6754e688e1) was introduced in response to infantile over-weight and obesity rates above the national average. In 2013, 27,000 children were overweight or obese, including 21.0% of under 18s in Amsterdam compared to 15.0% nationwide. These were spread unequally across the city. Children of low-income groups and low educational achievement, migrant and minority ethnic backgrounds were particularly affected. In 2012, for instance, 21.8% of children from the poorest areas were overweight compared to 9.6% in the wealthiest areas. From 2012 to 2015, the number of overweight and obese children dropped by 12%, with the biggest fall amongst the lowest socio-economic groups.

From the outset, it was determined that the response would have to be structured (enabling long-term commitment), interventionist (providing a disciplined framework), focused in the local area (noting different responsibilities at a national level) and integrated. The focus on the city region was because a managed project would be most successful at this size, not least because local government powers could affect the necessary changes. The key objectives of the AAGG were to:

- Reduce obesity by enabling children to eat and drink healthy foods
- Increase their physical activity
- Enable good quality sleep. The links between poor patterns of sleep and obesity have been well established (Miller et al. 2015).

AAGG recognised that eliciting behaviour change in a population required consideration of the complex and multi-factorial determinants of childhood obesity, aiming to:

- Understand the causes of obesity in context, that is the structural determinants within which psychological mechanisms, individual lifestyle factors and living and working conditions, are worked through
- Stimulate cultural change through addressing these factors through a 'whole-systems approach', that is, an approach which flows through the different contexts. Critical here is the idea of behaviours being reinforced by different environments. In effect, the programme looked to establish positive environments to empower the children, turning the obesogenic environment on its head.
- Enable the healthy choice to be the easy choice. In effect this meant enabling good deliberation.

This involved agencies across the city taking joint responsibility for the project, including Health, Housing and Social Support, Sports and Work and Income, coordinated by the Department of Social Development. Professional collaboration was cross-sector including schools, medical professionals, planning bodies, sports organisations, communities, charities and industry. AAGG established seven guiding principles and 10 pillars of action as the focus of coordination, building on previous work in France and the Netherlands (Hawkes and Halliday 2017, p. 44).

The principles included:

- Eradicating overweight and obesity is a long-term task that will take a generation
- The programme, actions and activities must be sustainable
- The programme is inclusive of all people and across all policy areas
- Addressing childhood obesity is a matter of shared responsibility
- The approach is evidence-based – 'learning by doing, doing by learning'
- Choices must be made to focus efforts
- The primacy of prevention.

TEN PILLARS OF ACTION

Each pillar was mapped to an inter-departmental working party with responsibility for its implementation. The first six were aimed at preventing children from becoming overweight or obese, the seventh pillar is 'curative' and the final three were secondary or facilitative.

A. Preventative, focusing on:

- The start of pregnancy until age 2, including screening of infants for risk of obesity, counselling for expectant mothers, information provided to pregnant women about healthy diets and mothers supported to breastfeed. This also included provision of a smartphone app to monitor baby development, and the provision of coaching.
- Schools (pre-schools and primary schools). This included setting parameters such as nutrition taught in class, healthy birthday treats and water or milk only to be drunk (with no fruit juice brought in). Extra gym classes were developed focused on children's motor skills and development. In addition, 'prevention scans' were instituted to assess schools against core requirements, enabling the school to develop its strategies. As school meals were not provided, the scheme worked with parents to encourage them to provide a healthy packed lunch, typically one that was cheaper than processed food.
- Neighbourhood and community, including after-school activities for children, subsidies for sports club memberships for low-income families, assigning community health ambassadors linking to welfare organisations, civil society, minority ethnic organisations and local shops to promote healthy lifestyles.
- Healthy environment, including review of healthy urban design, such as making cycle routes safer, and health food environment.

B. Curative:

- Helping children who are overweight or obese to regain a healthier weight. This included assigning youth healthcare nurses, and developing care plans.

C. Facilitative:

- Learning and research approach
- Use of digital facilities
- Use of communications and methodologies for behavioural insights.

Examples of innovative digital tools included digital health coins earned by families and exchanged for a discount on health products. The on-line 'Living and Action Plan', was used to set achievable goals for parents and children. Ongoing research is focused on how such communication can be enhanced. The learning focus looked to coordinate care between relevant professionals and ensure communication of behavioural insights throughout the network. This allows ongoing action to be observed and managed (learning by doing), developing good practice or ending ineffective practice.

STRATEGIC ANALYSIS

The policy research unit (Hawkes et al. 2017) suggests several strategic lessons from this case, focusing on:

Strong vertical leadership, with the deputy mayor using local power to clear away unnecessary obstacles and secure commitment from the council. Management of the AAGG was initially placed in the Department for Social Development, taking it out of the remit of Public Health, a statement that obesity was an issue that extended beyond a narrow view of public health to include, amongst other things, social justice. The effect was to pave the way for leadership and commitment from across the city.

A collaborative, cross-departmental approach. Collaboration and how this could achieve objectives, rather than funding, was the starting point. Where funding has been secured, there has been a clear and specific use for it. Collaboration was focused on the support groups for the

10 actions (see above) and demanded an approach which was aware of tensions and possible conflicts, and developed strategies to resolve conflicts and focus on shared responsibility.

Strategic use of power and influence. This involved focusing on the local area where the council could exert power, working only with businesses who were signed up to the project and focusing on the areas of worst childhood obesity.

Clear parameters and expectations. This included good learning techniques, such as focusing both on the long-term purpose and on setting a series of short-term achievable objectives. Both contributed to the development of the overall narrative.

An academically rigorous basis for action, focused on the support of ongoing research which both contributed to the development of learning in the project and to wider debate and practice development.

A culture of reviewing, monitoring and reflective action. This included in-house teams regularly assessing the impact of the project, and community engagement which involved wider reflection and the development of greater community awareness.

A creative approach to addressing barriers. This included an openness to experiment and an openness to different perspectives, for example, in developing the business case for any aspect of the project.

ETHICAL ANALYSIS

The AAGG has had little ethical analysis to date. It is, however, focused on the core principles of respect and justice, attention to active deliberation and dialogue, increased awareness of the complex local environment and the effects on the different stakeholders. It provides a framework of values and actions, but these are not prescriptive. The framework is rather focused on learning, awareness and shared commitment over time. It is focused on developing narrative, at personal, family, institutional, community and regional levels. There is a strong sense of the principles of subsidiarity, that is, of appropriate responsibility being taken at different levels. It is focused on dialogue, including the communication of new learning points across all stakeholders. The stress is on cooperation focused on peacebuilding approaches, rather than competition. Throughout, the work focuses on taking responsibility for ideas, values and action; shared and individual responsibility; creative responsibility based on learning. Hence, the activity could be seen as dialogic paternalism. However, the key ethical focus was the supported development of responsibility across all stakeholders. We focus on two examples, parents (including work with schools) and business.

Parents

Parents were given the information to enable rational decision making and agency. This included what constitutes a healthy breakfast and how good sleep patterns affect health and well-being. It also included practical information such as: alternatives to feeding for calming a fussy infant (avoiding the use of food as a calming tool); recognising signals from the child of being hungry or full; ways to develop physical activities as a part of everyday life.

They were assisted in developing accountability and enabling their children to develop accountability. This included helping parents to provide a good decision-making framework about what foods could be eaten, and decisions about bedtime. The simple issue of ensuring that children got enough sleep involved empowering parents and children in approaches to bedtime that focused on choice and conflict resolution skills. Critically, it helped to develop parental confidence and mastery of the situation and offer pathways to achieving objectives, key aspects of the virtue of hope. The pathways were not simply techniques, but were focused on the parent-child relationship. Hence, whilst the objectives were to do with bringing down obesity, the focus was on responsibility and relationships. Eating together as a family was also encouraged, as a focus for dialogue.

This learning was supported by other stakeholders including: coaches, schools, business, researchers (including research on sleeping patterns in the area and the development interventions) and other parents, thus leading to dialogue which developed positive responsibility. One example of this was dialogue between the parents and schools when the parents initially chose not to reinforce the use of water rather than fruit juice. The dialogue involved both reflection on purpose and a successful negotiation of shared responsibility. This was also a good example of learning though focus on action. Another example (Hawkes and Halliday 2017, p. 48) involved one parent's question about activities for Mother's Day. This led to dialogue in the neighbourhood meeting, generating an 'oatmeal revolution', involving parents and organisations developing healthy fun centred around oat-based breakfasts and recipes with their children (extending to Ramadan dishes).

Business

AAGG worked with business in a number of different ways. It was important to work with business because they are part of the community and thus can radically affect how families develop their response to obesity. It was equally important that business was challenged to work with key principles and actions. Hence, AAGG developed genuine dialogue with business with the aim of developing a shared responsibility.

The process began with developing an active network between AAGG, the Amsterdam Health and Technology Institute, the Free University of Amsterdam and Albert Heijn, the largest supermarket chain in the Netherlands (34.1% of the market share). The network encouraged businesses involved in the production, supply and sale of food to make food products healthier. This included making smaller portions and reducing the amount of sugar, fat and salt in products. If a business wanted to be involved in the programme, it had to meet various requirements including: ensuring healthier checkout environments; displaying large traffic-light labelling posters in soft and alcoholic drinks aisles; clearer labelling as part of establishing a common standard with clear guidelines for healthy eating. The network recognised that business has a responsibility to shareholders to make sufficient profits. Hence, it helped business to develop strategies, such as smarter management of stocks, so that profits would not be adversely affected.

AAGG also addressed the issue of marketing. The local authority accepted that marketing regulations, such as banning child-centred food adverts before 9:00 p.m. was a responsibility for national government. Nonetheless, AAGG joined forces with the Stop Child Marketing Alliance making use of an established set of guidelines around appropriate marketing. This stimulated the local authority to develop several different actions, such as banning unhealthy food and drinks sponsorship of city sports events where more than 25% of the audience are children. There was also a campaign to restrict the advertising of unhealthy foods, such as chips or ice cream, in buildings owned by the council. AAGG is not unique. There are other similar efforts including successful work in the city of Leeds (Rudolph et al. 2019), previous developments in Amsterdam and research in areas such as sleep and obesity (Hawkes and Halliday 2017). However, it provides an integrated and holistic focus which brings together strategy and ethics. The basis of the integration is the integrity of the different stakeholders and of the overall project.

The different stakeholders continually reflect on their own role, the core purpose of the project and underlying values and the development of practice which embodies these. The process itself is one of ongoing learning and development. The different stakeholders develop their own agency, accountability and creativity, and feel responsible for the whole. The focus is on ongoing dialogue which both supports other stakeholders and is able to challenge them in the light of clear focus on health and well-being. Hence, business, families and schools are both challenged and supported.

The Social Ethics of Healthcare

The core tensions at the heart of healthcare are between care for all, a classic egalitarian position (Tawney 1930), and how we steward limited resources, and ensure choice (autonomy) as part of that process. These tensions are there at all levels of healthcare practice with clinical and management decisions about how we determine which areas will be targeted and given priority. Thompson et al. (2006) argue for five different approaches to making decisions: clinical, epidemiological, egalitarian/ecological, administrative and management. These frameworks are not mutually exclusive, or adequate in themselves. All try to work through different aspects of the core ethical principles in the provision of care.

CLINICAL APPROACH

From an ethical point of view, the clinical approach has traditionally emphasised the primacy of the health practitioner's duty of care to the patient, their duty of protective beneficence based on the paradigm of the extreme dependency and vulnerability of the patient. Historically, this approach has tended to focus on paternalistic, often authoritarian, attitudes of the medical profession, often underplaying the expertise of other professions. From a practical perspective, the strength of the clinical approach lies in being rooted in the direct experience of practitioners of the clinical needs of individuals. It emphasises the importance of curative and interventionist medicine and proof of what works, based on rigorous clinical research, rather than the more speculative benefits of health promotion, prevention and rehabilitation.

However, it tends to assume that the medical perspective (usually the doctor's or consultant's) should determine decision making about resources, with the doctor's clinical judgement authoritative. Moreover, it is individualistic in dealing with clinical and ethical problems which may have complex social origins and consequences. It tends to be crisis-oriented and focused on short-term crisis management, rather than on long-term strategic planning and the wider consideration of research evidence of trends in morbidity and mortality. In attempts at reform of the UK National Health Service, including negotiation of the new GP contracts, clinical audit has been made mandatory. This insistence on independent clinical audit in the interests of greater public accountability has given positive weight to the clinical approach.

EPIDEMIOLOGICAL APPROACH

The epidemiological approach emphasises the need for objective health data on which to base consideration of health priorities. What is required is the scientific study and statistical analysis of the changing patterns of mortality and morbidity in society, including the ability to demonstrate trends in the occurrence and recurrence of epidemics and the relative incidence and prevalence of different types of medical disorders. Typically, the epidemiological approach is that favoured by community medicine specialists and health policy advisers. Planning practical public health measures and directions for health policy involves more than individual clinical judgement and requires more objective and universal indicators of both morbidity and health. Their focus tends to be on planning healthcare systems to serve the needs of specific communities, developing health priorities on the basis of epidemiological evidence.

The main ethical focus of this approach is social justice in healthcare, and its object is to achieve equality of access to services and equitable outcomes for different groups within the population. This is often framed based on rights language, summed up in Article 25(1) of the UN Universal Declaration of Human Rights (see also WHO 2017) 'everyone has the right to a standard of living adequate for the health and well-being of himself and of his family, including food, clothing, housing and medical care and necessary social services, and the right to security in the event of unemployment, sickness, disability, widowhood, old age or other lack of livelihood in circumstances beyond his control.'

Understanding health as a human right creates a legal obligation on states to ensure access to timely, acceptable and affordable healthcare of appropriate quality as well as to provide the services noted above. This is reviewed through various international human rights mechanisms, such as the Universal Periodic Review or the Committee on Economic, Social and Cultural Rights. In many cases, the right to health has been adopted into domestic law or Constitutional law. In developing this focus, WHO (1986) set out to achieve the following objectives for the 'New Public Health', by a process of enabling, mediation and advocacy with other countries, with the following aims:

- to reorient public health services to better meet actual local needs,
- to create supportive environments in which healthy communities can flourish,
- to strengthen local community action for health promotion,
- to develop the personal skills of people to manage their own health.

Rights, in other words, are not treated simplistically. There is a strong emphasis on responsibilities at all levels. Hence, in some form, there is the acceptance of the principle of subsidiarity, that is, that all levels of society should take responsibility, from personal to political. WHO (2019) are now focused on the Sustainable Development Goals (SDGs) and carefully update progress globally in relation to these. The SDGs focus on the responsibility of all stakeholders, including business, for developing the goals, including key elements of healthcare (see UN 2019 for recent targets). For WHO, healthcare ethics is a matter of global ethics. At its heart is a holistic view of health, which suggests that health is related to a complex global environment.

The strength of the epidemiological approach is that it aims to achieve objective and universally valid criteria for planning health services and resource allocation. This approach has been criticised as tending to be too far removed from the emotive reality of individual suffering and the demands of individuals to have their rights respected. Moreover, in pursuit of rational criteria for decision making, it underestimates the power of medical vested interests. However, the emphasis by WHO on the SDGs and the interconnected nature of health and healthcare refocuses it on poverty, deprivation and ignorance and their relationship to ill health in contemporary society.

EGALITARIAN AND ECOLOGICAL APPROACH

The egalitarian also begins with a holistic and interconnected view of health which demands attention to the social environment. The Beveridge Report (Beveridge 1942), which served as the basis for the UK Welfare State and informed the planning of the National Health Service, was egalitarian. As Beveridge expressed it, the welfare state was to serve as a means of organising society to combat the 'Five Giants: Want, Disease, Ignorance, Squalor, and Idleness', in the interests of social justice and more equitable access for all to health, education and welfare. Such concerns cross all cultures (see Nursi 1992, who adds social conflict). This focus leads to the development of:

- Universal benefits that would cover old age, unemployment and sickness
- A comprehensive health service, free at the point of care
- Vastly expanded public sector housing
- Free and universal secondary education
- Measures for full employment.

All of these elements have an effect on health and well-being, but the UK then moved to develop a National Health Service, growing partly out of the Emergency Medical Service set up in the light of the impending war of 1939–45. The experience of 5 years of war reinforced the sense of solidarity and shared care which led to the final institution of the health service in 1948. Equality at the heart of this is not simplistic, but focused in equal consideration of particular need rather than quantitative equality, of equality of opportunity (Tawney 1930). In fact, the vision of the service was not one of provider and consumer. Bevan (1948), 3 months after the foundation of the NHS, noted 'I have been exhorting the general public in the last few weeks to make use of this National Health Service prudently, intelligently and morally, because if too great a strain is placed upon it at the beginning it might breakdown, and because things are free is no reason why people should abuse their opportunity' (Duncan and Jowit 2018). Bevan's (1948) words suggest several things about the nature of the NHS:

- The relationship of the NHS is not simply with the patient but with everyone in that society, that is, anyone may be in need at any time.
- The corollary of this is that the relationship of the individual is not simply to the NHS but to all the other 'owners' of the service.
- The implication of this is that the relationship between the people and the NHS is a moral one. The relationship can be abused and therefore requires careful, responsible behaviour. This is raised in the NHS Constitution, and we shall return to this below. In moral terms, this involves the practice of responsibility by patients as well as service providers. This, Campbell and Swift (2002) note, can include the development of related virtues of the patient. Campbell's work focuses on the virtues that may be needed for the patient to come to terms with and work with, especially those with chronic conditions. The Bevan's (1948) quote above suggests the practice of intellectual (*phronesis*) and ethical virtues.

This begins to move towards Titmuss's (1992) view of the welfare society, which he distinguishes from the welfare state not least through the practice of care and 'ultra obligations', which we will examine below. Many different reports have developed and to monitor the egalitarian approach (World Bank 1993: UN 1993; Illsley and Svensson 1984; DHSS 1980). This approach has not been without its critics. Wilkinson (1996), for instance, argued that there is no simple correlation between high mortality rates and unemployment or social deprivation in the United States, Hong Kong and eastern European countries, citing rapid social and economic change and loss of hope as the key drivers. Nonetheless, the integrated view of health and healthcare remains robust.

ADMINISTRATIVE APPROACH

The administrative approach is based on the traditional model of the welfare state where healthcare and welfare are provided by a largely state controlled and funded service industry, which has to be managed by rational and accountable processes in the public interest. Those employed in the state public sector are charged with the responsibility of providing cost-efficient health services to the community on behalf of the state, and are accountable to the public only indirectly through government ministers. Health service planners and managers have an implied social contract with the patient public or 'consumers' of health services, and are accountable for the whole range of medical treatment, rehabilitation and preventive services in return for the payment of tax and/or health insurance (Harrison 2004).

The ethic of public sector administration is one of public service for the common good. Although ostensibly governed by consideration of universal fairness and respect for the rights of patients or consumers, the lack of direct accountability to consumers or the public means that the pattern of management and planning tends to be paternalistic and non-consultative. The administrative model gives particular emphasis to organisational and scientific rationality and to the contractual rights of patients and the duties of health professionals to maintain standards and quality assurance, based on models of public accountability (Beauchamp and Steinbock 1999).

The strengths of this approach are that it encourages centralisation of management, rational planning, data collection, and record-keeping to ensure public and financial accountability to Parliament, or to the local health authority, through the health service bureaucracy. Supported by the medical model of applied scientific method, management is set up to monitor services using largely medical indicators of mortality and morbidity as measures of progress. The effectiveness of medical procedures will, according to this model, be based on proper scientific tests, randomised trials and controlled experimentation.

BUSINESS MANAGEMENT APPROACH

This approach emerged from two reports in the 1980s, the Griffiths Report (1983) and Enthoven's (1985) Nuffield Trust Report. Both focus on better management techniques, the second giving a little more emphasis to the community (Honigsbaum 1995). They represent 'The New Public Management' or 'New Managerialism', who used the slogan 'Let the managers manage!' as a basis for their criticism of the earlier approaches, which were seen as dominated either by conservative medical models or those of public sector bureaucrats. The argument was that, by the adoption of a business management approach, 'health organisations could be made more efficient and effective by downsizing and applying management techniques that were originally developed by manufacturing firms and mass retailers of goods and services. Introduction of these business techniques would yield tighter managerial control over healthcare practitioners' (Harrison and Pollitt 1994).

This approach adopted the model of the 'internal market', creating a new micro-economic framework within which health service planning, decision making and delivery was to be conducted. The assumptions of this approach are that, in the deregulated market for health service provision, there are 'providers' and 'purchasers' of services. This model argued that individual clients could negotiate their treatment requirements with their doctor and/or other health professionals, who would either provide the service directly themselves or act as brokers in obtaining services from other providers on behalf of their patient. Where not immediately available, service provision could be contracted out to private sector or voluntary service providers. It was further argued that the range and standard of health services provided would be determined not on the basis of a priori medical assumptions or the vested interests of established institutions, but by market forces and the laws of supply and demand. The tests of efficiency, from the health authority or state government point-of-view, would be decided on the relative costs and benefits of alternative procedures. These were to be measured, like levels of productivity or turnover in business or industry, by predetermined 'performance indicators', for example, the numbers of operations or treatment procedures given, and by bed turnover or discharge rates.

Morality and the Market

The debate amongst these five positions has now begun to crystallise around morality and the market. It is important to note from the outset that, whilst this is often characterised as a debate between an ethical and non-ethical position, both sides are making ethical arguments. Those who advocate the market in healthcare argue that it is the most effective way to allocate scarce resources (Wempe and Frooman 2018). This is based on three reasons:
- freedom of choice, with the patient engaged in voluntary exchange
- overall welfare is increased, with all participants gaining from the exchange
- the good of healthcare would be more effectively distributed.

Underlying these points is an economic argument often referred to as 'universal commodification' (Wempe and Frooman 2018; Sandel 2013; Arrow 1963). This is focused on the optimising of consumer preferences, and argues that, provided legal constraints are respected, in principle, any good or service is best distributed by the free market (Wempe and Frooman 2018). The Thatcher revolution spent a lot of time in developing the moral reasons behind policy. Novak (1993), for instance, argued that the market place brought the community together to supply needs. It emphasised the autonomy of patients and the objectivity of 'consumer' rights. It certainly gave increased impetus to the demand for evidence of what works, based on proven effectiveness, and factual data on cost efficiency of service delivery relative to targeted goals and outcomes, as critical factors in determining priorities for strategic planning and the allocation of resources.

In the last decade, however, there has been increased questioning of this position from ethicists and from professional bodies such as the British Medical Association (BMA). There are two broad arguments for the moral limits of markets. First, markets do not necessarily produce just or equitable results. A classic example of unequal markets is given by Titmuss (1992). He argues that commercialising the blood supply in America meant that more blood came into the healthcare system from those in economic hardship. One of the primary effects of this was a redistribution of blood 'from the poor to the rich' (Titmuss 1992, p. 31). The primacy of making a profit leads to a skewed market, not a free market. One BMA (2017) paper notes further arguments, including:

- The possibility of markets to fragment care pathways and to destabilise, through possible economic failure, local health economies
- The need for commercial organisations to maximise profitability will entail money being taken out of the health economy that could have been used for patient care
- Commercial organisations will always experience conflicts between obligations to shareholders and obligations to promote the best interests of patients. The core of this argument is that the primary concern of business is to make profits (explicitly spelled out in Friedman (1983)).
- The possibility that commercial organisations will cherry-pick the easier and more profitable areas of care, resulting in a 'two-tier' health service
- The lack of obligation on commercial organisations to participate in education and training to the detriment of the medical work force and patient care
- It leads to questions about the primacy of 'patient-choice' because it fails to give patients the choices they most value. In any case, patients were most likely to choose local access to good quality care from a known and trusted NHS provider.
- The administrative and transaction costs of developing internal markets and competitive tendering take huge resources away from patient care. In the UK and globally, there is little evidence that costs are contained or reduced through market mechanisms.

A good example of the lack of long-term commitment by the private sector is the case of Hinchingbrooke Hospital.

10.1 PAUSE FOR THOUGHT

The Hinchingbrooke Hospital

In November 2011, Hinchingbrooke Hospital in Cambridgeshire was taken over by a private company, Circle Health. Not long into the contract, reports suggested that Circle was facing finance problems and had not been able to make the cost savings anticipated. Such companies have other obligations, to ensure that their services are translated into profits and this, arguably, can create a conflict of interest for such organisations that could threaten patient care. This concern was realised at Hinchingbrooke when it was rated as 'inadequate' in 2014 by the Care Quality Commission (CQC) (who inspect health and social care to ensure appropriate standards), and the hospital was put on 'special measures': 'The inspection highlighted serious concerns and CQC has told the trust it must improve'. In January 2015, Circle Holdings announced that it would end the contract to run the hospital, citing problems with funding cuts and increased demand for accident and emergency services. While all these pressures are recognised, unlike publicly owned hospitals, private companies have the option to walk away from these difficult situations – under the terms of the 10-year contract, it could be ended once they had invested a specific amount of money (£5 million), a form of 'get out' clause (although reports suggest it has to date spent slightly less than this figure – £4.84m). When healthcare provision is owned and run by the NHS, these fluctuations can be weathered and continuity in organisation and patient care maintained (BMA 2017).

A further argument about the moral limits of markets is that the use of market logic and practice can degrade the value of a good. Sandel (2013, p. 125) argues 'it is about the corrosive tendency of markets. Putting a price on the good things in life can corrupt them. That's because markets don't only allocate goods; they also express and promote certain attitudes toward the goods being exchanged…Economists often assume that markets are inert, that they do not affect the goods they exchange. But this is untrue. Markets leave their mark. Sometimes, market values crowd out nonmarket values worth caring about'.

The corruption of these goods can happen in two ways. Firstly, it sets up a self-contradiction. Certain goods, such as friendship or care, cannot, by definition, be purchased. You cannot buy friendship. Secondly, the market is not neutral, it expresses a view of the value of goods as merchandise. However, not all goods can be valued meaningfully on the open market. At one extreme, we cannot buy or sell people, or social goods such as voting rights (Sandel 2013). Some goods are to do with the well-being of the person. Titmuss (1992) develops such arguments in the *Gift Relationship*, focusing on the example of blood donorship. Blood donation is a symbol of shared relationship of care, not a commodity. There is, in other words, a social good in the donation of blood (Titmuss 1992, p. 31). The commercialisation of the blood supply undermined what Titmuss called 'the gift relationship', replacing bonds of solidarity with commercial exchange, and 'the market values that suffuse the system exert a corrosive effect on the norm of giving' (Sandel 2013; Titmuss 1992).

But what is this norm of giving? Do we all focus on the practice of gift giving? Titmuss tries to give an empirical answer to this. He points to sociologists such as Lévi-Strauss (1971) who offer evidence of some cultures which are focused on the bonds of care, where society is kept together through these. For Titmuss, then, this is a social good, and one that needs to be sustained through shared practice. There are problems with that kind of argument. First, the examples set forward by Lévi-Strauss and others may be true for certain communities, but it is not certain that they apply to all. The history of the developed West is much more complex, with rival views of what constitutes society and how it is held together. The second problem is that Titmuss focuses on altruism as the key to the social bond. This is a major ethical idea that it is important to focus on, the good of the other. Titmuss refers to altruism in this contest as 'ultra obligation', going beyond concern for the self. He even argues that true altruism does not draw attention to the giver, hence the giver should be anonymous. This is reinforced by the focus on organ donation. However, the danger of altruism as a social norm is that it could lead to a sense of coercion of the donor, when the core dynamic of donation is freedom to decide.

Arrow (1963), in arguing for a market, accepts the importance of altruism, but argues that the market does not prevent gift giving. On the contrary, altruism can be practised within the context of the market. Novak (1993) writes of the freedom to do one's duty, in the context of a market. Arrow, of course, sees the choice of altruism as purely an individual exercise. Titmuss, on the other hand, is asking a different question, not are there any constraints to altruism, and not how can we increase individual choice, but rather what kind of country do we want? In this respect, he sees altruism as something that needs to be developed and encouraged, that is, fostered. This suggests an important development of Titmuss's view on altruism. His vision is not of a welfare state but rather a welfare society. A welfare society is less about individual altruism and more about a sense of shared responsibility for health and the practice of mutual care. The health service then becomes a symbol of that. In broader terms, this focuses on cooperation rather than competition as the basis of healthcare provision.

Of course, the debate does not have to be between absolute altruism on the one hand and the market on the other. The provision of medical and nursing care is not just a commercial transaction like that with any other service industry. The relationship between the contracting parties is an inherently unequal and asymmetrical one in power terms. The vulnerability and dependence of the patient demands a quality of trustworthy expertise and responsibility on the part of the health professional which is unique to human services – because people's lives and health are at stake. Furthermore, the 'internal economy' was not an example of a free market, because the budgets made available to health authorities or hospital trusts were limited by government and subject to its regulation, and the relationship between 'purchasers' and 'providers' in the health sector bore little resemblance to that between manufacturers, suppliers and retailers in the wider business economy.

This suggests that the primacy of professional values and objectives is key to any just distribution. Like the example of the AAGG in public health, the focus should be on integrated services, shared responsibility and on core purpose rather than simply funding issues. This does not take from the importance of focusing on funding but looks also to find ways of developing and refining integrated practice at the appropriate level. Sandel (2013), focusing on democracy and dialogue, argues that the development of the market mechanism has been one of stealth, with most debate going on in government. The result was that there has never been a genuine democratic debate across the country, and thus about what people actually wanted. The practice of citizens' assembly would well suit this (https://www.citizensassembly.ie/en/).

In all of this, the mixed economy of healthcare provision has been a mixed blessing for nursing. On the one hand, the competitive environment has encouraged the private sector to poach nurses from the state hospitals, and nursing agencies have been able to offer nurses the inducements of improved flexibility and better pay and working conditions (which have been particularly attractive to nurses with family commitments). In primary care, nurses have been given increased responsibility for a lot of work previously done in hospitals, for example, screening and treatment of diabetes, asthma and cardiovascular disease. This has created opportunities for new career paths for nurses on the primary care team, including the roles of practice nurses, treatment room nurses, nurse practitioners, besides expansion in the role of district nurses, health visitors and midwives. The debate will not go away, and the challenge for ethical imagination and strategic creativity is there in the dialogue and debate about the UK Health and Social Care Act 2012.

Health and Social Care Act 2012

The legislation aimed to extend the market mechanism more than ever before and increase privatisation. It changed the commissioning of healthcare through creating a national NHS Commissioning Board, NHS England, which would oversee clinical commissioning groups. These groups are now responsible for commissioning services for their local populations, replacing Primary Care Trusts and Strategic Health Authorities. These were, first, to give more local control and, second, to be more sensitive to market mechanisms. The first of these is based on the principle of subsidiarity, giving responsibility and with that freedom, to local groups. In turn, this would provide more choice (freedom) for the patient. The second was seen as essential in dealing effectively with local complexities and finding the best entrepreneurial practice. Key to this was to stimulate competition between the different providers. Hence the Act sought to encourage organisations outside the NHS to bid for services previously offered by the NHS, enabling patients to choose from different sectors: commercial, third sector and the NHS.

With responsibility focused locally, the Act also abolished the secretary of state for health's duty to provide comprehensive health services throughout England and Wales, replacing it with a duty to exercise other functions to secure provision. How is this to be judged? Some argue that this is driven by the neoliberal vision noted above, focused on rolling back the state and thus the beginning of the end of the idea of a national health service (Hunter 2013). Others argue that the health service has always had some degree of a mixed economy, with provision outside the service itself, and this change simply makes the most of that mixed economy, ensuring that responsibility for the service is genuinely shared (Frith 2016). In this view, the Act liberates all aspects of a national health service. Critical to this had to be the development of an integrated service, one which had to ensure better accountability and regulation, with Monitor (now part of NHS Improvement) of the NHS Commissioning Board (now NHS England).

The 2012 Act came a year before the Francis Enquiry (2013) which, as noted above argued, advised against any further attempts to change the way in which the health service was run. Such changes can both lead to loss of key narratives about purpose and organisational memory (Robinson 2016) and a focus on narrow and short-term ends (Francis 2013). Hence, there has been no rush to change the Act. Nonetheless, questions have been raised about it by both the then prime minster and the secretary of state for health and NHS England, arguing for more integrated care given the challenge of an ageing population that includes people with chronic conditions (Charles et al. 2018).

CRITICISMS

This has been extended to several criticisms which echo previous debates. First, the division of the service between the commissioning side (NHS England) and the provider side (NHS Improvement) sets in stone duties which are conflictual. In this, the focus on competition makes it more, not less, difficult to integrate. This raises questions about whether competition, *per se*, can be the most effective driver of change. Second, many trusts have experienced what they have perceived as conflicting instructions and expectations from the different parts of the regulatory structure. For instance, NHS Improvement have encouraged trusts to increase their workload to balance their finances, at the same time as being asked to help restrict unnecessary admissions and ensuring they are located in better settings. This sets out the stark financial responsibility alongside a responsibility for implementing a broader policy which improves integrated care, possibly having to move some services outside hospital whilst rationalising others within that sector.

At the heart of this is the conflicting imperatives of market and care; competition *and* cooperation. Providers may see the sense in other areas providing some of their work, thus contributing to greater integration. However, a clear risk in this would be to undermine their own finances. Balancing their books is their statutory responsibility, and opens them up to be accountable for any failures. Third, in addition to the expectations of regulation, there are increased demands for information from different groups, including Clinical Commissioning Groups (CCGs), commissioning support units, urgent care networks, local accident and emergency delivery boards, and any other local arrangements set up, for instance, to monitor waiting-time performance. Information is also required from the CQC, the inspector and regulator of quality and safety and others. It is not surprising that this has led to an increase in bureaucracy.

Fourth, the rules of procurement have led to a proliferation of contracts being put out for tender, leading to further expense and delay. It is not clear whether this is because the commissioning bodies are fearful of getting the process wrong and are thus working through the detail (not least in reflecting European law), or whether the increase of lawyers for the contract is increasing the burden. Fifth, the attempts to create better integration in the system have proved unsuccessful. The core means to this in the Act was the creation of 44 sustainability and transformation plans, which would then evolve into sustainability and transformation partnerships (STPs). These would lead to the integrated care system, and would be negotiated locally. However, the very fact that these will vary around the country raises questions about the equality of provision (Charles et al. 2018). Hence there has been limited development. Perhaps the challenge for these bodies is that they have no legal status or formal constitution. Without a budget, they have no formal accountability. All they can do is to persuade those involved to develop integrated care. Even when organisations do wish to co-operate, either by farming out services or merging their activities, there are limitations on how far NHS organisations can delegate their powers to create such an integrated system.

RESPONSES

These have broadly fallen into two types: changes to the system, or work through the issues about integration over time under the present Act. Two examples of the first are the House of Commons Health and Social Care Select Committee recommendations (Health and Social Care

Committee 2018), and from the Institute for Public Policy Research, with proposed legislation from Lord Darzi (Darzi et al. 2018). The Select Committee argued for:

- A statutory basis for system-wide partnerships between local organisations
- The potential to designate accountable care organisations (otherwise known as integrated care providers) as NHS bodies, if they are introduced more widely
- Changes to legislation covering procurement and competition
- The merger of NHS England and NHS Improvement
- Changes to the CQC's powers.

Lord Darzi's review went further, recommending:

- The creation of a single NHS headquarters through the merger of NHS England, NHS Improvement, Health Education England and Public Health England
- The creation of around 10 regional health and care authorities that could replace the STPs, the 195 CCGs, and the 7 regional organisations of NHS Improvement and NHS England
- The ending of compulsory competitive tendering for frontline services, with the health and care authorities (and NHS and care providers) able to commission services from any provider, but with this clearly becoming an option, rather than, as at present, it often being seen as a requirement.

These would point to major legislative changes, and further disruptions. The other option is simply to develop change within the present Act, through ministerial discretion and ongoing deliberation. The then UK health secretary, Jeremy Hunt, for instance, merged Monitor and the Trust Development Authority into NHS Improvement. This was achieved through 'a legal workaround', with both having the same chief executive and chair, while still technically operating with separate boards and producing separate accounts. In effect, this involves leadership at the national and local level taking responsibility for focusing on the core purpose of the organisation. The issue of over-assurance (too many demands for too much information in too many different ways) demands a focus on more integrated reporting and smart dialogue, without having to change legislation. Excessive tendering and procurement is partly to do with a culture of negative responsibility and the fear of reprisals if rules are not followed. This also raises questions about ensuring clear communication and dialogue.

It is clear from the ongoing debate that there can be no simple system that can have the effect of permanence that the original Secretary of State for Health, Andrew Lansley, strove for. Any system needs to have ongoing critical reflection locally and nationally, and be encouraging responsibility at all levels and amongst all stakeholders, including patients, involving clarity about purpose, value and objectives of health care services, mutual accountability and shared responsibility for ongoing learning and developments. In line with this thinking, Gilbert et al. (2014) argue for a values-explicit approach that uses values as a means of regulating market forces. This means placing purpose and ends of care before means. As the AAGG case showed, putting this first led to better learning and more creative practice.

In some respects, this process is already underway in the UK with the NHS Constitution. Lord Darzi's review of the NHS in 2008 recommended that the NHS should make explicit its values and commitments to patients, and this should be enshrined in a Constitution: 'establish[ing] the principles and values of the NHS in England. [The Constitution] sets out rights to which patients, public and staff are entitled, and pledges which the NHS is committed to achieve, together with responsibilities which the public, patients and staff owe to one another to ensure that the NHS operates fairly and effectively' (Gilbert et al. 2014). The context for this is summed up by this statement from the NHS Institute for Innovation and Improvement: 'As our healthcare system becomes increasingly devolved, autonomous and entrepreneurial, there is a need for system-wide values, which reaffirm the social purpose of the NHS, to staff, patients and the public and inspire behaviours that put the needs of patients, staff and the public foremost in people's minds' (quoted in Frith 2015, p. 3). The Health Act 2009 (http://www.legislation.gov.uk/ukpga/2009/21/contents)

stipulated that all bodies providing NHS services (NHS, private and third sector providers) must 'have regard' to the Constitution in all their actions and decisions. The Constitution was updated in 2013, part of a drive to make organisations and patients more aware of the Constitution so that it can be used in deliberation at all levels. The Constitution spells out rights and responsibilities and the core character of the National Health Service, involving inclusive care and belonging to everyone.

10.2 PAUSE FOR THOUGHT

Constitutional matters – NHS Constitution 2019 (https://www.gov.uk/government/publications/supplements-to-the-nhs-constitution-for-england)

How often was the Constitution referred to in your professional training?

Do you think the character of the NHS is sufficiently developed in the document? Critically reflect on the lists of rights and responsibilities. Do they link effectively into the core purpose and principles?

How far are these actively focused on relationships with patients?

Are they brought as part of patient-centred decision making?

How would you develop the Constitution?

Frith (2015) questions how useful the Constitution is in practice, not least because it is not clear if the body which ensures healthcare providers will adhere to these values. The Constitution sets out rights of patients and responsibilities of providers, including pledges (non-legally binding 'goals') that independent organisations should have regard to, for example, that all employees should have rewarding jobs. The 2012 Health Act includes a provision that CCGs must have regard to the Constitution, stating that they will be held to account by NHS England for this. In practice, however, it is not clear what this means or how it can be achieved. The second suggestion of Gilbert et al. (2014) was to have a systems theory approach to the NHS. They suggest that the Principles and Rules for Cooperation and Competition could 'strike a balance between the benefits of co-operation and competition' (Gilbert et al. 2014, p. 5). In ethical terms, this involves two very different views of responsibility. Rules about competition seem to focus on negative responsibility, and the fear of not getting an action 'right'. The drive to integrate services and planning demands the practice of moral imagination, to develop creative approaches to service delivery which engage all stakeholders. This approach thrives on difference, dialogue and shared responsibility. Different perspectives provide challenge and ideas, whilst shared responsibility and dialogue provide commitment to core purpose and value, and the development of learning organisations.

The ethical and strategic question is which of these approaches will enable the practice of responsibility. Frith (2015), Gilbert et al. (2014), and others argue that the market focus is too narrow, and that it cannot drive the move to integrated services. Seddon (2014) additionally offers four arguments, that:

- The political focus on 'value for money' both narrows the accountability of politicians and leads to a form of teleopathy (see Chapter 1). Politicians are not simply accountable for the financing of the NHS, but also for maintaining the core character and purpose of the organisation.
- The focus on cutting costs often leads to the unintentional consequence of additional costs, citing the example of NHS call centres put in as a means of cutting costs, but actually leading to increased costs through an increase in A&E/ED patients
- The focus on targets encourages negative responsibility, leading to a climate of fear
- Focusing on care and integration of care is, in fact, the best way of achieving financial targets. This suggests the same dynamic as the AAGG, with funding to follow integration. The 'regulatory' framework then becomes focused at all levels on enabling and empowerment. As noted above, this also focuses on the motivations of agency, pathways and purpose, all connected to the value of the core purpose.

TABLE 10.1 ■ **Four Proposed Quality Indicators for the Creation of an Enabling Environment**

1. State how you will instruct, support and nurture all your staff to provide relationship-based person-centred medicine and person-centred healthcare.
2. Indicate how and when you will provide supervision from experienced mentors for all your staff.
3. Give details of the educational methods you will use to train all your staff in counselling and listening skills and compassionate empathy. Describe your strategy for Continuing Professional Development in person-centred care and state how and by whom this will be implemented.
4. Indicate how you will identify and support role models for the provision of person-centred healthcare and the implementation of a culture of intelligent kindness.

We may add to these the arguments that the trend towards metrics and 'league tables' places an emphasis on competition, not cooperation, that they lead to unrealistic expectations, and that the exposure of hospitals and health practitioners to public scrutiny and negative criticism simply increases staff stress, without addressing adequate criteria of care. Such arguments suggest that the focus of integration should be integrity, as with the AAGG example above. Integrity in this case demands that the core purpose is embodied in practice, in effect practising *phronesis*. This demands the development of reflective deliberation and learning at every level. Cox (2015) and Campling (2015) also argue that this takes us back to the principles, focused on compassion. This suggests that professional ethics, organisational ethics and social ethics should be focused on exactly the same principles and responsible practice. Cox and Gray (2015, p. 2) go further to suggest specific quality indicators (see Table 10.1).

Resource Allocation: Rationing

Other ongoing ethical questions include resource allocation and rationing in the public domain. As Edwards et al. (2015) note, rationing takes place whether we like it or not. There is a fixed budget and a need to prioritise funding. Use of the term rationing is often thought as problematic, based on the assumption that rationing involves a failure to provide a comprehensive service. In fact, there is good evidence that the public acknowledge that a 'comprehensive service' is not the same as a service that can solve all medical problems (Vize 2015; Maybin and Klein 2012). The dilemmas in resource allocation in healthcare management are of several kinds: practical dilemmas (about the use of resources), ethical dilemmas (handling conflicting principles) and policy dilemmas (summed up in the debate above). While we can distinguish these formally, it should be remembered, as we said in the book's introduction, that because all decisions we make in healthcare impact on people's quality of life, this means that no aspect of healthcare is morally 'neutral'. The ethics of resource allocation is not restricted to debate about issues like the expenditure of money on life-saving medical or surgical procedures for a small number of patients, or about equal rights of access to scarce high-technology equipment such as whole-body scanners or kidney dialysis machines. It refers also to expenditure on staff salaries, to the cost of building and equipping new hospitals or rebuilding and refurbishing old hospitals, to the cost of medical research, expenditure on drugs and disposable medical supplies, and on such homely things as furniture, fittings, decor and the quality of hospital food and how these are to be funded (e.g. by direct local fundraising, by 'public/private funding initiatives', or by the state).

Hence, the making of public health policy about these issues cannot be the exclusive preserve of doctors or bureaucrats, politicians or any particular class of 'experts'. Nurses not only have the same right to participate in public debate about these issues as any other citizens, but they also have a responsibility to do so, in view of their own front-line experience, professional expertise and academic excellence. In governance terms, they are key stakeholders, and should be involved in shared deliberation. Although less dramatic as resource issues than the challenges of transplants, in vitro fertilisation (IVF) or applications of genetic engineering or cloning to medicine, the issues of shortages of staff and equipment are likely to make a more direct impact on the morale and working conditions of nurses and other healthcare workers, and have direct relevance to the debate on the use of resources.

Some classic areas of ethical controversy about resource allocation which arise in clinical practice for nurses as well as doctors are, for example: the impact of staff shortages on the standards of care; the shortage of equipment for routine scanning leading to long delays for patients on waiting lists; the limited number of kidney dialysis machines relative to those needing urgent treatment while awaiting transplants; the limited number of organ donors relative to the need for liver, kidney and heart transplants; the ethical problems related to surrogacy or egg donation; the treatment of infertile couples by expensive and risky IVF; the justifiability of life-saving surgery for neonates who have severe disabilities, with possible long-term need for intensive care and the use of NHS facilities for cosmetic surgery, breast implants and invasive procedures such as liposuction and excision of fat to reduce obesity. Hard choices have to be made. The questions are, how are such choices to be made and who will make them? The underlying social ethical principle of the NHS is equality. To some degree, this is unconditional, at least in terms of treatment not being conditional upon payment, that is, free at the point of treatment. Equality also involves equality of respect; in effect, the principle of respect for persons and personal choice. This is not the same as equal resources given to every patient. The problems of each patient are different and thus 'equal attention' actually means appropriate attention, dependent on the need (Tawney 1930).

The principle of equality soon moves to the principle of justice, specifically justice as fairness. One audit (Fertility Fairness 2018) revealed that 87% of England's 195 CCGs failed to provide three full cycles of IVF treatment in line with the NICE guidelines. These guidelines also recommend that treatment should be available to the age of 40, and the audit found women over the age of 34 were refused IVF treatment on the NHS in 12 areas of England. Such examples suggest that regional decisions are skewing justice – treatment depends on post codes. At the very least, this suggests that there needs to be transparency about principles. Rumbold et al. (2012) argue that establishing such principles 'can shape how public money is spent in the NHS and, conversely, inform decisions about what will no longer be paid for'. They suggest principles such as clinical effectiveness, cost-effectiveness and equity. In ethical terms, the principle of equity needs to be given more weight for two reasons. First, it focuses on the principle of fairness/justice. Second, the principle of fairness, as noted in Chapter 2, is not simply about a cognitive principle. It focuses on relationships, in this case between the person and wider society and the health service, and thus upon the affective value of that relationship. Rumbold et al. (2012) suggest that the principles could be enshrined in the NHS Constitution and restated annually to remind NHS commissioners of what should underpin their decision making about resources and services. Hence, we are brought back to a shared focus on principles and transparent deliberation and accountability. Transparency about procedural fairness needs to be in place at national and regional levels. NICE does important work on:

- the use of health technologies within the NHS (appraising of new and existing medicines, treatments and procedures)
- clinical practice (guidance on the appropriate treatment and care of people with specific diseases and conditions)
- guidance for public sector workers on health promotion and ill health avoidance
- guidance for social care services and users.

However, the process of largely non-binding guidance from NICE and local autonomy is not transparent. Hence, CCGs are not fully accountable for their decisions on rationing. A careful balance is needed to ensure consistency at the national and CCG levels. This means that NICE has to give a clear account to justify their guidelines in relation to all the principles, and that CCGs also demonstrate to their stakeholders their method of deliberation about the rationing. This demands critical engagement with stakeholders in deliberation about rationing, that is, genuine dialogue and democracy. In that light, patients become involved in stating and accepting what the limitations of the service are. Klein and Maybin (2015) argue that this approach leads to both more effective and more ethical care.

Conclusion

This chapter has examined the ethics of public health and the social ethics of healthcare. The same principles examined in professional and organisational ethics inform both of these areas, with all levels of the healthcare project taking responsibility for the practice of care. Responsibility for care requires transparency, articulation of core purpose and value, critical dialogue and deliberation and shared development of practice.

References

Arrow, K. (1963). Uncertainty and the welfare economics of medical care. *The American Economic Review*, *53*(5), 941–973.

Berlin, I. (1969). Two concepts of liberty. In A. Quinton (Ed.), *Political philosophy* (pp. 141–155). London: Penguin.

Bevan, A. (1948). *Speech to the Executive Councils Association 7 October 1948*. Online available: Online avaiable: https://www.sochealth.co.uk/national-health-service/the-sma-and-the-foundation-of-the-national-health-service-dr-leslie-hilliard-1980/aneurin-bevan-and-the-foundation-of-the-nhs/bevans-speech-to-the-executive-councils-association-7-october-1948/.

Beveridge, W. (1942). *Social insurance and allied services*. London: HMSO.

Beauchamp, D., & Steinbock, B. (1999). *New ethics for the public's health*. Oxford: Oxford University Press.

British Medical Association. (2017). *The ethical implications of the use of market-type mechanisms in the delivery of NHS care*. London: British Medical Association.

Campbell, A., & Swift, T. (2002). What does it mean to be a virtuous patient? *Scottish Journal of Healthcare Chaplaincy*, *5*(1), 39–45.

Campling, P. (2015). Reforming the culture of healthcare: the case for intelligent kindness. *BJPsych Bulletin*, *39*(1), 1–5.

Cancer Research UK. (2019). *Obese people outnumber smokers two to one*. London: Cancer Research UK. Online available: https://www.cancerresearchuk.org/about-us/cancer-news/press-release/2019-07-03-obese-people-outnumber-smokers-two-to-one.

Chadwick, R., & Gallagher, A. (2013). *Nursing ethics*. London: Palgrave.

Charles, A., Wenzel, L., Kershaw, M., Ham, C., & Walsh, N. (2018). *A year of integrated care systems: reviewing the journey so far*. London: The Kings Fund. Online available: https://www.kingsfund.org.uk/publications/year-integrated-care-systems.

Cox, J. (2015). NHS values, compassion and quality indicators for relationship based person-centred healthcare: comment on "morality and markets in the NHS". *International Journal of Health Policy and Management*, *4*(6), 407.

Cox, J. L., & Gray, A. (2015). NHS at the Hustings: four quality indicators for a person-centred medicine. *European Journal for Person Centered Healthcare*, *3*, 1–3.

Darzi, A., Quilter-Pinner, H., & Kibasi, T. (2018). *Better health and care for all: a 10-point plan for the 2020s*. London: Institute for Public Policy Research – IPPR.

Department of Health and Social Security (DHSS). (1980). *Report of the Working Group on Inequalities in Health (Black Report)*. London: Department of Health and Social Security.

Duncan, P., & Jowit, J. (2018). *Is the NHS the world's best system?* London: The Guardian. Online available: https://www.theguardian.com/society/2018/jul/02/is-the-nhs-the-worlds-best-healthcare-system, 2 July.

Edwards, N., Crump, H., & Dayan, M. (2015). *Rationing in the NHS*. London: Nuffield Trust.

Enthoven, A. (1985). *Reflections on the management of the National Health Service*. London: Nuffield Trust.

Health and Social Care Committee. (2018). *Integrated care: organisations, partnerships and systems. Seventh Report of Session 2017–2019*. London: House of Commons Health and Social Care Committee.

Fertility Fairness. (2018). *Fertility fairness.* London: Progress Educational Trust. Online available: http://www.fertilityfairness.co.uk/.

Francis Report. (2013). *The Mid Staffordshire Foundation Trust Public Enquiry.* London: The Stationery Office. Online available: http://www.midstaffspublicinquiry.com/.

Friedman, M. (1983). The social responsibility of business is to increase its profits. In T. Donaldson, & P. Werhane (Eds.), *Ethical issues in business* (pp. 239–243). New York: Prentice-Hall.

Frith, L. (2015). The changing national health service: market-based reform and morality; comment on "morality and markets in the NHS. *International Journal of Health Policy and Management, 4*(4), 253–255.

Frith, L. (2016). The changing face of the English National Health Service: new providers, markets and morality. *British Medical Bulletin, 119*(1), 5–16.

Gilbert, B., Clarke, E., & Leaver, L. (2014). Morality and markets in the NHS. *International Journal of Health Policy and Management, 3*(7), 371–376.

Griffiths Report. (1983). *NHS management inquiry.* London: Department of Health and Social Security. Online available: https://navigator.health.org.uk/theme/griffiths-report-management-nhs

Habermas, J. (1992). *Moral consciousness and communicative action.* London: Polity.

Hafez, N., & Ling, P. (2005). How Philip Morris built Marlboro into a global brand for young adults: implications for international tobacco control. *Tobacco Control, 14*(4), 262–271.

Harrison, M. (2004). *Implementing change in health systems.* London: Sage.

Harrison, S., & Pollitt, C. (1994). *Controlling health professionals.* Buckingham: Open University.

Häyry, H. (1991). *The limits of medical paternalism.* London: Routledge.

Hawkes, C., & Halliday, J. (2017). What makes urban food policy happen: insights from five case studies. *International Panel of Experts on Sustainable Food Systems.* Online available: https://openaccess.city.ac.uk/id/eprint/19325/1/.

Hawkes, C., Russell, S., Isaacs, A., Rutter, H., Viner, R. (2017). Rapid response briefing paper 1: what can be learned from the Amsterdam Healthy Weight Programme to inform the policy response to obesity in England. *Obesity Policy Research Unit,* (OPRU). Health and Social Care Act 2012. http://www.legislation.gov.uk/ukpga/2012/7/contents/enacted.

Honigsbaum, F. (1995). *Priority setting processes for health care in Oregon USA; New Zealand; the Netherlands; Sweden and the UK.* Oxford: Radcliffe Medical Press.

Hunter, D. J. (2013). A response to Rudolf Klein: a battle may have been won but perhaps not the war. *Journal of Health Politics, Policy and Law, 38*(4), 871–877.

Illsley, R., & Svensson, P. (1984). *The health burden of social inequalities.* Copenhagen: WHO.

Klein, R., & Maybin, J. (2015). *Thinking about rationing.* London: Kings Fund.

Lévi-Strauss, C. (1971). *Elementary structures of kinship.* New York: Beacon Press.

MacDonald, M. (2015). *Introduction to public health ethics 2: philosophical and theoretical foundations.* Quebec: Institute National de Sante Publique.

Maybin, J., & Klein, R. (2012). *Thinking about rationing.* London: Kings Fund.

Miller, A., Lumenga, J., & LeBourgeois, K. (2015). Sleep patterns and obesity in childhood. *Current Opinion Endocrinol Diabetes Obesity, 22*(1), 41–47.

National Health Service. (2019). *National Health Service Constitution.* London: HMSO. Online available: https://www.gov.uk/government/publications/supplements-to-the-nhs-constitution-for-england.

National Institute for Health and Care Excellence. (2014). Identification, assessment and management of overweight and obesity in children, young people and adults. (Clinical Guideline 189). London: National Institute for Health and Care Excellence. www.nice.org.uk/guidance/cg189.

Novak, M. (1993). *The Catholic ethic and the spirit of capitalism.* New York: The Free Press.

Nursi, S. (1992). Cited in Şükran Vahide, *Bediuzzaman Said Nursi,* Istanbul, p. 95.

Plummer, J. (2019). *Cancer research UK defends harmful and misleading campaign.* Third Sector. Online available: https://www.thirdsector.co.uk/cancer-research-uk-defends-harmful-misleading-obesity-campaign/communications/article/1590155. 05 July.

Ricoeur, P. (2000). *The concept of responsibility: an essay in semantic analysis in The Just. Translated by Pellauer.* D. Chicago: The University of Chicago Press.

Robinson, S., & Kenyon, A. (2009). *Ethics and the alcohol industry.* London: MacMilllan.

Robinson, S. (2016). *The practice of integrity in business.* London: MacMillan.

Rudolf, M., Perera, R., Swanston, D., Burbery, J., Roberts, K., & Jebb, S. (2019). Observational analysis of disparities in obesity in children in the UK: Has Leeds bucked the trend? Pediatric Obesity. *14*(9): e12529.

Rumbold, B., Alakeson, V., & Smith, P. (2012). *Rationing health care*. London: Nuffield Trust.

Swierstra, T. (2011). Behavior, environment or body. Three discourses on obesity. In M. Korthals (Ed.), *Genomics, obesity and the struggle over responsibilities* (pp. 27–38). Dordrecht: Springer.

Sandel, M. (2013). *What money can't buy: the moral limits of markets*. London: Penguin.

Seddon, J. (2014). *The Whitehall effect*. London: Triarchy Press.

Tawney, R. H. (1930). *Equality*. London: Allen and Unwin.

ten Have, M., De Beaufort, I. D., Teixeira, P. J., Mackenbach, J. P., & van der Heide, A. (2011). Ethics and prevention of overweight and obesity: an inventory. *Obesity Reviews*, *12*(9), 669–679.

Thomas, L. (2019). *An Open Letter to Cancer Research UK*. Online available: https://medium.com/@laura_86024/an-open-letter-to-cancer-research-uk-19ecaa71b263.

Thompson, I., Melia, K., Boyd, K., & Horsburgh, D. (2006). *Nursing Ethics*. Fifth edition. Edinburgh: Churchill Livingstone.

Titmuss, R. (1992). *The gift relationship*. London: Penguin.

United Nations. (1993). *United Nations Development Programme Human Development Report*. United Nations.

Vize, R. (2015). *Rationing is a fact of life for the NHS*. London: The Guardian. Online available: https://www.theguardian.com/healthcare-network/2015/apr/24/rationing-care-fact-of-life-nhs. 24 April.

Wanless, D. (2004). *Securing good health for the whole population*. London: HMSO.

Wempe, J., & Frooman, J. (2018). Reframing the moral limits of markets debate: social domains, values, allocation methods. *Journal of Business Ethics*, *153*(1), 1–15.

World Health Organisation. (2019). *Progress towards SDGs*. Geneva: World Health Organisation. Online available: https://www.un.org/sustainabledevelopment/progress-report/.

World Health Organisation. (2017). *Ending childhood obesity*. Geneva: World Health Organisation.

World Health Organisation. (1986). *The Ottawa charter for health promotion*. Geneva: World Health Organisation. Online available: https://www.who.int/healthpromotion/conferences/previous/ottawa/en/.

Wilkinson, R. (1996). *Unhealthy societies: the affliction of inequalities*. London: Routledge.

World Bank. (1993). *Investing in health*. Oxford: Oxford University Press.

Normative Ethics

LEARNING OUTCOMES

When you have read and worked through this chapter, you should be able to make a:

- Description, analysis and critique of rational theories of ethics
- Description, analysis and critique of non-rational theories of ethics
- Description, analysis and critique underlying cultural worldviews that influence how we see the good
- Description, analysis and critique of the use of religion in ethics
- Development of an ethics of care in nursing which will include all the different elements of normative theory

Introduction

As noted in the first part of the book, there are two different kinds of theory in ethics, descriptive and normative. The first looks to explain how we practice ethics. The second seeks to provide the basis for morality, for judging something to be right or wrong. Most of us tend to switch off at the mention of the word theory. As we noted in the first chapter, theory is often associated with abstract thinking and thus is seen as the opposite of practice. Properly understood, however, **theory is about providing meaning to experience or practice**. Scientific theories seek to provide convincing explanations about physical phenomena. The theory of evolution, for instance, seeks to explain how the animal world has developed. Such is its status that it has now become accepted by most scientists as fact (Dawkins 2010). Like any theory, however, it is conceivable that it could be disproved.

We began with descriptive theories of ethics because we wanted to focus on practice and how we do ethics. The danger of beginning with normative theories is that we can try to simply apply theory directly to practice, without full attention to the situation and with a concern more for justifying theory than informing practice. This chapter will focus on normative theories and how they explain ethical meaning and can inform practice. The West has been dominated by two rationalist theories, utilitarian and deontological. Strictly speaking, these are not discrete theories but rather two theoretical schools that have had different expressions down the history of ethics. For our purposes, we will sum up the major elements and critiques of these theories. We will then examine the so-called non-rational theories, in particular virtue ethics. We will also critically examine underlying worldviews that inform our idea of what is good, including cultural and religious views of ethics. This will bring us back to virtue ethics and, in particular, to the basis of nursing, compassion and an ethics based in care. We will begin with a case of a medical emergency *in extremis,* close to the peak of Everest.

Everest Emergency

In 2006, David Sharp returned to Everest, determined to conquer it. In 2003 and 2004, he had been part of unsuccessful attempts. The extent of Sharp's determination can be gauged by the fact that he lost several toes in his first attempt. The story of what happened to him in 2006 involves some speculation. It is believed that he did reach the top, climbing by himself and with a limited supply of oxygen. During the descent he ran out of oxygen, and eventually died from exhaustion and cold, whilst sheltering beneath a small outcrop on the crest of the northeast ridge. Sharp had collapsed while he was still clipped on to a fixed line used by climbers on that route, and he was just 3 feet from it. Before he died, as many as 40 people passed by him. Most of these were members of two climbing teams from Himex, a company specialising in mountain ascents, and a following Turkish team. A few members of these teams did stop to ascertain his condition, and to attempt either to comfort him or help him in some way. Reports suggest that the first ones to do this stopped on their descent. Some, in their ascent, claimed not have seen him, in some cases because of the effects of altitude. With the encumbrances of climbing gear and goggles, even things close might be missed. Others suggest that they may have thought that Sharp was in fact the corpse of an Indian climber who had died there in 1996, a well-known 'feature' of the climb. It would, however, have been difficult for climbers not to realise that something was wrong given his proximity.

11.1 PAUSE FOR THOUGHT

Considering the Climb of Everest

Each of the climbers had to make a decision as they unhooked themselves from their safety line to go round Sharp, and then rehook themselves.
- What would your decision have been?
- How would you have made that decision?

- When asked to an account of your thinking and actions, how would you justify them?
- Now compare your thinking with two of your student colleagues. Are you convinced with their argument? If not, why not?
- Finally, listen to your colleagues' assessment of your arguments. Do they confirm your thoughts and feelings?
- Do they challenge your thinking in any way, and if so, how?

Response

There was international outrage about the decision to leave Sharp to die. This was best expressed by Sir Edmund Hillary, leader of the first team to climb Everest, who argued that the culture of mutual care in the climbing community was being driven out by the combination of personal ambition in a high-risk pursuit and commercialisation (for a 2003 interview with Hillary on the commercialisation of climbing Everest, see http://news.bbc.co.uk/1/hi/world/south_asia/2938596.stm).

Faced by a dying man, most of the climbers thought it was more important to get to the top of the mountain. This would see the action as a 'bystander effect', with individuals not getting involved and not asking too many questions. McCoy (1983), in a similar case, argues that this can occur when ambitions to achieve an objective are such that they cloud ethical awareness. It is also argued that the highly successful commercial organisation Himex reinforced this. It was the firm's job to ensure that its customers achieved their ambition in safety, anything else is secondary.

Some journalists argued that a rescue could have been made had the Himex teams been stopped on the way up, in other words, had the head of Himex and his team leaders chosen not to give his customers what they had paid for.

In response, Brice, owner of Himex, and his medical advisors, argued that the proper thing to do was not to rescue Sharp. His argument calculated that if he were to try to rescue him, this might put his customers at risk. He prided himself on a strong safety record, having never lost a customer. Moreover, he calculated that rescue at the point of descent would not have been feasible. In any case, given the condition of the man, a rescue attempt would have been futile, and would have put at risk up to 20 people. The response of Brice suggests that there is a difference between personal and institutional ethics. The ethical choice of the individuals faced with Sharp was direct and immediate. The choice in one respect was simple, to do what one could or to walk on by. It could be argued, then, that the role of the institutional leaders was more complex, involving responsibility for the safety of several different stakeholders, not just the one man mutely appealing for help. The response of Hillary, of course, suggests otherwise. His argument is that there is a simple choice. You either do the right thing, respond to the dying man, or you do the business thing. By definition, he suggests, business avoids doing the right thing. It is primarily concerned with making money and will do whatever it takes to achieve that. The suggestion is that business is either value neutral or that its objectives do not take account of ethical issues. Hence, the ethical issues are always secondary, something that you can attend to if you have time and resource. However, this is a false dichotomy, in that Himex also focused on ethical theory, in their case, the first of two rational theories, utilitarianism.

Utilitarian Theory

This theory suggests that we find the meaning of ethics by looking at the consequences. In particular, something is right if it maximises the good, producing the greatest good for the greatest number (Mill 1993). The greatest good is the greatest happiness. The stress in all this is the maximisation of social goods and, in particular, happiness. In the case above, Brice and his medical advisors rely heavily on this theory. The consequences of the different stakeholders were potentially several. The safety of the customers, the guides and any rescue team was at stake if a major operation was organised – the future of the firm itself, and all those who depended on it. There are two major kinds of utilitarianism, act and rule:

- Act utilitarianism focuses on the individual act which is likely to produce the most good. The case above is broadly of this type.
- Rule utilitarianism focuses on sets of rules or codes that would maximise the good. Much of public health ethics falls into this category, such as a regulation for wearing seat belts in cars. The case above does not have such specific rules. However, at various points, the debate about the case referred to the climber's code, that is a set of unwritten rules that climbers accepted (https://www.pbs.org/wgbh/pages/frontline/everest/etc/roundtable.html). This included the idea that each climber was responsible for his or her self and their group. Especially in the so-called death zone (final 1000 ft), the conditions are such that it becomes physically very difficult to offer help, or even to remain focused. The implication of this focus on responsibility is that if a climber does not take care of, for instance, his oxygen (which Sharp did not), then he should accept the responsibility of his death. Such a thought might be interpreted as a 'rule' for climbers which leads to the maximisation of the good for most people on the mountain.

DIFFICULTIES WITH UTILITARIAN THEORY

There is no doubt that consequences need to be examined in any attempt to decide what is right to do. Trying to base all ethical judgements solely on this theory, however, is problematic.

- What is the happiness that Mill argues for? He suggests that the good of happiness involves the higher, not the base pleasures. But what are the criteria for deciding what a higher pleasure is, and why is it good? In any case, who decides? The theory does not help in actually defining what is good. A higher pleasure might be defined by some as high culture, by others as survival and others as psychological well-being. This is exemplified in the case above. Candidates for happiness included the climbing groups' desire to get to the top. Should this be respected or is it a 'base' pleasure? Hillary argued that a much higher pleasure is precisely found in doing all that was possible to save Sharp. This would have required a full medical assessment. A short while after Sharp's death, an American team close to the peak of Everest came across an abandoned Australian climber (https://www.nytimes.com/2012/03/25/world/asia/lincoln-hall-australian-mountaineer-dies-at-56.html). Lincoln Hall had been left by two sherpa's for dead the night before, having suffered high-altitude cerebral oedema. Fortunately, there had been no rocks at that point to bury him. The team called off its ascent to bring the climber down. Behind Hillary's argument was the idea that avoiding responsibility for climbers could lead to an erosion of concern for the self or others.
- Any definition of happiness or good may well depend on different cultural views, and how do you decide between them? What is good for one group may not be good for another, exemplified in this case.
- The stress on consequences can easily lead to the end justifying any means. Can it be right to have killed so many people in Hiroshima and Nagasaki in order to end the Second World War? Can it be right to accept or give bribes to keep a work force employed? Can it be right to use torture in order to save lives? In the last example, Walzer (1973) offers the ticking bomb scenario, where a terrorist knows where a bomb, due to go off shortly, is in a populous city. Many would argue that torture was right if it saved several thousand people. One person suffers, but many live more happily as a result.
- Torture might be justified in such an extreme case, but, argues Walzer, torture remains wrong. Defence against torture remains enshrined in human rights codes across the globe,

because it says something about how we should treat human beings, regardless of consequences. Hence, it is often argued that torture is one of the few things that cannot have exceptions. It is always wrong. Ironically, this could give rise to another level of utilitarian argument, along the lines that unless we make a stand on torture, this could give a sign globally that it is acceptable, leading to increased suffering. At the very least, such examples raise real problems for the theory.

- The stress on good for the majority can easily lead to the oppression of the minority. Just because something will benefit 50.5% of the population does not make it good, and might in any case disadvantage the 49.5%.
- It may not be possible to assess the consequences with any precision. One of the problems about the global warming arguments, for instance, is that science cannot give an absolute picture of the consequences. Hence, Sarewitz (2004), in relation to climate change, argues that politicians should not rely simply on science to tell them what to do. The politicians have to take responsibility for settling on the values they believe are critical for the good stewardship of the environment, one of the most important being the precautionary principle. This means that even if you are not sure about precise consequences, you take the precaution of trying to sustain the environment.

It is important to estimate consequences, but we cannot rely entirely on utilitarian arguments. The stress on utilitarianism in the climbing arguments is important, but does not take account of wider issues, core moral intuitions and core questions about how we handle responsibility. Because of the uncertainty about defining what is good, it could be argued that utilitarianism is not a stand-alone ethical theory at all, but rather an important element in ethical decision making.

Deontological Theories

The theory that most immediately stands against a simple utilitarianism is the deontological theory (*deon* is Greek for duty). The deontological approach to ethics argues that duty or principles is the base of ethics rather than consequences. Right actions, according to Kant (1964), are prescribed by principles, such as: keep promises, be truthful, be fair, avoid inflicting suffering on others, return the kindness of others. Kantian ethics is thus about doing the right thing regardless of whether it makes one happy – quite the opposite of Mill's view. Kant also sees duties specific to the self, such as do no harm to the self and develop one's character and skills. Kant suggests that these duties:

- embody respect for persons
- apply without qualification to all rational persons
- are universal principles.

What makes a person worthy of respect for Kant is the capacity to be rational (see Chapter 2), to develop the good that will enable the person to do his or her duty and to fulfil key purposes. This respect involves treating people as ends in themselves, with their own purpose and capacity. This in turn means treating people not as a means to our ends. Coercion and manipulation of different kinds exhibit disrespect in these terms, such that the other is only useful for what they can do for you. This leads to certain key moral imperatives. Kant contrasts these, referred to as categorical imperatives, with non-moral imperatives, which he refers to as hypothetical. *Hypothetical imperatives* are commands which are based on a condition, such as, 'If you want to get fit, then exercise regularly'. *Categorical imperatives* have no such conditions. It is simply wrong to cheat or break a promise. These are basic principles which are true without any reference to conditions or consequences. Such principles also have to be able to apply universally, and Kant argues that most common principles pass this test. 'Promises should be kept', for example, applies in all situations. If we did not keep promises, then the very meaning of the word would be brought into question (ironically, a utilitarian argument).

For Kant, this points to a view of ethics which is based upon absolute principles. The authority for such principles does not come from some outside source, such as God, but from their rational foundation. As we noted in the first part of this book, Beauchamp and Childress (1994) suggest four major principles in professional ethics: respect for the autonomy (self-governance) of the client, justice (treating all parties fairly), beneficence (working for the good of the client) and non-maleficence (avoiding harm to the client). A deontological approach to the case above is precisely what Hillary argues for. For him, this is based on the nature of humanity and always being open to the needs of the other. Key principles in the case then include:

- Compassion. In terms of Sharp, this would involve being with him in his situation. If he were approaching death, this would include staying with him whilst he was dying, and trying at least to engage him, to understand what had happened and what his desires and feelings were.
- Respect. This would involve a broader respect both for Sharp and the others involved in the situation.

CRITIQUES OF DEONTOLOGICAL THEORY

11.2 PAUSE FOR THOUGHT

Considering Principles
- What are the principles that inform your practice?
- What are the principles that inform the practice of your workplace?
- What are the principles embodied in the planning and practice of your management?
- Can you think of any principle that has no exception, one that can apply in every situation?

Principles provide a powerful basis to ethics. Once again, however, it is difficult to see this as an exclusive foundation. It makes sense to stress the duty of the person. However:
- It is difficult to see how principles can be absolute, that is, without exception. The principle of promise keeping is justified by saying that if people do not keep promises, then the meaning of promise keeping is eroded. But this is only true if promises are broken regularly. It is possible to say that, all things being equal, promises should be kept, the reasons being that they form the basis of a relationship or contract. However, it may be possible that a person has to break a promise, because of some greater concern. For example, a person may have promised to maintain confidentiality, only to realise that the person involved is a murderer who could kill again. Equally, it could be that a person is not able to keep a promise. For example, a person may promise to support a particular project but lose the resources, personal or financial, to do this. In both those situations, it could be argued that it is wrong to keep a promise. This applies to any great principle. It is very difficult to find any principle that does not have an exception to it.
- Absolute principles have the danger that they discourage the taking of responsibility for working things out in context. This can lead to a lack of awareness of the situation.
- The idea of reason as the basis for respecting another person excludes human beings who are unable to reason intellectually, not least the severely learning disabled. The very word 'person' is as much a word which expresses value, as it is a description. Hence, there is real danger of excluding some humans from that respect if it is at all conditional, that is, if respect is based upon some particular aspect or property of the person. It would, for example, exclude people with more severe learning disabilities from respect.
- The general nature of principles requires that details be worked through in practice. In other words, it is hard to know just what they mean until one can see how they relate to a

case. This could mean that any principle might have very different meanings. A good illustration outside the world of business is the case of the conjoined twins in Chapter 3.

- Just as the principles of respect for life can lead to different conclusions in practice, principles such as equality or freedom can have different meanings. Often the key ethical debate is about what they do mean (see Chapter 2).

11.3 PAUSE FOR THOUGHT

Considering the Theory Underpinning Practice
- Which of the two major ethical theories informs your ethical practice?
- Which of the two might best inform ethics in healthcare and why?

Summing Up So Far

Utilitarianism and deontological theories are important perspectives about ethics, and must be involved in ethical decision making. Hence, for instance, it is possible to accept fundamental principles without making them absolute (applicable in the same way in all situations). However, taken as single ethical theories, offering one narrative to explain ethics, they raise more questions than they offer answers. Hence, philosophers have turned to other theories to supplement these.

Non-Rationalist Theories

Several non-rationalist approaches to ethics stress additional aspects to be taken into account, in particular, intuitionism, feminism, discourse ethics and virtue ethics. Non-rational means that they involve more than simply rational calculation.

INTUITIONISM

Ranged against the two examples of rational foundations to ethics, Hume (1975) had little time for the place of reason as a foundation of ethics. We must rather look to the heart, the passions. Reason could provide the rational justification of means, but nothing can provide a rational justification of ends. The promptings of the heart are no excuse for ignorance, and reason has to guide our understanding of the world and the possibilities of that world, but intuition is very much at the base of what we determine to be good. Hume's position suggests that reason and emotion are critical parts of any foundation of ethics. The importance of acknowledging feeling in decision making is reinforced with the work on emotional intelligence (Solomon 2007). Nonetheless, intuitionism does have its problems. It is hard to build ethics purely on feelings. How would we distinguish which feelings were right and which wrong without rational criteria?

FEMINIST ETHICS

This approach has close parallels with the feminist ethics of care and much pastoral theology over the last two decades, which stresses care, empathy and trust as the basis of the ethical response (Robinson 2008). It is not simply about women's rights. Feminist writers contrast justice with care (Koehn 1998). Justice, they argue, is solution-driven and based upon power. It assumes there is 'right' solution to any ethical dilemma. In contrast, care as the foundation of ethics is concerned not simply with solving ethical dilemmas, but rather with understanding the underlying relationships and what is needed to bring people together. Hence, feminist ethics has a lot in common with conflict resolution approaches, looking to involve all parties in working out the ethical response. This is an ethics which looks to develop trust and is dependent upon key attributes such as empathy and care. Feminist ethics shares with critical theory (Western 2007) a concern to analyse the power dynamic of any ethics. It is sometimes expressed as a justice versus care debate. In fact, feminism emphasises restorative rather than retributive justice.

DISCOURSE ETHICS

Awareness of this reflection and plurality has also led to a greater stress on the need for dialogue as essential for discovering ethical meaning. Habermas (1992) suggests that ethical meaning emerges from dialogue, enabling reflection on values and the discovery of shared norms. Getting the process right for such dialogue is thus of the highest importance, and Habermas suggests basic conditions for this, including respect for the other. Benhabib (1992) goes further, noting that, whilst the dialogue may reveal shared moral meaning, the conditions of dialogue themselves already embody moral meaning, not least respect for those we are in dialogue with (Benhabib 1992). Hence, whilst dialogue is important in sharing and testing ethical meaning, the dialogue itself depends upon core principles.

VIRTUE ETHICS

Perhaps the most important ethical theory to challenge the two rationalist ones in the last three decades has been virtue ethics. MacIntyre (1981) was responsible for the re-emergence of ethics built around virtue. He argues that we must choose between Aristotle and Nietzsche. Aristotle places ethics in a community of shared meaning (Aristotle 2004). Nietzsche (2003) suggests that the traditional moral language no longer binds us. Indeed, he argues, such language tended to impose meaning on society, robbing the individual of the freedom to determine his or her own values. Hence, he argues that it *should* no longer bind us.

McIntyre argues for Aristotle. Ethical meaning, he suggests, is situated in a community of practice, and is communicated not through principles but stories, including community ritual, which sum up the key virtues of the community. And it is virtues which are at the heart of ethical meaning. As we noted in Chapter 3, Aristotle sees virtues as dispositions for action which occupy the mean, or middle, not the extreme. Underlying the virtues is the *telos*, purpose or end, which involves well-being or happiness. In all this, the approach is to get the character right and good ethical practice follows from this. Unlike Kant, who saw the good decision as a matter of the will, not a matter of emotions and therefore of inclinations, Aristotle saw the ethically correct person acting out of the inclinations that the virtues gave him. Such virtues are learned through practice.

Virtue ethics is an important ethical theory, but also has its problems. First, it does not really get over the problem of how to handle ethical relativity, the idea that there is no shared understanding of ethics. If each community is the basis for ethical meaning, then there can be no sense of shared ethics beyond that community. There has to be dialogue to develop virtues across different interconnected groups. Second, and connected, community-based ethics excludes any sense of justice that applies to all. This is exemplified by universal human rights, the belief that certain rights apply to all regardless of their culture or community. Action which abuses those rights is seen as unjust. Third, virtue ethics assumes a community which has a single voice and view of the good. In fact, all communities have many voices, with very different perspectives. Again, the meaning of these is accessed through dialogue between members of the community. Nonetheless, virtue ethics takes us beyond the unthinking use of principles or consequences to owning how we think, what our identity is and what this requires of us. The practice of core virtues in enabling reflection and dialogue then becomes critical. All of this points to an ethics which is about thinking flexibly, not simply about applying principles or finding clear solutions.

Worldviews

Most of the rational ethical theories are dominated by the question 'what is right or wrong?' Underlying that is another question – what is good? And the answer to that depends upon the worldview that one holds. Worldviews are simply views of the world that give an explanation of what life is about and what is of value in that world. It might involve a view of how the world was created (cosmology), of the nature of the world as it is and how all the different parts relate (ecology) or of the role and value of humanity in that world (anthropology). In recent years, the global warming debate has been dominated by a worldview that stresses the interconnectedness of the social and physical environment. This in turn has concluded that humanity has to take more responsibility for the environment and the view that it is not ethical to waste resources (Jonas 1984). Feminist ethics is based on a view of the world that has similar interconnectedness. The ethics itself then stresses people working together for the good.

Murdoch (1972) argued against ethics as focusing simply on narrow views of obligation, that is, 'what it is right to do' in any situation. It also has to articulate what the good life is, 'what it is good to be' (Taylor 1989, p. 5). And this requires not just reason but a vision of the good, and thus imagination. Critical moral consciousness, a real awareness of all who were involved in any situation and of the issues that came from those relationships, was a key part of this. Murdoch stressed the importance of the person taking responsibility for their ethical reflection and decision making, and argued this needed more focus on the underlying meaning and how that connected to broader view of the good. Hence, for her, narrative becomes a key vehicle for ethical reflection. All this places value, and an awareness of what values one holds and why, before reasoning and action.

11.4 PAUSE FOR THOUGHT

Worldview/s

- What is/are your worldview(s)?
- How does it inform your view of the good?
- What are the dominant worldviews in the developed world?
- What are dominant worldviews in the developing world?
- What might be the worldview underpinning the nursing profession of healthcare in general?

Often worldviews are implicit or assumed. In the West, for instance, there is a strong consumerist worldview (Miles 1998). This is built around individual choice and the freedom to choose. The worldview of nature as interconnected stresses rather a view of community, or people working together to pursue sustainability (Jonas 1984). Hence, worldviews are not simply statements of fact. They involve major ethical values such as freedom, community or equality. They provide the value framework through which we view the world, what we believe about the world. Any person or group may have several different worldviews or may have worldviews that appear to conflict with other worldviews. So how do we judge between different worldviews? The worldview has to be tested against reality.

- Does it lead to harm, physical or psychological? Some worldviews, for instance, lead to the exclusion of others who do not agree.
- Does it lead to good ends, such as resolving conflict? As noted above, there is good evidence, for instance, that genuine working together leads to positive workplaces and greater productivity.
- How far is the worldview engaging the major values, such as freedom, equality and community? Stress on simply one of these will tend to lead to a narrow worldview, such as individual freedom against equality.

Worldviews are, then, not right in themselves. Simply because I believe something about the world does not make this view good. It is possible for any worldview to be used to a bad end, and therefore, as Bauman (1989) notes, it is important to be aware of different worldviews and to critically engage them. To illustrate this, we turn at this point to perhaps the most prevalent basis for worldviews globally – those involving transcendence, religions.

Transcendent Worldviews

Transcendent worldviews are mostly expressed in religion. Some would argue that religion has no place in applied ethics. However, the majority of the world in some way bases its ethics on religion.

11.5 PAUSE FOR THOUGHT

Spirituality

The term spirituality is often associated directly with religion. However, it is not exclusive to religion. It involves:

- An awareness and appreciation of the social and physical environment. From this can emerge a belief system which includes an awareness of our dependency on others. This may or may not involve belief in a god of established religions. It is possible, for instance, to believe in the earth as a synergistic and self-regulating, complex system that helps to maintain and perpetuate the conditions for life on the planet, that is, the Gaia principle (Lovelock 2016).
- The capacity to relate and respond to this environment
- The development of significant life meaning and purpose based on this response (Robinson et al. 2003)

    Do you have a developed spirituality? If so, how does it relate to your professional practice?

The first thing to say is that religion, like ethics, has many different approaches. The two broad theoretical bases are natural law and care (ethics based on love, care or compassion), and these provide what is sometimes a competing view of ethics, even within religion.

NATURAL LAW

Natural law is based on the idea of creation. In the Abrahamic religions (Christian, Jewish and Islamic), it is argued that God created the world and his purposes are revealed in that creation. Those purposes are what show us the good at the base of ethics. One obvious example is to do with sexuality. Natural law argues that God created man and woman as sexual beings for the purpose of procreation. From that, it is argued by some religions (see Sherwood 2020) that homosexuality, for instance, does not fulfil God's purposes and is therefore ethically wrong. There are, however, real problems with natural law. Hume (1975) argues we cannot simply say that something is right or wrong because of what it is. You cannot base a prescription about what you should do on a description of how things are. It is an important example of an ethical fallacy (see Chapter 3). It makes a logical leap without any real evidence of what is good or bad. Of course, natural law thinkers would argue that they are not basing their ethics on a description but rather on the purpose behind the description, that is God's purpose in creation. But who decides what God's purpose is? Historically, it has been those in power who have decided what is good. At different points in the history of religion, those in power have decided that order is paramount, allowing them to accept slavery, exclusively male leadership and so on. In all this, religions have often simply used transcendent worldviews as the basis for defending their own institutional power.

CARE

The second stress in most religions is some form of care, summed up in love and respect for common humanity, the so called 'golden rule'. Some of the versions of that include:

- *Christian.* 'Treat others as you would like them to treat you' (Luke 6, 31). 'Love your neighbour as yourself' (Matthew 22, 39).
- *Hindu.* 'Let not any man do unto another any act that he wishes not done to himself by others, knowing it to be painful to himself' (Mahabharata, Shanti Parva).
- *Confucian.* 'Do not do unto others what you would not want them to do to you' (Analects, Book xii, 2).
- *Buddhist.* 'Hurt not others with that which pains yourself' (Udanavarga, v.18).
- *Jewish.* 'What is hateful to yourself do not do to your fellow man. This is the whole Torah' (Babylonian Talmud, Shabbath 31a).
- *Muslim.* 'No man is a true believer unless he desires for his brother what he desires for himself' (Hadith Muslim, imam 71–2).

All of these expressions of care involve inclusiveness, mutuality and related aspects such as unconditional love and empathy. This does not actually tell us what is right in any situation. It is rather the starting point for working this out, through commitment to people and projects over time.

However, there is little argument for religion as the basis of all ethics. Any religious imperatives need to be interpreted and critically tested, not accepted regardless of context or reason. Plato (2005) pointed to this in the dialogue *Euthyphro.* He asks is something right because God says so, or is it right independently of God's command? If it is the first, then how do we know that is not simply based upon the whim of the divine? If it is the second, then judgements about what is ethically right depend upon rational criteria, and ethics becomes independent from God. Of course, the power of this dilemma is only a problem if you believe that ethics should be based upon obeying God's commands uncritically.

Much of religious worldviews are based in key religious texts. However, it is not easy to discern the voice of God in Scriptures which are a product of their culture, expressed through laws, rules, songs, and stories. Once again, critical dialogue becomes essential, as in the conjoined twin's case of Chapter 3. Markham (1994) and Ramadan (2009) argue that both secular and religious ethics involve a plurality of cultures, with differences and the need for dialogue as much within religions as between religions and wider society. See Chapter 5 for how a religious view, in this case Jehovah's Witnesses, might be carefully challenged.

Integrating Different Normative Theories

There are several different normative ethical theories, all of which have limitations, all of which connect to some broader view of the good. Given that all of them also have some convincing elements, it is important to recognise those elements in a theoretical overview. There are two ways in which that might be achieved in nursing and in wider healthcare – in the context of practical decision making (see Chapter 2) and in a normative view of care ethics which brings all of these elements together.

All of the ethical theories inform the practice of deliberation. Utilitarian theory informs the need to both find out about the situation (gathering data) and consider the possible consequences to all the stakeholders. Deontological theory involves the importance of the key principles. Hence, there is a rational framework. The non-rational theories then remind us that decisions are always affected by relationships and feelings, and therefore require a wider view of rationality than simple exercise of the intellect or empirical skills. This inevitably takes us back to the psychology of decision making. Intuition is precisely a form of affect which causes the person to think about what one is doing (Solomon 2007; 1992). Decisions have to feel right. That could be a feeling generated by a professional code, a relationship with a colleague or patient, a more established relationship with family and so on. The feeling then has to be questioned – what does it mean, how will it be worked through into practice? The feeling might be very positive, that is, this is the right thing to do. This too has to be questioned. Negative feelings may entirely dominate any attempt to deliberate. Hence, in the Mid Staffs case, fear generated by a culture of harassment literally caused professionals across all sectors to avoid deliberation. Effective professional decision making was made difficult if not impossible.

Feelings may be conflicted, leading to the kind of moral distress noted in Chapter 5. In all this, feelings are central to ethical practice but have to be interrogated and understood. To engage feelings demands the practice of the virtues, as noted in Chapter 3. Courage, as the leadership foundation argued, is necessary if the nurse is to face up to pressure from her leadership. Courage is necessary but not sufficient. *Phronesis* is critical, both to reflect on the core purpose of the nurse but also to reflect on the core communities she is part of which share that purpose. Reflection is then not simply on purpose or principle but their embodiment. In a summary and analysis of research on drug taking in sport, and the motivations of athletes who came off drugs, one of the most powerful motivations was not principles or concepts of value and purpose, but rather situations in which the offender felt strong dissonance because of a significant relationship (Backhouse et al. 2006). The persons gained distance from the self, saw themselves in relation, for instance, to their open and caring wider family and began to take responsibility for their actions.

The virtue of temperance is critical to the very practice of deliberation, enabling a person or group to reflect without being drawn into extreme positions. This allows the person or group to be able to imagine and assess consequences more effectively. Dialogue is critical to this process. First, it assists reflection more effectively, internally and externally. This is because dialogue engages difference, leading to mutual challenge and widening perception and awareness. Literally, the more we are in dialogue, the more we develop self-awareness and awareness of our social and physical environment. Second, the practice of dialogue in itself enables the formation of character through the practice of the virtues. Dialogue, opening up what we think and feel, and listening to what others think and feel, demands courage, temperance and *phronesis*, so that we can develop our understanding of core values and purpose, stand up for these and work together with others who share those values. Key to integrating these different theories is an ethics of care. This enables engagement with religions and their stress on care seen in terms of love, with virtue and dialogic ethics and with the professional ethics focus on holding together justice and respect.

An Ethics of Care

Care can be said to provide the commitment that enables this learning dialogue to continue, enabling trust. It is this commitment to the other which enables mutuality, even when there is asymmetricality: junior doctor and senior nurse; ward cleaner and staff nurse; senior doctor and nurse; administrator and nurse leader; nurse and patient; nurse lecturer and student and so on. In a sense, asymmetricality of power, knowledge (academic, practical, relational), experience and so on, is written into all relationships. Hence, as Habermas (1992) noted, mutual respect has to be the foundation of and the means to developing dialogue. Mutual and equal respect, as well as love, then are often seen as elements of the concept of care (Outka 1972). The concept of care brings together four elements:

- Moral. It is both a principle and a virtue, the ground and meaning of ethics
- Epistemic. It's about knowledge, a way of knowing
- A way of empowering. This focuses on the practice of care
- Focused on community not on the individual, and connects the virtues.

THE GROUND AND SUBSTANCE OF ETHICS

Care provides grounds for ethics and the ethical content. This is focused on an inclusive responsibility that transcends rules, an appreciation of the particular other and mutuality that includes care for self and others. Such content informs principles, rules and practice.

Inclusive

Care is unconditional and thus sets up an inclusivity. From a Christian perspective, Schotroff (1978) reminds us that this is partly an attitude of inclusivity, but that it must lead to a concrete social event, something summed up in the command to go beyond love of neighbour to love of enemy: 'the Christian is challenged to include the persecutor in his own community even the enemies of the community are to be given a place in its common life and in the kingly rule of God' (Schotroff 1978, p. 23). This is not a make-believe world in which the enemy suddenly becomes one of us. It may be that the enemy remains the enemy, but we nonetheless have to love her, to use moral imagination in seeing how she can be worked with. This sets up the extent of responsibility for the other in every situation. For healthcare workers, this includes providing care for everyone, regardless of one's feelings about them.

Care as Non-Directive

Care cannot be precise in ethical guidance. Indeed, Bauman (1993) suggests that it demands careful consideration of any situation to see how it might be embodied. The responsibility to do something about this, to respond, nonetheless remains with the individual. Bauman contrasts the precise order or rule with the ethical demand, which is 'abominably vague, confused and confusing, indeed barely audible. It forces the moral self to be her own interpreter' (Bauman 1993). Faced by this demand, Bauman suggests two dangers. First, the demand can be defused by narrowing its focus. Hence, as Schrage notes, the Hebrew command to love the neighbour (Leviticus 19:18) was originally inclusive but over time was narrowed down to Israelites (Scharge 1988, p. 73). Bauman reminds us that the key dynamic of the Nazi Holocaust was to see the Jews and others as outside the moral claims of humanity (Bauman 1993; see also Gaita 2000). The second danger is to use codes and regulations as means of avoiding responsibility for working out the ethical response in practice. The responsibility of care exactly has no limits, and 'does not reach a boundary beyond which nothing is required' (Scharge 1988, p. 74).

Beyond Simply Fairness

Care ethics always exceeds a narrow justice or rights morality (Woodhead 1992, p. 64). This is a difficult position, though as Oppenheimer (1983) notes, it is embodied to some degree in human practice, not least in the example of parenting. Importantly, this means that the ethical attitude is not rational or simply calculative. Indeed, Bauman argues that it is 'endemically and irremediably *non rational*' (Bauman 1993, p. 60). Rationality can easily be seen as about survival and the capacity to calculate one's interest, something essentially defensive. In this light, the attitude of care precedes any use of rules in ethics. Woodhead contrasts this with the view of morality which is concerned 'with the regulation of the competing claims of individuals rather than with the establishment of loving personal relationships' (Woodhead 1992, p. 60). The first of these is achieved by 'a formal hierarchy of moral laws or rights'. The laws apply to all people and rights are possessed by all. Underlying this view is a concern for justice and fairness, and an attempt to apply ethics in a discernibly consistent, and even objective, way. However, as Simone Weil notes, any rights have to be founded themselves on some sense of prior obligation, and this is an obligation to the other which must be based upon need (Woodhead 1992, p. 63). Hence, the ethical impulse, the impulse to see the other as invaluable, precedes any attempt to calculate ends. The critical underlying point is that care moves the person away from the role of spectator, or as Bauman suggests 'tourist', to direct relationship, direct awareness of the other as kin (Ballatt and Campling 2011) and therefore to a sense of responsibility which precedes any reflection on the particular moral response.

Appreciation

Care as unconditional is based on the sameness of the other, recognition and acceptance of common humanity. Hence, Kierkegaard can write of the 'common mark' illuminated by 'the light of the eternal' (Kierkegaard 1946, p. 73). Care's focus is the value of the particular, in which light Tawney was able to see equality not as equal treatment for everyone but rather different treatment based on different need and capacity (Tawney 1930).

Mutuality

The dynamic of empathy, as noted above, assumes mutuality not least because, just as empathy enables the other to disclose herself, at the same time it involves a disclosure of the one who offers empathy. Such mutuality also raises the importance of self-love.

Self-Love

The self is an 'other' (Ricoeur 1992). To exclude the self would therefore be inequitable. As Oppenheimer puts it, 'if any creature is to be loved and cherished, then sooner or later we ourselves are likewise to be loved and cherished' (Oppenheimer 1983, p. 103).

Such care is both unconditional, remaining committed to the self and conditional in the sense of recognising particular worth of the self. The balanced care that is given to the self by another, precisely enables the person to treat his or her self in the same way. Hence, Jackson (2003, p. 11) can write of a 'proper self-love'. Importantly, self-love which is both inclusive and also conditional provides the moral basis for the self-critique at the heart of the ethical process. It invites the person both to accept that he or she is of worth intrinsically, and also invites them to consider their worth in practice, in what they create and how they relate. This is no cosy care, but one which sets up a tension between the self as experienced by the self and the self in relationship and response. It calls forth a response that has to reflect on purpose, practice and the relational context of both, and it gives value to and recognises value in all of this. Hence, at the heart of care is challenge. Self-care and worth which is based purely on unconditionality, which does not challenge the person to respond, and in particular to contribute to community, thus confirming worth in action, can easily move into non-reflective self-esteem. As Erikson notes, the global goal of enhancing self-esteem 'on the assumption that happiness, success and responsible behaviour will automatically follow' leads to a confused ethic that does not begin to engage with the challenges and demands of the relational network (Erikson 1987, p. 163).

11.6 PAUSE FOR THOUGHT

Self-Interest as the Basis of Ethics – Isn't Self-Interest Bad?

There are several ethical theories which argue that the very basis of ethics is, and should be, self-interest. Broadly, these fall under four headings:

Enlightened self-interest, which argues that if we act to serve the interests of others, this will be in our own interest.

Ethical egoism, arguing that self-interest is the prime obligation of ethics.

Hedonism, involving a school of ethics which argues that pleasure is the only intrinsic good and therefore must always be pursued.

Rational egoism, which argues that rational decisions are made in one's own interest. In other words, rationality is, itself, self-interest. You do something because it is good for you.

It is important to be aware of these aspects of ethical theory, not least because in some countries these views form the basis of how they develop health care. Paul Ryan, a former speaker of the House of Representatives was heavily influenced by rational egoism and proposed a market approach to healthcare which focused on self-reliance and choice (https://eu.usatoday.com/story/opinion/2017/03/07/health-care-obamacare-replacement-paul-ryan-column/98858696/). Making healthcare an entitlement, so the argument goes, would simply stop both of these. This is based on the philosophy of Ayn Rand (1964), focusing on the virtue of selfishness.

There is not the space to critique her views in detail. However, the major critique is that most forms of the primacy of self-interest are built around a false dichotomy. You must choose either altruism (concern purely for the other) or self-interest. Altruism destroys individual responsibility, and self-interest is the most effective motivator of responsibility, which is, it is argued, for the good of everyone (Rand 1964).

Against this, first, an ethics of care argues that individualism cannot be sufficient grounds for ethics. Humanity is interdependent, with mutual interests and needs. Second, this demands concern for both the self and others, and thus ways of working that will allow such mutuality to flourish. Mutual flourishing then becomes a key end of ethics, not competition.

The characterisation of care as simply or primarily other oriented (altruistic) also tends to stress what is often seen as encouraging sacrifice. Feminists note the way in which such a view has led to oppression (Woodward 1992). Women historically were given the role of carer, kept in place by guilt for the woman who tries to break out of such sacrifice and look to fulfilment beyond the family. Underlying views of love in theology and philosophy show rather a balanced perspective, with different views being held together (Robinson 2008):

- *Agape*, unconditional love which is other-centred
- *Eros*, love based in conditions (such as attraction for person or project), often seen as self-centred
- *Philia*, love of friendship, found in different contexts.

Care, in its inclusive sense, brings all of these together. It provides a basis of mutuality, which focuses on the other and the self, being concerned for the other and also taking pleasure (*eros*) in the purpose of caring (including research that furthers care, and public health innovations) and in the act of care. Florman (1994, p. 147), in writing about the passion for creative practice of the engineering profession, refers to 'existential pleasure'. *Philia* extends care to patients and colleagues. This is friendship offered 'on the way'; a companion who is with you on the journey, however brief (Vanier 2001), in which responsibility is discovered, shared and practised.

Care, Principles, Rules and Worldview

Though the concept of care is broad, it does, in fact, have substantive meaning that can be expressed in general principles. The stress on inclusivity, that sees the other as part of common humanity, leads to the principles of *community* or *fellowship* – something which fits into the basic human need of belonging. Concern for particularity of the other leads to the principle of *freedom* and diversity. Commitment to the other naturally leads to the principle of *equality of respect*. Arising from these are a number of other principles such as participation and mutual responsibility.

These principles are not of themselves axiomatic in the sense of commonly defined or accepted. The term equality, for instance, has at least 100 logically distinct meanings (Rae 1981). Hence, there is no simple meaning which all might agree upon prior to 'application'. More importantly, each of these general principles is informed by care, and by each other. Community is not about the solidarity of a community against others and the rest of the world, but rather about an inclusiveness which opens communities to others, and which is thus outward looking and self-critical. The idea of freedom is not simply negative freedom (freedom from oppression or constraint) or positive freedom (freedom which enables), but involves freedom to learn, to develop, to take responsibility for the self and for the other.

In all this, it is important to note that care holds together all these, almost as a community of principles. The principle of care enables a constant dialogue with other principles, questioning and clarifying each other. Such principles then remain constant, applying to all situations, but never absolute in the sense of being applied in the same way *to* all situations. They enable a consistency of meaning but at the same time can only fully discover ethics *in* the situation, through reflection on practice (van der Ven 1998, p. 260). Care ensures that all principles are tested. Underlying all this is the worldview of human life as interdependent and interactive. The individual is not isolated but comes to fruition in community and learns autonomy through relationships.

A WAY OF KNOWING

Care has an epistemic function. It is the way of revealing the other, both to the self and to the other. This implies that the 'other' is not instantly accessible. Weil (1977), indeed, argued that the other is often invisible, with many factors, from prejudice to fear, causing this. Hence, she writes, 'If you want to become invisible, there is no surer way than to become poor'. She goes on to say, 'Love sees what is invisible' (both quoted in Gaita 2000, p. xvi). Care goes beyond artificial boundaries to reveal the humanity of the other. This is what Levinas (1998) means by ethics beginning with the face of the other. In the Mid Staffs case, we saw other concerns getting in the way of knowing the other – patient, family, colleagues. The dynamic of this is expressed in the idea of empathic care. Kohut characterises empathy as follows:

> *(1) the recognition of the self in the other, is an indispensable tool of observation, without which vast areas of human life remain unintelligible, (2) the expansion of the self to include the other, constitutes a powerful psychological bond, (3) the accepting, confirming, and understanding human echo evoked by the self, is a psychological nutriment without which life as we know it could not be sustained.*
> (Kohut 1982, p. 398)

Scheler (quoted in Campbell 1984, p. 77) notes it is more than fellow feeling, describing it as 'a genuine reaching out and entry into the other person and his individual situation, a true and authentic transcendence of oneself'. It is a movement beyond the concerns for the self, including fear and guilt, and with this, an expansion or reaching out of the self. This involves not taking the self too seriously, and thus Scheler can write of abandoning 'personal dignity'. Caring, then, is not a self-conscious process. Self-conscious concern for the other is when a person wants to communicate their identity as a carer, allowing the self to intrude into the care.

This movement towards the other does not lose the individuality of the one who cares. Indeed, the movement away from focus on self enables distance which allows her to see herself more clearly. It also enhances the value of the other, bringing out the value they possess and enabling them to disclose what is unique about themselves to themselves and to the other. The second part of Kohut's description of empathy clearly signals this inclusive acceptance of the other and the psychological bond which this provides. Empathy is very much a working out of, and a sign of, care. Without an assurance of this acceptance, it would be difficult for the person to disclose any thing of herself. Indeed, without that care, it would be impossible to see the truth of the other. The natural human dynamic is to keep hidden that which is imagined as not acceptable. Hence, there is always a wariness about possible judgement from the other. Margulies suggests four components of empathy:

- *Conceptual empathy*, stressing cognitive understanding of the other
- *Self-experiential empathy*, referring to memories, affects and associations which are stirred in the listener, thus causing her to identify with the experience of the other

- *Imaginative – imitative empathy*, involving imagining oneself into a model of the other's experience
- *Resonant empathy*, the experience of 'affective contagion', where the listener feels the feeling of the other (Margulies 1989, p. 19).

Empathy involves an interplay of all of these aspects, leading to an openness to the self and others and to the different aspects of the self – affective, cognitive and somatic. This openness and reaching out to the other means that the empathic engagement does not deal in static truth, looking behind the other to reveal *the* truth. On the contrary, if, reaching out to the other enables her to reveal something of herself, then the truth about the other, our awareness of the other, is continuously evolving. Facts and truth are 'a creation of the relationship itself, a continuous coming into being of possibilities requiring further exploration' (Margulies 1989, p. 12). In the light of this, empathy is both open to difference and sameness in the other. Openness to difference is characterised by wonder, surprise, curiosity and astonishment. Berryman (1985) notes that it is in childhood where this sense of surprise and wonder is at its height, not least because young children live at the limit of their experience most of the time. The de-centring of the self that Scheler refers to ensures that the listener does not assert her truth on the other but is genuinely open to and surprised by the other. At the same time, the listener comes to know the sameness in the other. Gaita notes that this is not the cognitive recognition of some generalised common humanity, but rather the recognition of what he refers to as the 'preciousness' of the other. This is a recognition that the other is one with you. Shared humanity is found in the particular, local story of the other (Gaita 2000). Every narrator needs an 'address', needs roots and we see our common humanity as we experience those roots, and begin to understand the roots of others in their terms and translate that story into our language (Gaita 2000, p. xxix).

In this movement, empathy involves mutuality, an ongoing revelation of the self and other. The dynamic of this lies at the heart of genuine dialogue, dialogue which can begin to understand the other in their terms and which can both enable and allow the challenge that comes from difference, and also enjoy the support and acceptance which comes from sameness. This mutual disclosure is not necessarily symmetrical. On the contrary, any relationship involves differences which lead to different aspects of the self being revealed. In the caring relationship, for instance, the carer may not reveal intimate details of her life. She will nonetheless reveal, in body language and in words, her attitude and her values, aspects of herself, how she feels about the other. For the person being cared for this becomes a critical narrative that she is reading from the other, as to whether she is accepted or not. For someone who comes to that relationship from a world of conditional value, they are already faced with something new. Hence, part of the mutuality in that relationship begins to emerge through the testing of the carer's narrative. The mutuality of empathy is such that Augsburger (1999) prefers to use the word interpathy (Swinton 2001; Margulies 1989; Campbell 1984).

Empathy then is at the heart of awareness of the 'other', and it is precisely this that is able to hold together the different and often ambiguous aspects of the other: good/bad; same/different; particular/universal; supportive/dangerous; autonomous/part of community. Schlauch (1990) notes that this enables other tensions to be held together in knowing the other, between:

- believing and doubting. The doubting leads to the testing, and testing to a form of belief
- separated and connected (Belenky 1986). Care enables the person to see the other as both different and the same
- understanding and explaining. The first involved empathic awareness, the second looks at underlying causal dynamics.

The capacity to hold together and thus accept ambiguity enables both carer and patient not to be drawn into polarised perceptions or attempts to end uncertainty too quickly. It is important to stress the connection of empathy to care. Empathy of itself, apart from care, cannot be a base of ethics. As Kristjansson (2004) notes, 'the same capacity to discern or event identify with another's feelings is also a necessary condition for taking pleasure in, rather than bemoaning the suffering, for example through pure malice or *Schadenfreude*' (p. 298). Perhaps the best example of this in literature is the villain of Shakespeare's *Othello*, Iago. What makes Iago in one sense the ultimate villain is precisely that he understands the emotional world of all the other characters so well, and indeed is felt by all to be a true friend who listens and counsels. This is why he is so successful at manipulating the other characters. What he lacks is care. Othello himself is the total opposite. He cares a great deal but has little empathy. Hence, he does not fully understand Desdemona, and has little self-understanding, characterising himself, naively, as 'one who loved not wisely, but too well' (*Othello*, act 5, scene 2).

In the light of all this, empathic care is essential to working through the core ethical principles of decision making (see Chapter 2). It is also essential to the professional delivery of care, be that in nursing or in the boardroom, precisely because the epistemic element enables the practitioner to maintain the necessary distance that ensures the best direction in care. Through dialogue, face to face or across the organisation, authentic trustworthy care is revealed.

A WAY OF EMPOWERING

The nature of care is to share power and not to take away from the other the responsibility for 'seeing' for themselves. Much that is done in the name of care and love ends up as manipulation. The lover is unable to wait and wants to see the outcome now. Professional carers are very prone to this, not least because professionalism looks for evidence of a successful outcome. Such a care might involve doing things for the other and once more the danger of a patronising love which cares for the other *in spite of* her failings (Bauman 1993, p. 97). This is a love which actually retains the power of conditionality and thus of judgement. It wants to be good to the other but also wants the other to know this. Inclusive care, on the other hand, involves a natural openness and is essentially vulnerable, partly because you have to wait and partly because you cannot know the outcome when you share that care. Hence, this takes one beyond the comfort zone into risk. W. H. Vanstone sums this up well: 'the power which love gives to the other is the power to determine the issue of love – its completion or frustration, its triumph or its tragedy. This is the vulnerability of authentic love – that it surrenders to the other power over its own issue, power to determine the triumph or tragedy of love' (Vanstone 1977, p. 67).

The dynamic of care, however, is more than simply one of caring and waiting. It involves the proactive reaching out with positive concern for the other, enabling response in terms of revelation of the self and testing of the other. It is this dynamic which enables the development of power (Kohut 1982). Care empowers the other through enabling the articulation of narrative, reflection on meaning and the embodiment of response. The very presence of the carer then is key (Fahlberg and Roush 2016). Technical skills enhance this but cannot be a substitute (Kohut 1982).

NARRATIVE

Care provides the safe environment within which the person can begin to develop her narrative. Narration is critical to the development of the character, which, as van der Ven notes, is refigured 'in the twofold sense of uncovering its concealed dimensions and transforming its experienced dimensions' (van der Ven 1998, p. 358). Narration is a complex function that brings together all levels of awareness and meaning. It enables the person to gain distance from the self, and so begin to become aware of experience, the effect of experience on the self and the meaning and feelings which shape that experience. Freeman (1993, p. 45) refers to this as a stage of *distanciation*, which achieves differentiation, 'a separation of the self from the self, such that the text of one's experience becomes the object of interpretation'. In this, the self becomes both subject and object, leading to the possibility of dialogue *with* the self *about* the self. Articulation of narrative in this sense is not simply a bilateral communication with the other. Yes, it is transmitted to the other, the listener, but it also involves the relationship with the self. The self can hear what is being said and often discovers something new about data, feelings or thoughts, something new about the self and the other. Hence, van der Ven (1998, p. 358) can speak of the development of the dialogic self, and of the self as both reader and writer. It is precisely this dynamic which can lead to surprises, and which enables clarification of the person's feelings and values, and thus empowerment.

REFLECTION

The more the story is articulated in the presence of another, the more it becomes reflective, and the more it focuses on the many different stories within that. As Bakhtin (1993) notes, these stories are filled with contradictions, creating not simply a universe but a 'pluriverse' or 'heteroverse', around significant others, wider communities, the environment and so on. This leads to many different dialogues, each with interactions which generate surprise, challenge and possibilities (van der Ven 1998, p. 359). Such surprise and challenge are the result of contradictions or connections that might be made between the different narratives and often lead to anxiety on the part of the person who is being cared for. Once more, the temptation is to reduce that anxiety through reassurance or attempt to resolve the issue for the patient. However, as Halmos and Freeman note, it is crucial that the carer first enables her to develop the dialogue so that the underlying dissonance can be seen and second enables her to face and work through the challenges (Freeman 1993; Halmos 1964). Only with the security and support of care can the person begin to take responsibility for what, for some, is a risky process. In more severe illness, this risk means working through what is important to the patient. This may involve working through several different conflicts and contradictions, including ones between:

- ideas/values and feelings
- attitude of the person to self and others
- differences between, values, beliefs and practice
- the view of the other and 'reality' of the other
- attitude and practice in the past and present
- care for others and care for the self. Often a person will show a strong narrative of concern for others and yet have quite a different narrative with regard to the self, seeing the self as not worthy of care.

The presence of the other then enables the person to examine the different narratives and the tensions between them, to test them, including the reality of any perceptions of the other and to either affirm meaning or work through to new meaning.

LIFE MEANING

The development of life meaning is critical to empowerment. It is connected to the development of identity and thus the development of the agent. As noted in Chapter 2, this in turn is connected to questions of self-worth and value. This in turn depends upon both a sense of unconditional and conditional worth, a sense of being accepted for the self and also accepted because of the contribution of the self to the community and a recognised purpose. Both of these can be seen as basic human needs, set out by Kaufman as:

- A close interpersonal relationship which provides an environment of unconditional care. The experience of being nurtured.
- The experience of nurturing. This involves the practice of care for others and the assurance that this is a task of value (Kaufman 1980, p. 65).

Care addresses the need for unconditional acceptance experientially. Because it leads to reflection on the different narratives, it also enables the person to see the nature and value of those relationships. Nurturing enables the different people involved, patient or colleague, to take responsibility for decision making. As Taylor (1989) notes, decision making is perhaps the most empowering activity because it both confirms and develops identity and sets out possibilities to commit to. Enabling decision making is not simply about giving choices, but rather enabling careful deliberation. This may be straightforward, with limited issues, or complex, as in facing terminal illness. The full weight of care's empowering presence is that it is directly calling the other to respond empathetically, both by being open to her network of relationships and discovering meaning, and being open to the self and so responding in a way that affirms unconditional value and the value of the response (McFadyen 1990). Such empowerment then is not simply about 'giving power' to the other. It is about both a sharing of power, and in some respects, a taking of power. The carer recognises the power of the other and enables her to use that power in the process of mutual testing. The context of that is that the caring relationship is already one in which power is imbalanced, in which the person is already in the role of 'failure', 'stranger', 'person in need'. Sharing of power in that context is about breaking down the barriers of those roles, and offering a respect that accepts the other as equal. In that relationship, the person can then begin to take and practice power.

Care then finally empowers the person to move from the values to the new possibilities, the sharing of responsibility and the creating of new practice. In this, it is not simply the unconditional concern for the person that gives them the power, it is also the concern for their creative capacity which empowers, focusing on practice that makes a difference, further creating meaning in and through action. Once more this applies to co-professionals. The absence of the practice of purpose prevents the kind of existential pleasure of care that we referred to in Chapter 3, disempowering the organisational leader as much as the nurse. The Mid Staffs case showed how this led to poor deliberation and practice.

CARE AND COMMUNITY

Care develops in a community. The limitation of Kohlberg's and Kant's view of respect is its focus on the individual. However, the responsibility of and for care is both individual and communitarian. Hence, as noted in Chapter 3, the nurse is both responsible for her practice of care and for the care of the whole healthcare community. The leader is responsible for the quality of care across the piece, and thus is as much a carer as the nurse. The quality of care is about the existential nature of care, not simply the delivery of a product. That existential nature finds meaning in the culture of the organisation. This means that the organisation itself is not simply a means of 'delivery' but a community which reflects on and expresses the meaning of care in action. This community provides:

- The framework of care, one which is concerned about the health and well-being of all in the community. The ethics focuses on shared and creative responsibility, and this dovetails in with the practice of care
- The priorities of care, people not products
- The focus of deliberation and dialogue about the practice of care
- The narrative of care
- The shared responsibility of care.

Autonomy and Patient-Centred Care

The outline of an ethics of care provides a way of viewing ethics in any context. It is, however, particularly applicable to nursing and healthcare. It is important here to underline how this affects the concept of patient-centred care. As we have noted in the text, there is a danger of seeing person-centred care as focused on the protection of choice, in effect a form of consumer care. At its best, this is focused on respect for the consumer, giving a chance for feedback and enabling options to be examined. In many cases, that is sufficient, and the feedback can also contribute to the development of organisational culture. However, the danger of this approach is an underlying dynamic being content if various boxes have been ticked… 'Yes, we did check with the patient, we did see if they would recommend this service to their friends and family, and look at the feedback….an average of nine out of ten, we must be doing a good job'.

An ethics of care suggests that to limit patient-centred care to such a consumer model is to miss the point of care and above all to misunderstand choice, and with it, the underlying ethical principle of respect for autonomy. Autonomy is at the centre of empowering care, because it enables the patient and often the family to focus on their situation and what means most to them, and to find meaningful ways of responding. It is not just about giving hope, through information, but about enabling the patient to *be* hopeful, feeling a mastery of the situation, seeing pathways even when the biggest avenues are closing and coming to terms with the limitations an illness may impose. It enables patients in more difficult situations to develop virtues such as mindfulness and metacognition, the capacity to see themselves and their situation more clearly. This dynamic of care provides the basis for good ethical deliberation.

Conclusion

Care provides the basis for a normative practical ethics – bringing together normative and descriptive ethical theory. It provides the basis for the practice of integrity, integrating:

- The virtues. Empathy or *phronesis* without care can lose purpose. Courage without care can become imbalanced. Hope, truthfulness and trust without care can lose any sense of realism or commitment. Aquinas (1981) sees love (*caritas*) as the root of the virtues: progressively motivating and illuminating the practice of courage, self-mastery, justice, diverse social virtues and every exercise of intellectual and technical excellence.
- Significant meaning and practice, through the four elements of care noted above. In this, clear thinking and the development of psychological maturity are all part of a holistic view of ethics. Reaching a satisfying ethical judgement may demand change, moving away from earlier ethical assumptions.
- Different aspects of care, for self, other, community, project and purpose and wider environment. This integration is of particular importance because it recognises responsibility at all levels not just for individual actions and integrity but for the integrity of the wider project. The nurse is accountable to her patients, her profession, her healthcare institution and to the wider project of healthcare offered to society. She is also accountable for the integrity of each of these. And just in case this sounds like a burden too heavy to bear, ethics of care reminds us that we all share it, at different times and in different ways. At the centre of an ethics of care is dialogue and the growth of responsibility which enables that sharing.

In the end, an ethics of care focuses on identity, both individual and professional. Ethics built on who you are means that you own ethical meaning and practice (the basis of integrity), and don't have to bring in separate perspective or discrete skills. Hence, in focusing on the quality of care, in professional nursing, in the leadership of healthcare organisations and beyond, a normative ethics of care provides the bedrock of an ethical culture in which responsibility is articulated and practised by all.

References

Aquinas, T. (1981). *Summa theologica*. New York: Resources for Christian Living.

Aristotle. (2004). *Nicomachean Ethics*. London: London: Penguin.

Augsburger, D. (1999). *Pastoral counseling across cultures*. Westminster: John Knox.

Backhouse, S., McKenna, J., & Robinson, S. (2006). *International literature review: attitudes, behaviours, knowledge and education – drugs in sport: past, present and future*. Montreal: World Anti-Doping Agency – WADA.

Bakhtin, M. M. (1993). *Towards a philosophy of the act*. Houston: University of Texas Press.

Ballatt, J., & Campling, P. (2011). *Intelligent kindness: reforming the culture of healthcare*. London: RCPsych Publications.

Bauman, Z. (1993). *Postmodern ethics*. Oxford: Blackwell.

Bauman, Z. (1989). *Modernity and the Holocaust*. London: Polity.

Beauchamp, T., & Childress, T. (1994). *Principles of biomedical ethics*. Oxford: Oxford University Press.

Belenky, M. (1986). *Women's ways of knowing*. New York: Basic Books.

Berryman, J. (1985) Children's spirituality and religious language. *British Journal of Religious Education, 7*(3): 120–127.

Benhabib, S. (1992). *Situating the self*. London: Polity.

Campbell, A. (1984). *Moderated love: a theology of professional care*. London: SPCK.

Dawkins, R. (2010). *The greatest show on earth*. London: Black Swan.

Erikson, R. (1987). The psychology of self-esteem: promise or peril. *Pastoral Psychology, 35*(3), 163–171.

Fahlberg, B., & Roush, T. (2016). *Mindful presence: being "with" in our nursing care Nursing, 46*(3), 14–15.

Florman, S. (1994). *The existential pleasures of engineering*. New York: St Martins Press.

Freeman, M. (1993). *Rewriting the self*. London: Routledge.

Gaita, R. (2000). *A common humanity*. London: Routledge.

Habermas, J. (1992). *Moral consciousness and communicative action*. London: Polity.

Halmos, P. (1964). *The faith of the counsellors*. Constable: London.

Hume, D. (1975). *Enquiries concerning human understanding and concerning the principles of moral*. Oxford: Oxford University Press.

Jackson, T. (2003). *The priority of love*. Princeton, NJ: Princeton University Press.

Jonas, H. (1984). *The imperative of responsibility: in search of an ethics for the technological age*. Chicago: University of Chicago Press.

Kant, I. (1964). *Groundwork of the metaphysics of morals*. Translated by Paton, J. New York Harper and Row.

Kaufman, G. (1980). *Shame: the power of caring*. Washington: Schenkman.

Kierkegaard, S. (1946). *Works of love*. Princeton: Princeton University Press.

Koehn, D. (1998). *Rethinking feminist ethics*. London: Routledge.

Kohut, H. (1982). Introspection, empathy and the semi-circle of mental health. *International Journal of Psychoanalysis, 63*, 395–407.

Kristjansson, K. (2004). Empathy, sympathy, justice and the child. *Journal of Moral Education, 33*(3), 291–306.

Levinas, E. (1998). *Entre nous: on thinking-of the-other*. New York: Columbia University Press.

Lovelock, J. (2016). *Gaia: a new look at life on earth*. New York: Oxford University Press.

McFadyen, A. (1990). *The call to personhood*. Cambridge: Cambridge University Press.

MacIntyre, A. (1981). *After virtue*. London: Duckworth.

Margulies, A. (1989). *The empathic imagination*. New York: W.W. Norton.

Markham, I. (1994). *Plurality and Christian ethics*. Cambridge: Cambridge University Press.

McCoy, B. (1983). The parable of the sadhu. *Harvard Business Review, 61*(5): 103–108.

Miles, S. (1998). *Consumerism: as a way of life*. London: Sage.

Mill, J. S. (1993). *Utilitarianism*. Oxford: Oxford University Press.

Murdoch, I. (1972). *The sovereignty of the good*. New York: Schucker.

Nietzsche, F. W. (2003). *Beyond good and evil*. London: Penguin.

Oppenheimer, H. (1983). *The hope of happiness*. London: SCM.

Outka, G. (1972). *Agape: an ethical analysis*. New Haven: Yale University Press.

Plato. (2005). *Euthyphro*. London: Penguin.

Rae, D. (1981). *Equalities*. Cambridge, MA: Harvard University Press.

Ramadan, T. (2009). *Radical reform: Islamic ethics and liberation*. Oxford: Oxford University Press.

Rand, A. (1964). *The virtue of selfishness: a new concept of egoism*. New York: New American Library.

Ricoeur, P. (1992). *The self as another*. Chicago: Chicago University Press.

Robinson, S., Kendrick, K., & Brown, A. (2003). *Spirituality and the practice of healthcare*. London: MacMillan.

Robinson, S. (2008). *Spirituality, ethics and care*. London: Jessica Kingsley.

Scharge, W. (1988). *The ethics of the New Testament*. Edinburgh: T. and T. Clark.

Schlauch, C. R. (1990). Empathy as the essence of pastoral psychotherapy. *Journal of Pastoral Care, 44*(1), 3–17.

Schotroff, L. (1978). Non-violence and the love of one's enemies. In R. H. Fuller (Ed.), *Essays on the love commandment* (pp. 9–39). Minneapolis: Fortress.

Sarewitz, D. (2004). How science makes environmental controversies worse. *Environmental Science and Policy*, 7(5), 385–403.

Sherwood, H. (2020). Sex is for married heterosexual couples only, says Church of England. Online available: https://www.theguardian.com/world/2020/jan/23/sex-married-heterosexual-couples-church-of-england-christians.

Solomon, R. (1992). *Ethics and excellence*. Oxford: Oxford University Press.

Solomon, R. (2007). *True to our feelings*. Oxford: Oxford University Press.

Swinton, J. (2001). *Spirituality and mental health care*. London: Jessica Kingsley.

Tawney, R. H. (1930). *Equality*. London: Allen Unwin.

Taylor, C. (1989). *Sources of the self*. Cambridge: Cambridge University Press.

van der Ven, J. (1998). *Formation of the moral self*. Grand Rapids: Eerdmans.

Vanier, J. (2001). *Becoming human*. London: DLT.

Vanstone, W. H. (1977). *Love's endeavour, love's expense*. London: Darton, Longman and Todd.

Walzer, M. (1973). Political action: the problem of dirty hands. *Philosophy and Public Affairs*, 2(2), 160–180.

Weil, S. (1977) *The Love of God and Affliction*. In: Panichas, G.A. *The Simone Weil Reader*. New York: David McKay. pp.475–495.

Western, S. (2007). *Leadership: a critical text*. London: Sage.

Woodhead, L. (1992). Feminism and Christian ethics. In L. Daly (Ed.), *Women's voices: essays in contemporary feminist theology* (pp. 59–68). London: Marshall Pickering.

Resources

There are extensive resources for follow up debates regarding issues raised in this text and for guidance on professional standards. We have set them out under journals, books and websites. Most of the journals are available on the web, through universities or direct.

Journals

JOURNAL OF ADVANCED NURSING

The Journal of Advanced Nursing (*JAN*) is a world-leading international peer-reviewed journal. *JAN* targets readers who are committed to advancing practice and professional development on the basis of new knowledge and evidence. This includes nursing ethics, for example, Kanganiemi, M., Pakkanem, P., Korhonen, A. (2015). Professional ethics in nursing: an integrative review. *Journal of Advanced Nursing*, 71 (8).

https://onlinelibrary.wiley.com/page/journal/13652648/homepage/productinformation.html

AMA JOURNAL OF ETHICS

The *AMA Journal of Ethics* exists to help medical students, physicians and all health care professionals navigate ethical decisions in service to patients and society. The journal publishes cases and expert commentary, medical education articles, policy discussions, peer-reviewed articles for the journal based on audio CME, visuals and more. Its March 2020 issue, for instance, examines organisational ethics: https://journalofethics.ama-assn.org/home

See the following web sites for religion and spirituality in healthcare practice: https://journalofethics.ama-assn.org/issue/religion-and-spirituality-health-care-practice

AMERICAN JOURNAL OF NURSING

This includes evidence-based clinical application papers and descriptions of best clinical practices, original research and QI reports, case studies, narratives, commentaries and other manuscripts on a variety of clinical and professional topics, including nursing ethics.

https://journals.lww.com/ajnonline/Fulltext/2015/03000/Ethical_Issues.5.aspx

See for example:

http://ojin.nursingworld.org/MainMenuCategories/ANAMarketplace/ANAPeriodicals/OJIN/TableofContents/Vol-23-2018/No1-Jan-2018/Ethical-Awareness.html

CLINICAL ETHICS

This is devoted to the discussion of key issues surrounding the application of ethics in clinical practice, research and policy. Published quarterly, the journal contains articles under the headings of Case Studies, Public Policy and Law, Empirical Ethics and Papers. Additional material is included to help develop cross-disciplinary debate and increase the understanding of the complex ethical issues.

https://journals.sagepub.com/home/cet

ETHICS AND BEHAVIOUR

This includes the exercise of social and ethical responsibility in human behaviours; ethical dilemmas or professional misconduct in health and human service delivery; the conduct of research involving human and animal participants; fraudulence in the management or reporting of scientific research and public policy issues involving ethical problems.

Data based, theoretical and particularly instructive case analyses, as well as brief summaries of problem cases are also published.

https://www.tandfonline.com/toc/hebh20/current

LEADERSHIP

This is designed to provide an ongoing forum for academic researchers to exchange information, insights and knowledge on both theoretical development and empirical research on leadership.

https://journals.sagepub.com/home/lea

JOURNAL OF MEDICAL ETHICS

It features articles on ethical aspects of healthcare relevant to healthcare professionals, members of clinical ethics committees, medical ethics professionals, researchers and bioscientists, policy makers and patients.

https://jme.bmj.com/

NURSING ETHICS

Nursing Ethics takes a practical approach to this complex subject and relates each topic to the working environment. The articles on ethical and legal issues are written in a comprehensible style, and official documents are analysed in a user-friendly way.

https://journals.sagepub.com/home/nej

PUBLIC HEALTH ETHICS

Focuses on a systematic analysis of the moral problems in public health and preventive medicine. It contains original articles, reviews and case studies about the nature of public health and related concepts (e.g. population, public, community, prevention); discussions of values in public health and ethical issues in relation to all aspects of public health policy and practice. This includes normative issues in epidemiological research, health promotion, infectious diseases control, screening, population genetics, resource allocation, healthcare system reform, vaccinations, environmental and lifestyle factors relevant to health, equity, justice and global health. *PHE* combines theoretical and practical work from different fields, notably philosophy, law and politics, but also epidemiology and the medical sciences.

https://academic.oup.com/phe

JOURNAL OF RELIGIOUS ETHICS

Aims to foster new work in neglected areas and to stimulate exchange on significant issues. Emphasising comparative religious ethics, foundational conceptual and methodological issues in religious ethics. It includes work on medical ethics, such as euthanasia and abortion.

https://onlinelibrary.wiley.com/journal/14679795

RESEARCH ETHICS

Focuses on ethical issues in the conduct of research, the regulation of research, the procedures and process of ethical review, as well as broader ethical issues related to research such as scientific integrity and the end uses of research. The journal aims to promote, provoke, host and engage in open and public debate about research ethics on an international scale but also to contribute to the education of researchers and reviewers of research.

https://uk.sagepub.com/en-gb/eur/journal/research-ethics#aims-and-scope

JOURNAL OF SOCIAL POLICY

It places particular emphasis upon articles which seek to contribute to debates on the future direction of social policy, to present new empirical data, to advance theories or to analyse issues in the making and implementation of social policies, including health policies across the world.

https://www.cambridge.org/core/journals/journal-of-social-policy

ETHICAL SPACE: THE INTERNATIONAL JOURNAL OF COMMUNICATION ETHICS

Provides a space for both academics and practitioners to reflect on and critique the ethics of communication. It contains news, views, interviews and peer-reviewed papers on ethical matters in journalism, public relations, marketing, health communication, information science, organisational and management communication and related fields.

www.abramis.co.uk/ethical-space/feature.php

ORGANIZATION

This is the major forum for dialogue and innovation in organisation studies, addressing significant current and emergent theoretical, meta theoretical and substantive developments in the field. It includes work on culture, ethics and healthcare.

https://uk.sagepub.com/en-gb/eur/journal/organization

Other Nursing Journals

These journals cover a wider spectrum of governance, leadership, management, public health, health and social policy:

Public Health Nursing
https://onlinelibrary.wiley.com/journal/15251446
Journal of Community & Public Health Nursing
https://publons.com/journal/43783/journal-of-community-public-health-nursing
Policy, Politics, & Nursing Practice
https://journals.sagepub.com/home/ppn
Journal of Nursing Management
https://onlinelibrary.wiley.com/journal/13652834
Nursing Outlook
https://www.journals.elsevier.com/nursing-outlook
Nursing Inquiry
https://onlinelibrary.wiley.com/journal/14401800
Worldviews on Evidence-Based Nursing
https://sigmapubs.onlinelibrary.wiley.com/journal/17416787

International Journal of Nursing Studies
   https://www.journals.elsevier.com/international-journal-of-nursing-studies
Journal of Nursing Scholarship
   https://sigmapubs.onlinelibrary.wiley.com/loi/15475069
International Journal of Health Policy and Management
   http://www.ijhpm.com/

Books

Graham Avery. (2014). *Law and ethics in nursing and healthcare: an introduction.* London: Sage.

Sarah Banks & Ann Gallagher. (2008). *Ethics in professional life: virtues for health and social care.* London: Palgrave

Alastair Campbell. (2017). *Bioethics: the basics.* London: Routledge.

Dee Danchev & Alistair Ross. (2013). *Research ethics for counsellors, nurses & social workers.* London: Sage.

Patrick Davey, Anna Rathmell, Michael Dunn, Charles Foster, Helen Salisbury (Editors). (2018). *Medical ethics, law and communication at a glance.* London: Wiley

Ann Gallagher & Christopher Herbert. (2019). *Faith and ethics in health and social care: improving practice through understanding diverse perspectives.* London: Jessica Kingsley.

Gay Haskins, Michael Thomas & Lalit Johri (Editors). (2018). *Kindness in leadership.* London: Routledge.

Stephen Holland. (2014). *Public health ethics.* London: Polity Press

Peter Jenkins. (2007). *Professional practice in counselling and psychotherapy: ethics and the law.* London: Sage.

Graeme Laurie, Shawn Harmon & Edward Dove. (2019). *Mason and McCall Smith's law and medical ethics.* Oxford: Oxford University Press

Catarina Morais & Georgina Randsley de Moura. (2018). *The psychology of ethical leadership in organisations: implications of group processes.* London: Palgrave

Peggy Morgan & Clive A. Lawton. (2007). *Ethical issues in six religious traditions.* Edinburgh: Edinburgh University Press.

Michael J. Sandel. (2012). *What money can't buy: the moral limits of markets.* London: Allen Lane

Websites

AAFP ETHICS AND ADVANCE PLANNING FOR END-OF-LIFE CARE

Covers the core principles for end-of-life care, experimentation, unethical life-prolonging treatment, foregoing life-sustaining treatment, medical orders for end-of-life care and post-mortem decisions.

AAFP Ethics and Advance Planning for End-of-Life Care https://www.aafp.org/home.html

ACTIVE CITIZENSHIP NETWORK

The Active Citizenship Network (ACN) website hosts a section dedicated entirely to the European Charter of Patients' Rights. The section aims to enhance the Charter in all its forms. In addition, to inform the public of initiatives, involving the Charter, taken to increase the civil participation of all citizens, such as: what is a "Charter of Rights" and what is needed for; sites which host the Charter; the Charter in several languages; publications of the Charter; from the Charter to the Charters; the Forerunners of the Charter; clippings, web and press articles; videos; public events.

Active Citizenship Network http://www.activecitizenship.net/

AMERICAN NURSES ASSOCIATION

This includes the Code of Ethics and the Revision with interpretive statements. Also see ANA position statements here on ethics and human rights.
American Nurses Association https://www.nursingworld.org/

AMERICAN ASSOCIATION OF CRITICAL CARE NURSES

This includes the fours A's, to rise above moral distress, affirm, assess, act. It also includes the position statement on moral distress.
Association of Critical Care Nurses https://www.aacn.org/

BMA ETHICS

This includes an extensive ethics toolkit.
https://www.bma.org.uk/advice/employment/ethics

CENTER FOR PRACTICAL BIOETHICS

This includes case studies and work on public health ethics and COVID-19.
https://www.practicalbioethics.org/resources/case-studies

ESRC RESEARCH ETHICS FRAMEWORK

Excellent overview of principles, case studies and research ethics governance.
https://esrc.ukri.org/funding/guidance-for-applicants/research-ethics/

EUROPEAN NETWORK OF RESEARCH ETHICS COMMITTEES

Includes a link to TRREE, Training and Resources in Research Ethics Evaluation.
http://www.eurecnet.org/information/uk.html

GMC ETHICAL GUIDANCE

Includes an extensive ethical hub on different ethical issues.
https://www.gmc-uk.org/ethical-guidance

HASTINGS CENTER

The Hastings Center was important in establishing the field of bioethics. It is a non-partisan, non-profit organization of research scholars from multiple disciplines, including philosophy, law, political science and education. The websites offer different resources on bioethics.
https://www.thehastingscenter.org/publications-resources/

INTERNATIONAL COUNCIL OF NURSES (ICN)

The ICN Code of Ethics for Nurses, most recently revised in 2012, is a guide for action based on social values and needs. The Code has served as the standard for nurses worldwide since it was first adopted in 1953.
International Council of Nurses (ICN)

INTERNET ENCYCLOPAEDIA OF PHILOSOPHY

Extensive sections on all aspects of ethical theory and practice, including healthcare ethics.
https://www.iep.utm.edu/h-c-ethi/

JOHNS HOPKINS BERMAN INSTITUTE OF BIOETHICS

Wide ranging resources, including work on COVID-19.
https://bioethics.jhu.edu/
This also links to the Johns Hopkins School of Nursing:
https://nursing.jhu.edu/excellence/quality-safety/ethics/

KING'S FUND

The King's Fund is an independent charitable organisation working to improve health and
care in England. The Fund initiates frequent reports and focuses on health policy, values,
leadership and organisational governance.
https://www.kingsfund.org.uk/

MEDLINEPLUS

MedlinePlus is a service of the US National Library of Medicine, part of the National Institute of Health.
It includes practical tools for medical ethics.
https://medlineplus.gov/medicalethics.html

NATIONAL INSTITUTE FOR HEALTH AND CARE EXCELLENCE

Ethical guidelines here:
https://www.evidence.nhs.uk/search?q=ethical+guidelines
General guidelines here:
https://www.nice.org.uk/about/what-we-do/our-programmes/nice-guidance/nice-guide-
lines/making-decisions-using-nice-guidelines
Extensive ethics references here:
https://www.evidence.nhs.uk/search?q=values+and+ethics

NHS EDUCATION FOR SCOTLAND: LAW AND ETHICS. ADVANCED PRACTICE TOOLKIT

This includes implications of ethics for advanced nursing practice, and issues such as consent
and duty of care.
http://www.advancedpractice.scot.nhs.uk/law-ethics.aspx?tab=TabResources

NHS RESEARCH ETHICS COMMITTEES

Core governance of research ethics in the NHS.
https://www.hra.nhs.uk/about-us/committees-and-services/res-and-recs/

NUFFIELD COUNCIL ON BIOETHICS

Informs policy and public debate through timely consideration of the ethical questions raised by biological and medical research so that the benefits to society are realised in a way that is consistent with public values. Frequent reports.
https://www.nuffieldbioethics.org/

NUFFIELD TRUST

The Nuffield Trust is an independent health think tank, aiming to improve the quality of health care in the UK by providing evidence-based research and policy analysis, informing and generating debate.
It includes reports, papers and blogs on ethics and healthcare policy.
https://www.nuffieldtrust.org.uk/search?search=ethics

NURSING AND MIDWIFERY COUNCIL (NMC)

This includes the code of professional standards.
https://www.nmc.org.uk/

NURSING AND MIDWIFERY BOARD OF IRELAND (NMBI)

Includes extensive discussion and guidance on the Code and related areas such as trust and confidentiality.
https://www.nmbi.ie/Home

ROYAL COLLEGE OF NURSING

This includes and ethical impact assessment tool, ongoing debate about ethical issues and the development of the professional code and the ethics of different aspects of care, including end-of-life care.
https://rcni.com/hosted-content/rcn/fundamentals-of-end-of-life-care/ethics
https://www.rcn.org.uk/professional-development/publications/pub-006499

STANFORD ENCYCLOPAEDIA OF PHILOSOPHY

An excellent reference work on both ethical theory and ethical issues such as abortion and end-of-life treatment. It gives summaries of the key arguments and philosophical positions.
https://plato.stanford.edu/contents.html

UK GOVERNMENT PUBLICATIONS

Public health ethics in practice, overviews.
https://www.gov.uk/government/publications/public-health-ethics-in-practice

WORLD HEALTH ORGANIZATION

For global and public health ethical issues.
https://www.who.int/health-topics/ethics

SUBJECT INDEX